The Prescription Drug Abuse Epidemic

The Prescription Drug Abuse Epidemic

Incidence, Treatment, Prevention, and Policy

Ty S. Schepis, PhD, Editor

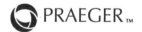

PRAEGER™

An Imprint of ABC-CLIO, LLC

Santa Barbara, California • Denver, Colorado

Library of Congress Cataloging-in-Publication Data

Names: Schepis, Ty S.
Title: The prescription drug abuse epidemic : incidence, treatment, prevention, and policy / Ty S. Schepis, PhD, editor.
Description: Santa Barbara, California : Praeger, an imprint of ABC-CLIO, LLC, [2018] | Includes bibliographical references and index.
Identifiers: LCCN 2018010856 (print) | LCCN 2018011814 (ebook) | ISBN 9781440852657 (ebook) | ISBN 9781440852640 (set : alk. paper)
Subjects: LCSH: Medication abuse—United States. | Opioid abuse—United States. | Drug abuse—United States. | Drug abuse—Treatment—United States. | Drug abuse—Political aspects—United States.
Classification: LCC RM146.7 (ebook) | LCC RM146.7 .P76 2018 (print) | DDC 362.29/90973—dc23
LC record available at https://lccn.loc.gov/2018010856

ISBN: 978-1-4408-5264-0 (print)
          978-1-4408-5265-7 (ebook)

22 21 20 19 18   1 2 3 4 5

This book is also available as an eBook.

Praeger
An Imprint of ABC-CLIO, LLC

ABC-CLIO, LLC
130 Cremona Drive, P.O. Box 1911
Santa Barbara, California 93116-1911
www.abc-clio.com

This book is printed on acid-free paper ∞

Manufactured in the United States of America

Contents

Acknowledgments

It should probably go without saying that the completion and publication of a book such as this is impossible without a host of individuals who contribute, and no one is more aware of this than I am, as editor. Nonetheless, please allow me to reiterate: the completion and publication of this book would not have been possible without the authors who submitted thoughtful and well-researched chapters, the editorial and production staff at Praeger/ABC-Clio, and the support of colleagues and family. I am truly indebted to each of them for their help with this project.

First, I am grateful for the contributions of every author to this volume. Enclosed within this book is the work of a truly staggering number of talented researchers and clinicians who work daily to reduce the societal toll of prescription misuse. Perhaps more importantly, every author I interacted with was helpful, thoughtful, and quick to reply—all of which are appreciated by a stressed editor. While easy to overlook, I would strongly urge you to spend some time reading the author biographies in the "About the Authors" section of this book. It was particularly gratifying to me that individuals were included from such a variety of academic and clinical disciplines and across a wide span of career stages. Chapter authors are not just the current authorities on prescription misuse, as many students, who are the future of the field, were included as coauthors on chapters. For their time and effort, I want to sincerely thank the authors of the chapters in this book. I believe our book (and it is most certainly our book) is a substantive contribution to the emerging literature on prescription misuse.

In addition, I want to thank Praeger/ABC-Clio for approaching me to serve as the editor of this book. When I accepted this challenge over two years ago, I had little idea of what I was truly getting into. The fact that I both survived and helped produce a strong book is due in no small part to the help and guidance I received from the staff at Praeger/ABC-Clio. My thanks also go out to these staff members for their help in shepherding a novice editor through his first book.

I am also fortunate to work in a wonderful department, Psychology, at Texas State University. My departmental colleagues are a great source of support, and they almost certainly (and patiently) listened to me complain in the times I was having unanticipated difficulty finding authors for chapters or was dealing with a crisis or two related to this book. I am quite lucky to work in such a collegial and academically diverse department.

Most importantly, I want to dedicate this book to my very understanding and supportive family. I spent the good part of many evenings seeking authors, editing chapters, and completing the chapters for which I was an author. Throughout it all, my wife did not complain—in fact, she was a sympathetic and helpful ear throughout the process. Making time to play with our two wonderful sons, William and Daniel, was also a very important way for me to cope during frustrating times. Finally, I would not be here (nor would this book) without my mother's patient and probably exhausting parenting. She was both parents in one, and I am forever grateful to her for that.

CHAPTER ONE

Introduction

Ty S. Schepis

From a variety of public health, medical, and other clinical experts (Cobaugh et al., 2014; DeVane, 2015; Kanouse & Compton, 2015; Kolodny et al., 2015) to the executive branch of the U.S. government (Newman, 2017) and the president of the United States (Ford, 2017), a consensus has emerged that prescription opioid misuse in the United States is an epidemic and a national crisis. While the attention to the topic has accelerated greatly in the past year, misuse of opioid medications, such as oxycodone (e.g., OxyContin), hydrocodone (e.g., Vicodin or Lortab), and fentanyl, and the consequences of such misuse have been increasing since the early 2000s in the United States. Increases in opioid misuse have occurred concomitantly with increases in emergency department visits (Substance Abuse and Mental Health Services Administration (SAMHSA), 2012), the number of individuals enrolling in addiction treatment (SAMHSA, 2014), and overdoses related to opioids (Rudd, Aleshire, Zibbell, & Gladden, 2016). More recent evidence points to an increase in heroin use driven by individuals who had previously misused opioids transitioning to heroin (Compton, Jones, & Baldwin, 2016) and continuing to use heroin (Palamar & Shearston, 2017). Furthermore, the United States is not the only country affected by opioid misuse, as commentators in Canada (Fischer, Gooch, Goldman, Kurdyak, & Rehm, 2014), Europe (Morley, Ferris, Winstock, & Lynskey, 2017), and Australia (Roxburgh et al., 2017) and a chapter of this volume can attest.

Opioid misuse is not the only form of prescription misuse to be concerned about, however. Stimulant medications that are often used to treat attention-deficit/hyperactivity disorder, including methylphenidate (e.g., Ritalin or

Concerta), lisdexamfetamine (e.g., Vyvanse), and various amphetamine formulations (e.g., Adderall) and benzodiazepine medications used in the treatment of anxiety and insomnia, including alprazolam (Xanax) and lorazepam
(Ativan), are also commonly misused medications and the source of great
potential harms to those engaged in misuse (Weaver, 2015; Weyandt et al.,
2016). Although the rates of misuse of these medications have been more
stable than the rates of opioid misuse, emergency department visits and the
number of individuals enrolling in addiction treatment have increased over
the past 15 years (SAMHSA, 2012, 2014).

This book aims to introduce readers to the phenomenon of prescription
medication misuse by providing a broad perspective on this ongoing public
health crisis. The chapters primarily focus on opioid misuse, given its outsized role in the overall prescription misuse crisis, with coverage included of
stimulant, benzodiazepine, and over-the-counter medication misuse. Chapters on special populations (e.g., older adults), settings where prescription
misuse is likely to be a particular issue (e.g., emergency departments), prescription misuse outside of the United States, the U.S. legal and policy environments, and a pair of theories with potential utility in preventing misuse
are included herein. While not exhaustive, this work will grant readers a
strong base of knowledge with which to engage policy makers and elected
representatives and serve as a starting point for further study of the scientific
literature.

Before proceeding into an overview of the chapters to follow, a pair of
points need to be addressed. First, readers may note that the terminology in
the chapters varies somewhat from author to author. In part, this is because
of an unfortunate lack of consensus regarding prescription misuse terminology that other commentators have been noting for years (Barrett, Meisner, &
Stewart, 2008; Boyd & McCabe, 2008; Compton & Volkow, 2006). While I
considered imposing external specific definitions for such terms as *misuse*,
abuse, and *nonmedical use*, the authors were free to choose their preferred
terms. Unless otherwise specified, the definitions of *misuse* and *nonmedical
use* basically correspond with the definition offered by Compton and Volkow:
"any intentional use of a medication with intoxicating properties outside of a
physician's prescription for a bona fide medical condition, excluding accidental misuse" (Compton & Volkow, 2006, p. S4). Use of the term *abuse* was
generally discouraged because of potential confusion with the DSM-IV psychiatric diagnosis of substance abuse; this diagnosis does not correspond
with the definition offered above, though use of the *abuse* label as a stand-in
for *misuse* or *nonmedical use* is seen in the literature.

Second, all terminology in this volume was written in a person-centered
fashion. In simpler terms, the use of potentially stigmatizing labels such as
misuser, *addict*, and *abuser* was avoided in favor of such terms as *person
engaged in misuse* or *person endorsing nonmedical use*. As noted by Becker and

Starrels in chapter 9 of this volume, there is ample reason to believe that the use of potentially stigmatizing labels does just that: it places a negative value judgment on a person. The use of these labels has inherent ethical problems, conflicting with the important principles of beneficence and respect for persons, and there is evidence that such labeling is counterproductive, as it discourages people from seeking treatment or taking other steps to cease prescription misuse (Kelly, Wakeman, & Saitz, 2015; Scholten et al., 2017).

Chapter Overview

The initial four chapters cover the background material on the medication classes of interest: opioids (chapter 2), stimulants (chapter 3), benzodiazepines (chapter 4), and other misused over-the-counter medications (chapter 5). The first three chapters examine the medical uses and pharmacological properties of the medication classes, and the fourth covers such risks as misuse, intoxication, and consequences of inappropriate use. The chapter on over-the-counter medications takes a brief look at a variety of medications, including antihistamines and laxatives.

The next three chapters examine populations of special interest for prescription misuse: adolescents and university students (chapter 6), young adults (chapter 7), and older adults (chapter 8). For younger individuals, focus is warranted due to the uniquely elevated rates of misuse in university students and young adults and, in all cases, due to the potential for misuse to adversely affect both neurobiological and psychosocial developmental trajectories. After the chapters on populations of interest, the next two chapters focus on prescription misuse through the lens of two particularly impacted medical settings: primary care pain management (chapter 9) and the emergency department (or emergency room; chapter 10).

The next two subsections of the book cover prescription misuse on national scales. First, chapters 11, 12, and 13 examine policy, law, and public health related to prescription misuse in the United States. Specifically, chapter 11 addresses federal law and policy, chapter 12 addresses the use of prescription drug monitoring programs (or PDMPs) to reduce prescription misuse, and chapter 13 addresses a variety of harm reduction approaches to reduce the opioid epidemic. Chapter 14 examines prescription misuse outside the United States, in the United Kingdom.

Finally, two chapters consider larger theories that may be relevant to prescription misuse. Chapter 15 describes and applies three health behavior theories to prescription misuse, while chapter 16 describes criminological theory and applies it to misuse. The book ends with a final and brief chapter that points toward future directions for research and policy that may help reduce rates of both prescription misuse and the associated consequences that have so significantly affected tens of millions or more worldwide.

References

Barrett, S. P., Meisner, J. R., & Stewart, S. H. (2008). What constitutes prescription drug misuse? Problems and pitfalls of current conceptualizations. *Current Drug Abuse Reviews, 1*(3), 255–262.

Boyd, C. J., & McCabe, S. E. (2008). Coming to terms with the nonmedical use of prescription medications. *Substance Abuse Treatment, Prevention, and Policy, 3*, 22. doi:10.1186/1747-597X-3-22.

Cobaugh, D. J., Gainor, C., Gaston, C. L., Kwong, T. C., Magnani, B., McPherson, M. L., . . . Krenzelok, E. P. (2014). The opioid abuse and misuse epidemic: Implications for pharmacists in hospitals and health systems. *American Journal of Health-System Pharmacy, 71*(18), 1539–1554. doi:10.2146/ajhp140157.

Compton, W. M., Jones, C. M., & Baldwin, G. T. (2016). Relationship between nonmedical prescription-opioid use and heroin use. *New England Journal of Medicine, 374*(2), 154–163. doi:10.1056/NEJMra1508490.

Compton, W. M., & Volkow, N. D. (2006). Abuse of prescription drugs and the risk of addiction. *Drug and Alcohol Dependence, 83 Supplement 1*, S4-7.

DeVane, C. L. (2015). An epidemic of opioid prescriptions. *Pharmacotherapy, 35*(3), 241–242. doi:10.1002/phar.1571.

Fischer, B., Gooch, J., Goldman, B., Kurdyak, P., & Rehm, J. (2014). Non-medical prescription opioid use, prescription opioid-related harms and public health in Canada: An update 5 years later. *Canadian Journal of Public Health, 105*(2), e146–149.

Ford, M. (2017, Aug 10). Trump informally declares the opioid crisis a national emergency. *The Atlantic.* https://www.theatlantic.com/politics/archive/2017/08/president-trump-declares-the-opioid-crisis-a-national-emergency/536514/.

Kanouse, A. B., & Compton, P. (2015). The epidemic of prescription opioid abuse, the subsequent rising prevalence of heroin use, and the federal response. *Journal of Pain & Palliative Care Pharmacotherapy, 29*(2), 102–114. doi:10.3109/15360288.2015.1037521.

Kelly, J. F., Wakeman, S. E., & Saitz, R. (2015). Stop talking "dirty": clinicians, language, and quality of care for the leading cause of preventable death in the United States. *American Journal of Medicine, 128*(1), 8–9. doi:10.1016/j.amjmed.2014.07.043.

Kolodny, A., Courtwright, D. T., Hwang, C. S., Kreiner, P., Eadie, J. L., Clark, T. W., & Alexander, G. C. (2015). The prescription opioid and heroin crisis: a public health approach to an epidemic of addiction. *Annual Review of Public Health, 36*, 559–574. doi:10.1146/annurev-publhealth-031914-122957.

Morley, K. I., Ferris, J. A., Winstock, A. R., & Lynskey, M. T. (2017). Polysubstance use and misuse or abuse of prescription opioid analgesics: A multilevel analysis of international data. *Pain, 158*(6), 1138–1144. doi:10.1097/j.pain.0000000000000892.

Newman, K. (2017, Aug 8). Health Secretary Tom Price calls opioid epidemic "an emergency." *U.S. News and World Report.* https://www.usnews.com/news/national-news/articles/2017-08-08/tom-price-vows-to-treat-opioid-epidemic-as-an-emergency.

Palamar, J. J., & Shearston, J. A. (2017). Nonmedical opioid use in relation to recency of heroin use in a nationally representative sample of adults in the United States. *Journal of Psychoactive Drugs,* 1–8. doi:10.1080/02791072.2017.1368747.

Roxburgh, A., Hall, W. D., Dobbins, T., Gisev, N., Burns, L., Pearson, S., & Degenhardt, L. (2017). Trends in heroin and pharmaceutical opioid overdose deaths in Australia. *Drug and Alcohol Dependence, 179,* 291–298. doi:10.1016/j.drugalcdep.2017.07.018.

Rudd, R. A., Aleshire, N., Zibbell, J. E., & Gladden, R. M. (2016). Increases in drug and opioid overdose deaths—United States, 2000–2014. *MMWR: Morbidity and Mortality Weekly Report, 64*(50–51), 1378–1382. doi:10.15585/mmwr.mm6450a3.

Scholten, W., Simon, O., Maremmani, I., Wells, C., Kelly, J. F., Hammig, R., & Radbruch, L. (2017). Access to treatment with controlled medicines rationale and recommendations for neutral, precise, and respectful language. *Public Health, 153,* 147–153. doi:10.1016/j.puhe.2017.08.021.

Substance Abuse and Mental Health Services Administration. (2012). *Drug Abuse Warning Network, 2010: National Estimates of Drug-Related Emergency Department Visits.* Rockville, MD: Substance Abuse and Mental Health Services Administration.

Substance Abuse and Mental Health Services Administration. (2014). *Treatment Episode Data Set (TEDS): 2002–2012. National Admissions to Substance Abuse Treatment Services* (BHSIS Series S-71, HHS Publication No. (SMA) 14-4850). Rockville, MD: Substance Abuse and Mental Health Services Administration.

Weaver, M. F. (2015). Prescription sedative misuse and abuse. *Yale Journal of Biology and Medicine, 88*(3), 247–256.

Weyandt, L. L., Oster, D. R., Marraccini, M. E., Gudmundsdottir, B. G., Munro, B. A., Rathkey, E. S., & McCallum, A. (2016). Prescription stimulant medication misuse: Where are we and where do we go from here? *Experimental and Clinical Psychopharmacology, 24*(5), 400–414. doi:10.1037/pha0000093.

CHAPTER TWO

Opioids

Gregory B. Castelli and Winfred T. Frazier

Opioids are a class of medications that have been widely used to relieve acute and chronic pain for millennia. *Opioid* is the modern term used to describe all substances that bind to opioid receptors, including agonists and antagonists (Hemmings & Egan, 2013). *Narcotics* describe medications with the potential for abuse. Both terms are routinely used interchangeably in the clinical setting, with opioids as the overarching label for the entire class. *Opiate* is a less frequently used term that describes drugs directly derived from the opium poppy plant. As it is all encompassing, opioid is the most accurate nomenclature. For more on the history of opioids, see chapters 9 and 13.

Opioids are divided into several different chemical and structural classes; each opioid is available in various doses and delivery modalities (Ballantyne & Mao, 2003). Table 2.1 provides an overview of major opioid analgesic products. Commercially available products have different rates of onset and durations of action, which is important for clinicians to be aware of when prescribing these medications for patients (DiPiro et al., 2017). In addition to various dosage forms, rates of onset, and durations of action, prescription opioids come in several formulations, including immediate- and extended-release preparations, and various routes, including oral, transdermal, intravenous, and intramuscular.

Opioids have a high abuse and misuse potential, with some (e.g., heroin) commonly used illegally despite lacking clinical indications (Jamison & Mao, 2015). Opioid use and misuse is a major public health concern in the United States, with many federal agencies noting that the deleterious consequences of opioid misuse, including death, have reached epidemic proportions.

Pharmacology

Opioids that are used clinically share many structural features. Morphine and codeine are naturally occurring opioids. They are both found in *Papaver somniferum*, which is commonly known as the poppy plant (Thorn, Klein, & Altman, 2009). A methyl group contained in codeine is the only structural difference between these two opioids. Many semisynthetic opioids are created through modification of the morphine molecule (see Table 2.1). Synthetic opioids, while clinically active, do not occur in nature and have been engineered for medical purposes.

Opioids simulate the properties exerted by endogenous chemicals of pain perception. Endogenous opioids, including enkephalins, endorphins, and dynorphins, are chemicals found in the human body that act on opioid receptors. In addition to the body's natural pain response, these chemicals have been implicated in many neurological and psychological conditions, including anxiety, legal and illegal drug use, reward pathways, and the body's response to pain (Vallejo, Barkin, & Wang, 2011). This effect on the body's reward pathway may help explain the negative effects of long-term prescription opioid use, such as dependence and hyperalgesia.

Opioids exert their main pharmacologic pain effects through interacting with opioid receptors found primarily throughout the body's nervous system, including the brain, spinal cord, peripheral sensory nerves, and autonomic nerves. Three main classes of opioid receptors have been identified: mu (μ), kappa (κ), and delta (δ). Opioid receptors are also widely distributed in other tissues, including cardiovascular, pulmonary, and gastrointestinal; the activation of receptors at these sites can lead to the adverse effects discussed later in this chapter. These receptors are guanine (G) protein-linked receptors; agonists binding to these receptors will activate G-protein pathways to produce an inhibitory effect (Pardo & Miller, 2018). Adenylate cyclase of the cyclic AMP pathway and influx of calcium are inhibited, and potassium efflux and production of prostaglandins and leukotrienes are increased, causing hyperpolarization of presynaptic cells and reduced excitability of neurons. In addition to opioid receptor binding, opioids have effects at multiple other sites in the body, attenuating the pain response. Opioids inhibit the release of the neuromodulator substance P, producing a diminished pain stimulus that travels through the spinal cord and dorsal horn (De Felipe et al., 1998).

Physical dependence and tolerance are two important and characteristic traits of opioids (Vallejo et al., 2011). Physical dependence is the need to keep using a drug to avoid withdrawal syndrome. Tolerance, where larger doses are needed to provide similar analgesia, develops after chronic exposure to opioids. Tolerance can also be defined as a diminished analgesic effect to the same dose of an opioid following extended use. Tolerance is an innate and

Table 2.1 Commonly Used Opioid Analgesic Products

Medication: Generic (Brand)	Chemical Source	Equianalgesic Dose		Typical Starting Doses		Onset	Duration	Available Formulations	Available Routes of Administration
		Parenteral Onset 15–30 min	Oral Onset 30–60 min	Parenteral	Oral				
Phenanthrenes (morphine-like agonists)									
Morphine (Embeda, MS Contin, Kadian)	Naturally occuring	10 mg	30 mg	1–5 mg IV/IM q3–4h	5–15 mg q3–4h	10 min	ed	Capsule (ER); oral solution; tablet (IR, ER); tablet (ER); suppository; IV solution	IV, PO
Oxycodone (Oxycontin, Roxicodone, Percocet)	Semisynthetic	N/A	20 mg	N/A	10 mg q4–6h	30–60 min	4–6h 12h (ER)	Capsule (IR, ER); tablet (IR, ER) oral solution; tablet (IR with APAP)	PO
Oxymorphone (Opana, Numorphan)	Semisynthetic	1 mg	10 mg	1–1.5 mg q4–6h	5–10 mg q4–6h	10–20 min	3–6h	Tablet (IR, ER); IV solution	IV, PO
Hydromorphone (Dilaudid, Exalgo)	Semisynthetic	1.5 mg	7.5 mg	0.5–1 mg IV/IM q3–4h	2–4 mg q3–4h	10–20 min (IV) 6h (Oral ER)	4–5h 13h (ER)	Tablet (IR, ER); oral solution; IV solution; suppository	IV, PO
Hydrocodone (Norco, Hysingla, Zohydro)	Semisynthetic	N/A	20 mg	N/A	5–10 mg q4–6h	30–60 min	2–4h 12–24h (ER)	Capsule (ER); tablet (ER); tablet (IR with APAP)	PO
Codeine	Naturally occuring	120 mg	200 mg	30 mg IM q3–4h	30–60 mg q3–4h	30–60 min	4–6h	Tablet (IR); oral solution; tablet (IR with APAP)	PO

8

Phenylpiperidines (meperidine-like agonists)

Drug	Type			Parenteral dose	Oral/other dose	Onset	Duration	Formulations	Routes
Fentanyl (Duragesic, Fentora, Lazanda)	Synthetic	*Varies	50–100 mcg	25–50 mcg IV q1–2h	Transdermal: 25 mcg/h q72h	7–15 min (IV) 6h (transdermal)	1–2h (IV) 72–96h (transdermal)	Buccal film; IV solution; sublingual/buccal products; patch; intranasal solution; tablet	IV, transdermal, sublingual, buccal
Meperidine (Demerol)	Synthetic	300 mg	75–100 mg	50–100 mg IV/IM q2–3h	Not Recommended	10–15 min	4–6h	Tablet (IR); oral solution; IV solution	IV, PO

Diphenylheptanes (methadone-like agonits)

Drug	Type			Parenteral dose	Oral/other dose	Onset	Duration	Formulations	Routes
Methadone	Synthetic	*Varies	*Varies	2.5–10 mg IV/IM q8–12h		30–60 min	4–8h	Tablet (IR); oral concentrate; IV solution;	IV, PO

Agonist-antagonist derivatives

Drug	Type			Parenteral dose	Oral/other dose	Onset	Duration	Formulations	Routes
Buprenorphine (Buprenex, Butrans)	Synthetic	*Varies	*Varies	0.3 mg IM q6–8h	75 mg q12–24h Transdermal: 5 mcg/h q7d	10–20 min	6h	Buccal film; patch; IV solution; tablet; implant	IV, sublingual, buccal, transdermal, subcutaneous

Central analgesics

Drug	Type			Parenteral dose	Oral/other dose	Onset	Duration	Formulations	Routes
Tramadol	Synthetic	N/A	N/A	N/A	50–100 mg q4–6h (max 400 mg daily)	60 min	4h 10h (ER)	Capsule (ER); tablet (ER, IR); oral suspension; cream	PO, transdermal

IR = immediate release, ER = extended release, IV = intravenously, PO = by mouth, APAP = acetaminophen hazardous property that can develop after only one dose of opioids (Kornetsky & Bain, 1968). Euphoria, commonly called a drug high, is the activation of reward pathways in the brain that underlines misuse and addiction. These concepts help describe the need for higher treatment doses, but they should not be confused with addiction or physical or psychological dependence.

Addiction is a primary chronic disorder of an individual pathologically pursuing reward or relief through substance use and other behaviors (American Society of Addiction Medicine, 2011). Addiction is the end result of neurochemical changes to the brain that create compulsive drug-seeking and drug-use behavior. The reasons why some people develop addiction to these inherently addictive medications while others do not are not clear. Addiction and overdose can occur in individuals with prescriptions for opioids to relieve pain and those who nonmedically use (i.e., those using medications that were not prescribed for them or were taken only for the experience or feeling that they cause). Almost 75 percent of all opioid misuse starts with people taking a medication that was not prescribed for them (Center for Behavioral Health Statistics and Quality, 2015). A study involving 136,000 opioid overdose patients treated in the emergency department in 2010 found that only 13 percent of those patients had a chronic pain diagnosis (Yokell et al., 2014). Predictors of overdose have been identified in the literature that can assist health care providers with targeting interventions for those at risk (Cochran et al., 2017; Rice et al., 2012; Sullivan & Fiellin, 2008).

Medical Uses

Virtually everyone experiences moderate or severe pain at some point in their lifetime. More than 30 percent of Americans have some form of chronic pain (Johannes, Le, Zhou, Johnston, & Dworkin, 2010), so it is unsurprising that opioids are the third most commonly prescribed class of medications in the United States, following antimicrobials and antidepressants (Zhong et al., 2013). According to the Centers for Disease Control and Prevention (CDC), 70.6 opioid prescriptions per every 100 persons were issued annually from 2012 to 2015 (Guy et al., 2017). This is approximately three times the number of prescriptions written in 1999. The average morphine milligram equivalent (MME) for each prescription is about 640 MME per person annually. Americans consume over 80 percent of the world's opioid supply, over 99 percent of all manufactured hydrocodone, and two-thirds of the world's illegal drugs (American Society of Interventional Pain Physicians, n.d.). It is estimated that 2 million people in the United States have a problematic pattern of opioid use that has led to clinically significant impairment, or opioid use disorder (OUD; American Psychiatric Association, 2013).

Opioids can be used for various types of pain, including pain caused by cancer and chronic noncancer pain (CNCP). Use of opioids for CNCP is controversial; the provider must carefully consider the risks and benefits of using this medication class before initiating opioid therapy (Von Korff, Kolodny, Deyo, & Chou, 2011). Medical and nonmedical use of opioids have increased dramatically over time due to several factors.

Opioid Prescribing: Past and Present

Opioid prescribing accelerated in the 1980s because of arguments made in the scientific literature and policy-driven influences. Low-quality studies published in prominent journals in the 1980s reported a minimal risk of addiction in patients using opioids (Portenoy & Foley, 1986; Porter & Jick, 1980). Another article published in 1990 reiterated the widespread belief that "therapeutic use of opiate analgesics rarely results in addiction" (Max, 1990). Pain was considered "the fifth vital sign," and relief of pain became one of the fundamental obligations of medical professionals. These studies and the growing pharmaceutical industry led to the liberalization of opioid use for the treatment of pain.

Opioid use increased greatly for treating CNCP. Welfare and health care reform in the 1990s also played a role in the overreliance on opioids (Coffin et al., 2016). Managed care organizations recognized that opioids were less expensive than comprehensive pain management clinics and consequently stopped reimbursement for those services (Schatman, 2011). Payers were unwilling to cover nonpharmacological interventions, leaving opioids as one of the few therapeutic options. In the early 2000s, the Joint Commission on Accreditation of Healthcare Organizations published a guide that stated that clinicians' concerns about opioid-related addiction were inaccurate and exaggerated. The embrace of opioids by the scientific community, in part due to these highly influential factors, led to changes in physicians' prescribing practices and a surge in opioid prescriptions (Franklin et al., 2005). This influx of opioid prescriptions is cited as a contributing reason for the opioid epidemic, which has led to opioid dependence and overdose deaths (Meldrum, 2016).

In recent years, the medical community has responded with tighter regulation of opioids, continuing medical education on the proper use of opioids, and increased availability of addiction treatment. Prescription drug monitoring programs (PDMPs) are widely utilized; 49 states have operational programs, except for Missouri (U.S. Drug Enforcement Administration, 2016). These changes have led to decreased opioid prescribing and decreased opioid-related morbidity and mortality. It is now more important for clinicians to be able to assess for appropriateness of opioid treatment and potential misuse and to communicate risks and harms than it is to understand the intricacies of opioid management. For more on PDMPs, see chapter 12.

The CDC released opioid prescribing guidelines for CNCP in 2016 to provide recommendations to clinicians (Dowell, Haegerich, & Chou, 2016). The report highlights twelve key recommendations that can be summarized in three groups (please see Table 2.2): (1) determining when to initiate or continue opioids for chronic pain; (2) opioid selection, dosage, duration, follow-up, and discontinuation; and (3) assessing risk and addressing harms of opioid use. In addition, the Department of Veterans Affairs and the Department of Defense have issued similar guidelines that mirror many of the CDC's recommendations (Department of Veteran Affairs and Department of Defense, 2017). Several strategies should be employed for managing chronic pain, with emphasis on nonpharmacological ones, such as physical therapy and psychological therapies, and nonopioid medication therapies, such as NSAIDs, acetaminophen, antidepressants, and topical lidocaine. If opioids are needed, the clinician and patient should engage in a shared decision conversation about the goals for pain management and the risks and benefits of opioid treatment. The dose and duration of opioids should be kept to a minimum and include frequent patient follow-up; preference should be given for immediate-release preparations (Dowell et al., 2016). Clinicians should also attempt to identify the potential of misuse prior to prescribing opioids through frequent PDMP use and urine drug testing.

Special Populations

Special consideration should be given prior to prescribing opioids for pain control in certain populations: older adults, patients with renal dysfunction, and patients with liver failure. Older adults have physiologic characteristics that affect the absorption, distribution, metabolism, and excretion of medications. In addition to renal and liver dysfunction associated with increased age, which can affect medication absorption and adverse medication effects, older adults have a higher fat-to-lean body weight ratio, potentially increasing drug duration of action (American Geriatrics Society Panel on Pharmacological Management of Persistent Pain in Older Persons, 2009). These adverse effects are discussed later in this chapter and, while they are pronounced in older adults, occur in patients regardless of age.

General approaches to using opioids in older adults should be employed: start therapy at lower doses; preferentially use products without active opioid metabolites (e.g., oxycodone, hydromorphone); and avoid long-acting agents. For more on prescription use and misuse in older adults, see chapter 8. Careful consideration should also be made when using opioids for patients with chronic kidney disease and chronic liver disease due to the potential of more frequent and severe adverse effects. The choice of opioid and small dose adjustments are important, as products vary on route of elimination (renal or hepatic), with some having active metabolites that can have effects on the body (Chandok & Watt, 2010; Dean, 2004).

Table 2.2   Centers for Disease Control and Prevention Recommendations for Prescribing Opioids

1. Nonpharmacologic therapy and nonopioid pharmacologic therapy are preferred for chronic pain. Clinicians should consider opioid therapy only if expected benefits for both pain and function are anticipated to outweigh risks to the patient. If opioids are used, they should be combined with nonpharmacologic therapy and nonopioid pharmacologic therapy, as appropriate.

2. Before starting opioid therapy for chronic pain, clinicians should establish treatment goals with all patients, including realistic goals for pain and function, and should consider how therapy will be discontinued if benefits do not outweigh risks. Clinicians should continue opioid therapy only if there is clinically meaningful improvement in pain and function that outweighs risks to patient safety.

3. Before starting and periodically during opioid therapy, clinicians should discuss with patients known risks and realistic benefits of opioid therapy and patient and clinician responsibilities for managing therapy.

7. Clinicians should evaluate benefits and harms with patients within 1 to 4 weeks of starting opioid therapy for chronic pain or of dose escalation. Clinicians should evaluate benefits and harms of continued therapy with patients every 3 months or more frequently. If benefits do not outweigh harms of continued opioid therapy, clinicians should optimize therapies and work with patients to taper opioids to lower dosages or to taper and discontinue opioids.

8. Before starting and periodically during continuation of opioid therapy, clinicians should evaluate risk factors for opioid-related harms. Clinicians should incorporate into the management plan strategies to mitigate risk, including considering offering naloxone when factors that increase risk for opioid overdose, such as history of overdose, history of substance use disorder, higher opioid dosages (50 MME/d), or concurrent benzodiazepine use are present.

9. Clinicians should review the patient's history of controlled substance prescriptions using state prescription drug monitoring program (PDMP) data to determine whether the patient is receiving opioid dosages or dangerous combinations that put him or her at high risk for overdose. Clinicians should review PDMP data when starting opioid therapy for chronic pain and periodically during opioid therapy for chronic pain, ranging from every prescription to every 3 months.

(continued)

13

Table 2.2 (*continued*)

4. When starting opioid therapy for chronic pain, clinicians should prescribe immediate-release opioids instead of extended-release/long-acting (ER/LA) opioids.

5. When opioids are started, clinicians should prescribe the lowest effective dosage. Clinicians should use caution when prescribing opioids at any dosage, should carefully reassess evidence of individual benefits and risks when increasing dosage to 50 morphine milligram equivalents (MME) or more per day, and should avoid increasing dosage to 90 MME or more per day or carefully justify a decision to titrate dosage to 90 MME or more per day.

6. Long-term opioid use often begins with treatment of acute pain. When opioids are used for acute pain, clinicians should prescribe the lowest effective dose of immediate-release opioids and should prescribe no greater quantity than needed for the expected duration of pain severe enough to require opioids. Three days or less will often be sufficient; more than 7 days will rarely be needed.

10. When prescribing opioids for chronic pain, clinicians should use urine drug testing before starting opioid therapy and consider urine drug testing at least annually to assess for prescribed medications as well as other controlled prescription drugs and illicit drugs.

11. Clinicians should avoid prescribing opioid pain medication and benzodiazepines concurrently whenever possible.

12. Clinicians should offer or arrange evidence-based treatment (usually medication-assisted treatment with buprenorphine or methadone in combination with behavioral therapies) for patients with opioid use disorder.

Adverse Effects

The rise in the number of prescriptions correlates with a rapid increase in opioid-related morbidity and mortality due to their intrinsic properties. It is estimated that 80 percent of patients who use opioids experience at least one adverse effect. Some of these adverse effects subside over time as the body becomes tolerant to opioids; others may be exacerbated as doses are increased and tolerance develops (Kalso, Edwards, Moore, & McQuay, 2004). Additionally, opioid overdose deaths are important to understand, as they are typically caused by an adverse effect. In 2015 alone, there were 20,101 overdose deaths related to prescription opioid medication, and 12,990 overdose deaths related to heroin (Rudd, Seth, David, & Scholl, 2016). Many factors exist that contribute to the likelihood of a patient experiencing an adverse effect, including age, other medications used concomitantly, genetics, and comorbid conditions. Prior to and following initiation of opioid therapy, clinicians should routinely evaluate and monitor patients for opioid-related adverse effects (Dowell et al., 2016). Patients experiencing adverse effects require changes to their treatment, which may include a dose decrease, an alternative opioid product, adding adjunctive treatment, or symptomatic management of a side effect. Adverse effects due to opioids are numerous.

Gastrointestinal Adverse Effects

Opioids can affect many aspects of gastrointestinal (GI) function. Between 40 percent and 95 percent of patients treated with opioids will experience constipation, with some incidents occurring after single doses. Opioid receptors are commonly found in enteric neurons, the neurons that affect GI absorption. When opioids are ingested, they bind to these receptors, leading to inhibition and decreased gastric motility. Additionally, opioids may act centrally, decreasing the activity of the autonomic nervous system (Yuan & Foss, 2000). Long-term consequences of opioid-induced constipation (OIC) include hemorrhoid formation, bowel obstruction, and potential bowel rupture and death.

Several prevention strategies exist for the management of OIC. As constipation is unlikely to improve over time, prevention is the goal for every patient being treated with opioids. Medications such as stool softeners, bowel stimulants, and osmotic agents are generally considered first-line treatments for prevention. Bulk-forming laxatives, such as psyllium, should not be used for OIC because these products can exacerbate abdominal pain and contribute to bowel obstruction in patients with advanced illness, poor functional status, and insufficient fluid intake (Rauck, 2013). A stimulant laxative (e.g., sennosides, bisacodyl), either alone or with a second agent, should always be used when preventing OIC as a means of counteracting the effects of opioids on GI motility (Kumar, Barker, & Emmanuel, 2014). If the response is insufficient after several classes of medications are used in combination, mu-opioid receptor antagonists may be employed, including methylnaltrexone, alvimopan, and naloxegol (Chey et al., 2014; Ford, Brenner, & Schoenfeld, 2013). These agents are specially formulated to not cross the blood-brain barrier, leading to peripheral opioid receptor antagonism without attenuating pain control.

In addition to constipation, opioids may also produce nausea and emesis by way of decreased gastric motility, stimulation of the chemoreceptor trigger zone, and enhanced vestibular sensitivity. Approximately 25 percent of patients treated with opioids will experience nausea and vomiting (Swegle & Logemann, 2006). Treatment for opioid-related nausea include antihistamines (e.g., diphenhydramine, hydroxyzine, promethazine); serotonin antagonists (e.g., ondansetron); prokinetic agents (e.g., metoclopramide); and antipsychotics (e.g., prochlorperazine).

Respiratory Adverse Effects

Although commonly discussed, respiratory depression generally does not occur when opioids are used appropriately at standard doses and titrated slowly. However, respiratory depression is the leading cause of opioid overdose deaths (Rudd et al., 2016). Respiratory depression caused by opioids is multifactorial. Opioids primarily depress the respiratory drive and rhythm generated in the medullary respiratory center (Pattinson, 2008). Additionally, opioids bind to opioid receptors in the pulmonary system, causing dampened respiratory activity, which leads to bradypnea (abnormally slow breathing), decreased volume, and decreased tidal exchange. Ventilatory response to carbon dioxide is decreased, leading to hypercarbia (elevated carbon dioxide levels in the blood) and hypoxemia (low oxygen levels in the blood; Lalley, 2008). While rare, respiratory depression may be increased due to several factors (Yaksh & Wallace, 2017).

Numerous depressant medications can have additive effects on opioid respiratory depression. Caution should be used in patients receiving sedatives, anesthetics, alcohol, and other central nervous system (CNS) depressants. Natural sleep can also contribute to respiratory depression due to a diminished sensitivity to carbon dioxide. Older adults are at greater risk due to changes in pulmonary physiology and an increased likelihood of drug interactions and comorbid conditions. Comorbid lung diseases, such as COPD, asthma, and sleep apnea, can contribute due to decreased hypoxic drive (Pattinson, 2008). Treatment requires opioid dose reduction, with severe respiratory depression requiring immediate administration of the opioid antagonist naloxone to reverse a potentially fatal overdose (see chapter 13 for more on naloxone and other harm-reduction approaches to opioid misuse).

CNS Depression and Somnolence

Central nervous system (CNS) depression leading to sedation is a common opioid side effect thought to be caused by the anticholinergic activity of opioids (Benyamin et al., 2008). Between 20 percent and 60 percent of patients will experience some sedation (Cherny et al., 2001). This sedation is the result of initiation or titration of opioid therapy or opioid use in combination with other medications, such as benzodiazepines, muscle relaxants, CNS depressants, anticholinergics, and alcohol. Although tolerance develops to these adverse effects, CNS depression may lead to increased morbidity, such as fatigue, memory loss, depression, and hallucinations (Reissig & Rybarczyk, 2005). Evaluating the current opioid regimen and making dose adjustments or medication changes where possible can help prevent these potentially dangerous side effects. Due to their potential for misuse, street value, and numerous adverse effects, using stimulants to treat CNS depression and somnolence caused by opioids should be reserved for special cases, such as patients with cancer pain.

Hyperalgesia

Opioid-induced hyperalgesia is defined as enhanced pain sensitization in patients receiving opioids (Yi & Pryzbylkowski, 2015). This phenomenon describes opioid-tolerant patients' increasing dose requirements to treat chronic pain and an inability to cope with pain stimuli that would be self-limiting in an opioid-naïve person. The current literature identifies several potential mechanisms of hyperalgesia, including central glutaminergic system response, spinal dynorphins, activation of descending pain pathways, genetic mechanisms, and enhanced nociceptive response (Lee, Silverman, Hansen, Patel, & Manchikanti, 2011; Yi & Pryzbylkowski, 2015). The best approach to treating opioid-induced hyperalgesia is weaning the patient off opioids completely. This is a conundrum for clinicians and patients, particularly because patients will perceive the need to increase pain treatment and not decrease it. Eventual opioid discontinuation requires patient education of hyperalgesia, a strong clinician-patient relationship, alternative pain treatment, and time to effectively taper opioid medication.

Pruritus (Itching)

Pruritus has an incidence of 2–10 percent in patients taking opioids (Cherny et al., 2001). Although a precise mechanism has not been identified, pruritus may be caused by central activation of the mu-opioid receptor (Ko, Song, Edwards, Lee, & Naughton, 2004). Additionally, opioid-induced histamine release from mast cells may play a role. Effective treatment strategies include antihistamine medications, moisturizers, opioid dose reduction, and switching opioid medications (McNicol et al., 2003).

Urinary Retention

Opioid-induced urinary retention is reported and can be especially problematic in postoperative patients. The precise mechanism of urinary retention is unknown, but decreased detrusor tone and force of contraction, decreased urge to void, and inhibition of the voiding reflex play a role (Benyamin et al., 2008).

Overdose

Morbidity and mortality due to opioids are one of the biggest public health issues affecting the United States today. Overdose death from prescription drugs is the leading cause of death in 17 U.S. states (American Society of Interventional Pain Physicians, n.d.), and opioid overdose deaths have increased 2.8-fold since 2002 (Rudd et al., 2016). The CDC and the White House have publicly stated that the effects of opioids have reached epidemic proportions (Rudd et al., 2016; White House, Office of the Press Secretary, 2016). Rates of opioid overdose deaths are also on the rise globally, which has raised concerns about a potential worldwide opioid pandemic (Martins & Ghandour, 2017). This epidemic has been building for decades, and it will take a coordinated systems approach to change the course of the crisis.

For every fatal overdose, up to 30 nonfatal overdoses occur (Darke, Mattick, & Degenhardt, 2003). Most individuals who engage in long-term heroin use experience at least one nonfatal overdose in their lifetime (Darke et al., 2014). Persons who experience nonfatal overdoses face high rates of chronic morbidity following injuries sustained during the overdose event, such as renal failure and anoxic brain injury (Warner-Smith, Darke, & Day, 2002). Furthermore, nonfatal overdoses are a predictor for future fatal overdoses (Coffin et al., 2007). Nonfatal overdoses are likely underreported due to the increasing public availability of naloxone, a medication that can reverse the effects of an opioid overdose (see chapter 13 for more).

The preventable nature of these overdoses represents opportunities for health care providers to intervene to mitigate risks of future overdoses. Most fatal overdoses occur when the patient is not enrolled in a long-term, stable drug treatment (Davoli et al., 2007). Potential responses include reassessing opioid prescribing and referring patients to addiction treatment. A study of commercially insured patients indicated that high rates of prescription opioid use occurred after a nonfatal overdose, suggesting that health systems could play a major role in informing opioid prescribers about a patient's addiction risk (Larochelle, Liebschutz, Zhang, Ross-Degnan, & Wharam,

2016). Understanding addiction risk could also lead to increased awareness and use of naloxone.

Risk Factors for Overdose

Several risk factors contribute to overdose, including prior overdose events, obtaining overlapping prescriptions from multiple providers and pharmacies, taking high daily dosages of prescription opioids, having mental illness or a history of alcohol or other substance abuse, and living in rural areas and having low income (Brady, Giglio, Keyes, DiMaggio, & Li, 2017). A prior overdose is the biggest risk factor for a future overdose (Stoové, Dietze, & Jolley, 2009). Higher dosages of opioids were associated with an increased risk of overdose compared to lower dosages (1 to <20 MME/day; Park et al., 2016). Use of extended-release (ER) or long-acting (LA) opioids were also associated with an increased overdose risk, compared with short-acting opioids. Having overlapping prescriptions was also strongly associated with increased risk of overdose (Paulozzi et al., 2012; Yang et al., 2015). Overdose risk also increases with the concomitant use of certain other medications, including muscle relaxants and benzodiazepines (Brugal et al., 2002).

Muscle relaxants, opioids, and benzodiazepines compose the "triple threat" of overdose. When combined, these medications are synergistic in their potential to cause respiratory depression, increasing the risk of death. It is well-known that opioid overdoses often involve more than one of these medications. Those using opioids often use muscle relaxants and benzodiazepines to augment the effect of euphoria. In those engaged in opioid use, combining the effects of benzodiazepines enhances the positive subjective effects of opioids (Jones, Mogali, & Comer, 2012).

Overdose risk increases with longer durations of benzodiazepine treatment (Turner & Liang, 2015). The use of four or more pharmacies or four or more prescribers in the past year were both associated with an increased overdose risk (Gwira Baumblatt et al., 2014). Opioid-related deaths are also higher in rural areas, even after adjusting for population density (Wunsch, Nakamoto, Behonick, & Massello, 2009), and white patients have almost twice the overdose rate as black patients (Chen, Hedegaard, & Warner, 2014). Inequity in pain management, with more restrictive use of opioids for black patients compared to white patients, can partly explain these racial differences (Becker et al., 2011; Kuo, Raji, Chen, Hasan, & Goodwin, 2016; Pletcher, Kertesz, Kohn, & Gonzales, 2008).

Substance use disorder diagnoses, including opioid use disorder (OUD), were associated with an increased risk of overdose. OUD is a problematic pattern of opioid use leading to clinically significant impairment or distress (American Psychiatric Association, 2013). This primary, chronic, and relapsing brain disorder currently affects 2.5 million Americans, and its prevalence continues to increase (Center for Behavioral Health Statistics and Quality, 2015; Martins & Ghandour, 2017). The chronicity and relapsing nature of OUD mirror other chronic conditions that are difficult to treat (e.g., hypertension, diabetes). Men have higher rates of OUD, as do patients ages 35–54 years, whites, and American Indians/Alaska natives (McCarberg, Hahn, Twillman, & Hodgkiss-Harlow, 2012). OUD is a clear predictor of overdose; therefore, it is important to look at all potential overdose factors for evaluating one's overdose risk, including socioeconomic status.

The opioid epidemic has had a disproportionate impact on Medicaid enrollees, as they are prescribed opioids at twice the rate of non-Medicaid enrollees (Coolen, Lima, Savel, & Paulozzi, 2009; Sharp & Melnik, 2015). These prescribing practices have led to a three times higher risk of overdose compared to non-Medicaid patients (Ghate, Haroutiunian, Winslow, & McAdam-Marx, 2010; Sharp & Melnik, 2015). In response to this disparity, Medicaid has implemented several national and statewide policies. Centers for Medicare and Medicaid Services (CMS) "best practice" policies for addressing prescription opioid overdose and misuse include such pharmacy benefit management strategies as reassessing preferred drug list (PDL) placement, introducing clinical criteria, prior authorization, step therapy, quantity limits, and implementing drug utilization review (DUR) processes. Some states have adopted new limits to the number of opioid pills that physicians can prescribe. Forty-six states have adopted quantity limits, and 45 states have adopted prior authorization targeted at opioid harm reduction (Smith et al., 2013). Medicaid is the single largest source of insurance for behavioral health services and OUD treatment, so improving and expanding treatment in the Medicaid population is crucial.

Heroin is a further major driver of the opioid epidemic. Heroin was a popular pain treatment in the late 1880s but was quickly found to be addictive. It is classified as a Schedule I drug under the Controlled Substances Act of 1970, making it illegal to prescribe. Despite these barriers, heroin use has continued to increase in the United States. The most common demographic of a person using heroin switched from a young urban African American male in the 1970s to a middle-aged white female from rural America more recently (Cicero, Ellis, Surratt, & Kurtz, 2014). In the United States today, heroin use is the highest it has been in the last 20 years (Jones, Logan, Gladden, & Bohm, 2015; United Nations Office on Drugs and Crime, 2017). Numerous studies indicate that prescription opioids serve as a gateway drug for subsequent heroin use, with four out of five individuals using heroin stating that their opioid use began with prescription opioids (Compton, Jones, & Baldwin, 2016; Muhuri, Gfroerer, & Davies, 2013).

Those who nonmedically use opioids have recently started shifting to heroin, which has a cheaper street value, higher purity, and is easier to obtain (Compton et al., 2016). Due in part to these factors, deaths due to heroin have been increasing precipitously in the last several years. In addition to the risk of overdose, intravenous (IV) drug use involving heroin has been implicated in many other medical conditions, including human immunodeficiency virus (HIV) and hepatitis C virus (HCV) infection. The relationship between heroin and prescription opioids highlights that neither issue should be addressed in isolation.

Fentanyl has played an increasing role in overdoses since 2013. Fentanyl is a synthetic opioid that is 50–100 times more powerful than morphine and 30–50 times more powerful than heroin, making it an extremely potent opioid. Fentanyl can rapidly suppress respiration, causing death more quickly than other opioids. From 2012 through 2014, the number of reported deaths involving fentanyl more than doubled, from 2,628 to 5,544 (Frank & Pollack, 2017). The relatively low production cost of fentanyl and increasingly high death toll poses a challenging problem in efforts to combat the opioid epidemic. Fentanyl is often mixed with heroin as a combination product, often without the knowledge of the person using it.

Finally, benzodiazepines and opioids taken together increase the risk the overdose by a factor of four (Park et al., 2016), and benzodiazepines are involved in 30 percent of opioid-involved drug overdoses (Chen et al., 2014). Although the benzodiazepine effect on respiratory depression in the brain is mild, the concurrent use with opioids has the potential to increase or prolong the respiratory depressant effect of opioids (Gudin, Mogali, Jones, & Comer, 2013). The number of individuals prescribed both an opioid and a benzodiazepine increased by 41 percent between 2002 and 2014 (Hwang et al., 2016), with approximately 50 percent of those coprescriptions from the same physician on the same day (Hwang et al., 2016). From 2004 to 2011, the rate of emergency department visits involving the nonmedical use of both drug classes increases significantly, and overdose deaths nearly tripled. In response, the Food and Drug Administration (FDA) released its strongest "box" warning on product labels that details the dangers of concomitant use of opioids and benzodiazepines in August 2016 (Food and Drug Administration, 2016).

Misuse

Unfortunately, opioid misuse is on the rise and is found in 21–29 percent of those using opioids (Vowles et al., 2015). Misuse, simply defined as not using a medication as prescribed or using it without a prescription, is increasing. This rise in opioid misuse has paralleled the dramatic rise in overall opioid prescription use. A shocking 59 percent of people who misuse opioids do not have a prescription for opioid medications (Compton et al., 2016). Excessive previous opioid prescriptions are a common culprit to future misuse. The unused opioid medication is left in the medication cabinet, which has the potential to be taken inappropriately by the original person who was prescribed the medication or by someone else. A staggering 40 percent of people who misuse opioids obtained them from friends or family (Han et al., 2017). Obtaining opioids from relatives is also very common in adolescents, with approximately 47 percent of adolescents receiving the medication for free from a friend or family member and about 13 percent purchasing an opioid from a friend or family member (Schepis & Krishnan-Sarin, 2009). Data from 2015 indicate that about 67 percent of adolescents at least 12 years of age obtained opioids from a family member or friend, whether for free or through a purchase (Center for Behavioral Health Statistics and Quality, 2016). There are several risk factors implicated in opioid misuse, including high daily MME use, people who obtain opioid from multiple providers and prescribers, and patients with mental health problems.

Evidence-based opioid prescribing, incorporating misuse screening tools prior to opioid prescribing, and frequent use of PDMPs can help curb misuse. The CDC guidelines on opioid prescribing described earlier in this chapter outline concrete steps for clinicians to use to reduce misuse and consequent morbidity. Screening tools aimed at identifying and preventing misuse prior to opioid prescribing include the validated opioid risk tool (ORT; Webster & Webster, 2005). This brief, self-administered tool can help identify patients who are potentially at risk for future misuse. Unfortunately, no single assessment can perfectly predict future opioid misuse. Urine drug screening prior to opioid prescribing and annually after opioid prescribing are essential in identifying misuse. Clinicians must use not only good history and physical exams to identify patient misuse, but also the numerous other tools in place to identify misuse.

Treatment of Opioid Use Disorder

Once OUD has been diagnosed, it is the clinician's duty to treat it safely and responsibly. Strategies must be both acute and long term to prevent morbidity and mortality. Treatment should be individualized and include both prescription medications and psychological interventions (Schuckit, 2016). Patients with OUD should be referred to proper treatment centers, including ones that offer medication-assisted therapy (MAT) augmented by psychological therapy. Use of long-acting oral opioids are the first-line treatment for opioid withdrawal. These include methadone and buprenorphine, with the goal of initially relieving symptoms and gradually reducing the dose to allow adjustment to the absence of an opioid (Schuckit, 2016). However, specialized licenses and training are required for providers before prescribing these medications (Sullivan & Fiellin, 2008), and these barriers can decrease patient access to treatment programs due to prolonged waiting lists and lack of availability in rural areas. The Substance Abuse and Mental Health

Services Administration provides training and resources for providers to assist with opioid use disorder. Psychological modalities should also be used to treat OUD, but they have been found to be inferior to medication therapy when used alone (Mattick, Breen, Kimber, & Davoli, 2009). Addiction counseling and support group meetings should also be considered (Jhanjee, 2014).

Conclusions

Opioid prescriptions have widely been used to manage various types of pain for the last several decades. There are many different products with various forms, doses, and routes of administration. However, opioid misuse leading to morbidity and mortality has reached epidemic levels. Easy access to opioids used for nonmedical use has contributed to the opioid problem. Unfortunately, deaths due to opioids continue to rise. To help prevent misuse and diversion of opioids, providers can engage in cautious and judicious prescribing by first trying alternative medications, using short courses of opioids (if warranted), and monitoring for signs of misuse or diversion. In addition, patient education is vital to prevent overdose deaths. Providers need to discuss the harms of opioids and provide resources to avoid adverse effects and death, including access to naloxone.

References

American Geriatrics Society Panel on Pharmacological Management of Persistent Pain in Older Persons. (2009). Pharmacological management of persistent pain in older persons. *Journal of the American Geriatrics Society, 57*(8), 1331–1346. doi:10.1111/j.1532-5415.2009.02376.x.

American Psychiatric Association. (2013). *Diagnostic and Statistical Manual of Mental Disorders* (5th ed.). Washington, D.C.: American Psychiatric Association.

American Society of Addiction Medicine. (2011). Public policy statement: Definition of addiction. http://www.asam.org/docs/publicpolicy-statements/1definition_of_addiction_long_4-11.pdf?sfvrsn=2.

American Society of Interventional Pain Physicians. (n.d.). The American Society of Interventional Pain Physicians (ASIPP) fact sheet. https://www.asipp.org/documents/ASIPPFactSheet101111.pdf.

Ballantyne, J. C., & Mao, J. (2003). Opioid therapy for chronic pain. *New England Journal of Medicine, 349*(20), 1943–1953. doi:10.1056/NEJMra025411.

Becker, W. C., Starrels, J. L., Heo, M., Li, X., Weiner, M. G., & Turner, B. J. (2011). Racial differences in primary care opioid risk reduction strategies. *Annals of Family Medicine, 9*(3), 219–225. doi:10.1370/afm.1242.

Benyamin, R., Trescot, A. M., Datta, S., Buenaventura, R., Adlaka, R., Sehgal, N., . . . Vallejo, R. (2008). Opioid complications and side effects. *Pain Physician, 11*(2 Suppl), S105–120.

Brady, J. E., Giglio, R., Keyes, K. M., DiMaggio, C., & Li, G. (2017). Risk markers for fatal and non-fatal prescription drug overdose: A meta-analysis. *Injury Epidemiology, 4*(1), 24. doi:10.1186/s40621-017-0118-7.

Brugal, M. T., Barrio, G., De, L. F., Regidor, E., Royuela, L., & Suelves, J. M. (2002). Factors associated with non-fatal heroin overdose: Assessing the effect of frequency and route of heroin administration. *Addiction, 97*(3), 319–327.

Center for Behavioral Health Statistics and Quality. (2015). *2014 National Survey on Drug Use and Health: Methodological Summary and Definitions.* Rockville, MD: Substance Abuse and Mental Health Services Administration.

Center for Behavioral Health Statistics and Quality. (2016). *Key Substance Use and Mental Health Indicators in the United States: Results from the 2015 National Survey on Drug Use and Health* (HHS Publication No. SMA 16-4984, NSDUH Series H-51).

Chandok, N., & Watt, K. D. S. (2010). Pain management in the cirrhotic patient: The clinical challenge. *Mayo Clinic Proceedings, 85*(5), 451–458. doi:10.4065/mcp.2009.0534.

Chen, L. H., Hedegaard, H., & Warner, M. (2014). Drug-poisoning deaths involving opioid analgesics: United States, 1999–2011. *NCHS Data Brief, 166*, 1–8.

Cherny, N., Ripamonti, C., Pereira, J., Davis, C., Fallon, M., McQuay, H., . . . Ventafridda, V. (2001). Strategies to manage the adverse effects of oral morphine: An evidence-based report. *Journal of Clinical Oncology, 19*(9), 2542–2554. doi:10.1200/jco.2001.19.9.2542.

Chey, W. D., Webster, L. R., Sostek, M., Lappalainen, J., Barker, P., & Tack, J. (2014). Naloxegol for opioid-induced constipation in patients with non-cancer pain. *New England Journal of Medicine, 370*(25), 2387–2396. doi:10.1056/NEJMoa1310246.

Cicero, T. J., Ellis, M. S., Surratt, H. L., & Kurtz, S. P. (2014). The changing face of heroin use in the United States: A retrospective analysis of the past 50 years. *JAMA Psychiatry, 71*(7), 821–826. doi:10.1001/jamapsychiatry.2014.366.

Cochran, G., Gordon, A. J., Lo-Ciganic, W. H., Gellad, W. F., Frazier, W., Lobo, C., . . . Donohue, J. M. (2017). An examination of claims-based predictors of overdose from a large Medicaid program. *Medical Care, 55*(3), 291–298. doi:10.1097/mlr.0000000000000676.

Coffin, P. O., Behar, E., Rowe, C., Santos, G. M., Coffa, D., Bald, M., & Vittinghoff, E. (2016). Nonrandomized intervention study of naloxone coprescription for primary care patients receiving long-term opioid therapy for pain. *Annals of Internal Medicine, 165*(4), 245–252. doi:10.7326/m15-2771.

Coffin, P. O., Tracy, M., Bucciarelli, A., Ompad, D., Vlahov, D., & Galea, S. (2007). Identifying injection drug users at risk of nonfatal overdose. *Academic Emergency Medicine, 14*(7), 616–623. doi:10.1197/j.aem.2007.04.005.

Compton, W. M., Jones, C. M., & Baldwin, G. T. (2016). Relationship between nonmedical prescription-opioid use and heroin use. *New England Journal of Medicine, 374*(2), 154–163. doi:10.1056/NEJMra1508490.

Coolen, P., Lima, A., Savel, J., & Paulozzi, L. (2009). Overdose deaths involving prescription opioids among Medicaid enrollees—Washington, 2004–2007. *MMWR: Morbidity and Mortality Weekly Report, 58*(42), 1171–1175.

Darke, S., Marel, C., Mills, K. L., Ross, J., Slade, T., Burns, L., & Teesson, M. (2014). Patterns and correlates of non-fatal heroin overdose at 11-year follow-up: Findings from the Australian treatment outcome study. *Drug and Alcohol Dependence, 144*, 148–152. doi:10.1016/j.drugalcdep.2014.09.001.

Darke, S., Mattick, R. P., & Degenhardt, L. (2003). The ratio of non-fatal to fatal heroin overdose. *Addiction, 98*(8), 1169–1171.

Davoli, M., Bargagli, A. M., Perucci, C. A., Schifano, P., Belleudi, V., Hickman, M., . . . Faggiano, F. (2007). Risk of fatal overdose during and after specialist drug treatment: The VEdeTTE study, a national multi-site prospective cohort study. *Addiction, 102*(12), 1954–1959. doi:10.1111/j.1360-0443.2007.02025.x.

De Felipe, C., Herrero, J. F., O'Brien, J. A., Palmer, J. A., Doyle, C. A., Smith, A. J., . . . Hunt, S. P. (1998). Altered nociception, analgesia and aggression in mice lacking the receptor for substance P. *Nature, 392*(6674), 394–397. doi:10.1038/32904.

Dean, M. (2004). Opioids in renal failure and dialysis patients. *Journal of Pain and Symptom Management, 28*(5), 497–504. doi:10.1016/j.jpainsymman.2004.02.021.

Department of Veteran Affairs, Department of Defense. (2017). Guideline summary: VA/DoD clinical practice guideline for opioid therapy for chronic pain. https://www.healthquality.va.gov/guidelines/pain/cot.

DiPiro, J. T., Talbert, R. L., Yee, G. C., Matzke, G. R., Wells, B. G., & Posey, L. M. (2017). *Pharmacotherapy: A Pathophysiologic Approach* (10th ed.). Columbus, OH: McGraw-Hill Education.

Dowell, D., Haegerich, T. M., & Chou, R. (2016). CDC guideline for prescribing opioids for Chronic Pain—United States, 2016. *JAMA, 315*(15), 1624–1645. doi:10.1001/jama.2016.1464.

Drug Enforcement Administration. (2016). State prescription drug monitoring programs. https://www.deadiversion.usdoj.gov/faq/rx_monitor.htm.

Food and Drug Administration. (2016). FDA requires strong warnings for opioid analgesics, prescription opioid cough products, and benzodiazepine labeling related to serious risks and death from combined use. https://www.fda.gov/NewsEvents/Newsroom/PressAnnouncements/ucm518697.htm.

Ford, A. C., Brenner, D. M., & Schoenfeld, P. S. (2013). Efficacy of pharmacological therapies for the treatment of opioid-induced constipation: Systematic review and meta-analysis. *American Journal of Gastroenterology, 108*(10), 1566–1574; quiz 1575. doi:10.1038/ajg.2013.169.

Frank, R. G., & Pollack, H. A. (2017). Addressing the fentanyl threat to public health. *New England Journal of Medicine, 376*(7), 605–607. doi:10.1056/NEJMp1615145.

Franklin, G. M., Mai, J., Wickizer, T., Turner, J. A., Fulton-Kehoe, D., & Grant, L. (2005). Opioid dosing trends and mortality in Washington State workers' compensation, 1996–2002. *American Journal of Industrial Medicine, 48*(2), 91–99. doi:10.1002/ajim.20191.

Ghate, S. R., Haroutiunian, S., Winslow, R., & McAdam-Marx, C. (2010). Cost and comorbidities associated with opioid abuse in managed care and Medicaid patients in the United Stated: A comparison of two recently published studies. *Journal of Pain & Palliative Care Pharmacotherapy, 24*(3), 251–258. doi:10.3109/15360288.2010.501851.

Gudin, J. A., Mogali, S., Jones, J. D., & Comer, S. D. (2013). Risks, management, and monitoring of combination opioid, benzodiazepines, and/or alcohol use. *Postgraduate Medicine, 125*(4), 115–130. doi:10.3810/pgm.2013.07.2684.

Guy, G. P., Jr., Zhang, K., Bohm, M. K., Losby, J., Lewis, B., Young, R., . . . Dowell, D. (2017). Vital signs: Changes in opioid prescribing in the United States, 2006–2015. *MMWR: Morbidity and Mortality Weekly Report, 66*(26), 697–704. doi:10.15585/mmwr.mm6626a4.

Gwira Baumblatt, J. A., Wiedeman, C., Dunn, J. R., Schaffner, W., Paulozzi, L. J., & Jones, T. F. (2014). High-risk use by patients prescribed opioids for pain and its role in overdose deaths. *JAMA Internal Medicine, 174*(5), 796–801. doi:10.1001/jamainternmed.2013.12711.

Han, B., Compton, W. M., Blanco, C., Crane, E., Lee, J., & Jones, C. M. (2017). Prescription opioid use, misuse, and use disorders in U.S. adults: 2015 national survey on drug use and health. *Annals of Internal Medicine, 167*(5), 293–301. doi:10.7326/m17-0865.

Hemmings, H., & Egan, T. (2013). *Physiology and Pharmacology for Anesthesia: Foundations and Clinical Application.* Philadelphia, PA: Elsevier.

Hwang, C. S., Kang, E. M., Kornegay, C. J., Staffa, J. A., Jones, C. M., & McAninch, J. K. (2016). Trends in the concomitant prescribing of opioids and benzodiazepines, 2002–2014. *American Journal of Preventive Medicine, 51*(2), 151–160. doi:10.1016/j.amepre.2016.02.014.

Jamison, R. N., & Mao, J. (2015). Opioid analgesics. *Mayo Clinic Proceedings, 90*(7), 957–968. doi:10.1016/j.mayocp.2015.04.010.

Jhanjee, S. (2014). Evidence based psychosocial interventions in substance use. *Indian Journal of Psychological Medicine, 36*(2), 112–118. doi:10.4103/0253-7176.130960.

Johannes, C. B., Le, T. K., Zhou, X., Johnston, J. A., & Dworkin, R. H. (2010). The prevalence of chronic pain in United States adults: Results of an Internet-based survey. *Journal of Pain, 11*(11), 1230–1239. doi:10.1016/j.jpain.2010.07.002.

Jones, C. M., Logan, J., Gladden, R. M., & Bohm, M. K. (2015). Vital signs: Demographic and substance use trends among heroin users—United States, 2002–2013. *MMWR: Morbidity and Mortality Weekly Report, 64*(26), 719–725.

Jones, J. D., Mogali, S., & Comer, S. D. (2012). Polydrug abuse: A review of opioid and benzodiazepine combination use. *Drug and Alcohol Dependence, 125*(1-2), 8–18. doi:10.1016/j.drugalcdep.2012.07.004.

Kalso, E., Edwards, J. E., Moore, R. A., & McQuay, H. J. (2004). Opioids in chronic non-cancer pain: Systematic review of efficacy and safety. *Pain, 112*(3), 372–380. doi:10.1016/j.pain.2004.09.019.

Ko, M. C., Song, M. S., Edwards, T., Lee, H., & Naughton, N. N. (2004). The role of central mu opioid receptors in opioid-induced itch in primates. *Journal of Pharmacology and Experimental Therapeutics, 310*(1), 169–176. doi:10.1124/jpet.103.061101.

Kornetsky, C., & Bain, G. (1968). Morphine: Single-dose tolerance. *Science, 162*(3857), 1011–1012.

Kumar, L., Barker, C., & Emmanuel, A. (2014). Opioid-induced constipation: Pathophysiology, clinical consequences, and management. *Gastroenterology Research and Practice, 2014*, 6. doi:10.1155/2014/141737.

Kuo, Y. F., Raji, M. A., Chen, N. W., Hasan, H., & Goodwin, J. S. (2016). Trends in opioid prescriptions among Part D Medicare recipients from 2007 to 2012. *American Journal of Medicine, 129*(2), 221.e21–30. doi:10.1016/j.amjmed.2015.10.002.

Lalley, P. M. (2008). Opioidergic and dopaminergic modulation of respiration. *Respiratory Physiology & Neurobiology, 164*(1-2), 160–167. doi:10.1016/j.resp.2008.02.004.

Larochelle, M. R., Liebschutz, J. M., Zhang, F., Ross-Degnan, D., & Wharam, J. (2016). Opioid prescribing after nonfatal overdose and association with repeated overdose: A cohort study. *Annals of Internal Medicine, 164*(1), 1–9. doi:10.7326/M15-0038.

Lee, M., Silverman, S. M., Hansen, H., Patel, V. B., & Manchikanti, L. (2011). A comprehensive review of opioid-induced hyperalgesia. *Pain Physician, 14*(2), 145–161.

Martins, S. S., & Ghandour, L. A. (2017). Nonmedical use of prescription drugs in adolescents and young adults: Not just a Western phenomenon. *World Psychiatry, 16*(1), 102–104. doi:10.1002/wps.20350.

Mattick, R. P., Breen, C., Kimber, J., & Davoli, M. (2009). Methadone maintenance therapy versus no opioid replacement therapy for opioid dependence. *Cochrane Database of Systematic Reviews, 3*, CD002209. doi:10.1002/14651858.CD002209.pub2.

Max, M. B. (1990). Improving outcomes of analgesic treatment: Is education enough? *Annals of Internal Medicine, 113*(11), 885–889.

McCarberg, B., Hahn, K. L., Twillman, R. K., & Hodgkiss-Harlow, C. J. (2012). A role for opioids in chronic pain management. *Archives of Internal Medicine, 172*(10), 824–825. doi:10.1001/archinternmed.2012.882.

McNicol, E., Horowicz-Mehler, N., Fisk, R. A., Bennett, K., Gialeli-Goudas, M., Chew, P. W., . . . Carr, D. (2003). Management of opioid side effects in cancer-related and chronic noncancer pain: A systematic review. *Journal of Pain, 4*(5), 231–256.

Meldrum, M. L. (2016). The ongoing opioid prescription epidemic: Historical context. *American Journal of Public Health, 106*(8), 1365–1366. doi:10.2105/ajph.2016.303297.

Muhuri, P. K., Gfroerer, J. C., & Davies, M. C. (2013). Associations of nonmedi-
cal pain reliever use and initiation of heroin use in the United States.
CBHSQ Data Review.https://www.samhsa.gov/data/sites/default/files/DR006
/DR006/nonmedical-pain-reliever-use-2013.htm.

Pardo, M., & Miller, R. (2018). *Basics of Anesthesia* (7th ed.). Philadelphia, PA:
Elsevier.

Park, T. W., Lin, L. A., Hosanagar, A., Kogowski, A., Paige, K., & Bohnert, A. S.
(2016). Understanding risk factors for opioid overdose in clinical populations to inform treatment and policy. *Journal of Addiction Medicine, 10*(6),
369–381. doi:10.1097/adm.0000000000000245.

Pattinson, K. T. (2008). Opioids and the control of respiration. *British Journal of
Anaesthesia, 100*(6), 747–758. doi:10.1093/bja/aen094.

Paulozzi, L. J., Kilbourne, E. M., Shah, N. G., Nolte, K. B., Desai, H. A., Landen,
M. G., . . . Loring, L. D. (2012). A history of being prescribed controlled
substances and risk of drug overdose death. *Pain Medicine, 13*(1), 87–95.
doi:10.1111/j.1526-4637.2011.01260.x.

Pletcher, M. J., Kertesz, S. G., Kohn, M. A., & Gonzales, R. (2008). Trends in
opioid prescribing by race/ethnicity for patients seeking care in US emergency departments. *JAMA, 299*(1), 70–78. doi:10.1001/jama.2007.64.

Portenoy, R. K., & Foley, K. M. (1986). Chronic use of opioid analgesics in nonmalignant pain: Report of 38 cases. *Pain, 25*(2), 171–186.

Porter, J., & Jick, H. (1980). Addiction rare in patients treated with narcotics.
New England Journal of Medicine, 302(2), 123.

Rauck, R. L. (2013). Treatment of opioid-induced constipation: Focus on the peripheral mu-opioid receptor antagonist methylnaltrexone. *Drugs, 73*(12),
1297–1306. doi:10.1007/s40265-013-0084-5.

Reissig, J. E., & Rybarczyk, A. M. (2005). Pharmacologic treatment of opioid-
induced sedation in chronic pain. *Annals of Pharmacotherapy, 39*(4), 727–
731. doi:10.1345/aph.1E309.

Rice, J. B., White, A. G., Birnbaum, H. G., Schiller, M., Brown, D. A., & Roland, C.
L. (2012). A model to identify patients at risk for prescription opioid abuse,
dependence, and misuse. *Pain Medicine, 13*(9), 1162–1173. doi:10.1111
/j.1526-4637.2012.01450.x.

Rudd, R. A., Seth, P., David, F., & Scholl, L. (2016). Increases in drug and opioid-
involved overdose deaths—United States, 2010–2015. *MMWR: Morbidity
and Mortality Weekly Report, 65*(5051), 1445–1452. doi:10.15585/mmwr.
mm655051e1.

Schatman, M. E. (2011). The role of the health insurance industry in perpetuating
suboptimal pain management. *Pain Medicine, 12*(3), 415–426. doi:10.1111
/j.1526-4637.2011.01061.x.

Schepis, T. S., & Krishnan-Sarin, S. (2009). Sources of prescriptions for misuse
by adolescents: Differences in sex, ethnicity, and severity of misuse in a
population-based study. *Journal of the American Academy of Child and Adolescent Psychiatry, 48*(8), 828–836. doi:10.1097/CHI.0b013e3181a8130d.

Schuckit, M. A. (2016). Treatment of opioid-use disorders. *New England Journal of Medicine, 375*(4), 357–368. doi:10.1056/NEJMra1604339.

Sharp, M. J., & Melnik, T. A. (2015). Poisoning deaths involving opioid analgesics—New York State, 2003–2012. MMWR: *Morbidity and Mortality Weekly Report, 64*(14), 377–380.

Smith, V. K., Gifford, K., Ellis, E., Edwards, B., Rudowitz, R., Hinton, E., . . . Valentine, A. (2013). *Implementing Coverage and Payment Initiatives: Results from a 50-State Medicaid Budget Survey for State Fiscal Years 2016 and 2017.* Menlo Park, CA: Henry J. Kaiser Family Foundation.

Stoové, M. A., Dietze, P. M., & Jolley, D. (2009). Overdose deaths following previous non-fatal heroin overdose: Record linkage of ambulance attendance and death registry data. *Drug and Alcohol Review, 28*(4), 347–352. doi:10.1111/j.1465-3362.2009.00057.x.

Sullivan, L. E., & Fiellin, D. A. (2008). Narrative review: Buprenorphine for opioid-dependent patients in office practice. *Annals of Internal Medicine, 148*(9), 662–670.

Swegle, J. M., & Logemann, C. (2006). Management of common opioid-induced adverse effects. *American Family Physician, 74*(8), 1347–1354.

Thorn, C. F., Klein, T. E., & Altman, R. B. (2009). Codeine and morphine pathway. *Pharmacogenetics and Genomics, 19*(7), 556–558. doi:10.1097/FPC.0b013e32832e0eac.

Turner, B. J., & Liang, Y. (2015). Drug overdose in a retrospective cohort with non-cancer pain treated with opioids, antidepressants, and/or sedative-hypnotics: Interactions with mental health disorders. *Journal of General Internal Medicine, 30*(8), 1081–1096. doi:10.1007/s11606-015-3199-4.

United Nations Office on Drugs and Crime. (2017). *World Drug Report 2016.* Vienna, Austria: United Nations Office on Drugs and Crime.

Vallejo, R., Barkin, R. L., & Wang, V. C. (2011). Pharmacology of opioids in the treatment of chronic pain syndromes. *Pain Physician, 14*(4), E343–360.

Von Korff, M., Kolodny, A., Deyo, R. A., & Chou, R. (2011). Long-term opioid therapy reconsidered. *Annals of Internal Medicine, 155*(5), 325–328. doi:10.7326/0003-4819-155-5-201109060-00011.

Vowles, K. E., McEntee, M. L., Julnes, P. S., Frohe, T., Ney, J. P., & van der Goes, D. N. (2015). Rates of opioid misuse, abuse, and addiction in chronic pain: A systematic review and data synthesis. *Pain, 156*(4), 569–576. doi:10.1097/01.j.pain.0000460357.01998.f1.

Warner-Smith, M., Darke, S., & Day, C. (2002). Morbidity associated with non-fatal heroin overdose. *Addiction, 97*(8), 963–967.

Webster, L. R., & Webster, R. M. (2005). Predicting aberrant behaviors in opioid-treated patients: Preliminary validation of the opioid risk tool. *Pain Medicine, 6*(6), 432–442. doi:10.1111/j.1526-4637.2005.00072.x.

White House, Office of the Press Secretary. (2016). Obama administration announces prescription opioid and heroin epidemic awareness week. https://obamawhitehouse.archives.gov/the-press-office/2016/09/19

/fact-sheet-obama-administration-announces-prescription-opioid-and
-heroin.

Wunsch, M. J., Nakamoto, K., Behonick, G., & Massello, W. (2009). Opioid
deaths in rural Virginia: A description of the high prevalence of accidental fatalities involving prescribed medications. *American Journal on Addictions, 18*(1), 5–14. doi:10.1080/10550490802544938.

Yaksh, T., & Wallace, M. (2017). Opioids, analgesia, and pain management. In L.
L. Brunton, B. A. Chabner, & B. C. Knollmann (Eds.), *Goodman and Gil-
man's: The Pharmacological Basis of Therapeutics* (12th ed.), 481–526. New
York: McGraw-Hill.

Yang, Z., Wilsey, B., Bohm, M., Weyrich, M., Roy, K., Ritley, D., . . . Melnikow, J.
(2015). Defining risk of prescription opioid overdose: Pharmacy shopping and overlapping prescriptions among long-term opioid users in
medicaid. *Journal of Pain, 16*(5), 445–453. doi:10.1016/j.jpain.2015.01.475.

Yi, P., & Pryzbylkowski, P. (2015). Opioid induced hyperalgesia. *Pain Medicine,
16 Suppl 1*, S32–36. doi:10.1111/pme.12914.

Yokell, M. A., Delgado, M. K., Zaller, N. D., Wang, N. E., McGowan, S. K., &
Green, T. C. (2014). Presentation of prescription and nonprescription opioid overdoses to US emergency departments. *JAMA Internal Medicine,
174*(12), 2034–2037. doi:10.1001/jamainternmed.2014.5413.

Yuan, C. S., & Foss, J. F. (2000). Antagonism of gastrointestinal opioid effects.
Regional Anesthesia and Pain Medicine, 25(6), 639–642. doi:10.1053/rapm
.2000.8658.

Zhong, W., Maradit-Kremers, H., St Sauver, J. L., Yawn, B. P., Ebbert, J. O., Roger,
V. L., . . . Rocca, W. A. (2013). Age and sex patterns of drug prescribing
in a defined American population. *Mayo Clinic Proceedings, 88*(7), 697–
707. doi:10.1016/j.mayocp.2013.04.021.

CHAPTER THREE

Stimulants

*Christian J. Teter, Marcus Zavala,
and Linh Tran*

Introduction and Therapeutic Uses

There have been recent increases in medical use, medical misuse, and non-medical misuse of prescription medications with abuse potential, such as central nervous system (CNS) stimulants (Chai et al., 2012; DEA, 2012; Fortuna, Robbins, Caiola, Joynt, & Halterman, 2010; McCabe, Knight, Teter, & Wechsler, 2005; McCabe, Veliz, Wilens, & Schulenberg, 2017; Safer, 2016), which are the focus of this chapter.

In regard to prescription stimulants, one of their primary uses is in the treatment of attention deficit/hyperactivity disorder (ADHD), which is characterized by the "classic triad" of impaired attention, impulsive behaviors, and excessive motor activity (Prince, Wilens, Spencer, & Biederman, 2017). The evidence base strongly supports both their safety and efficacy in the treatment of ADHD (Wolraich et al., 2011). Stimulants are generally considered to be first-line medication management for ADHD and demonstrate relatively large effect sizes for reducing ADHD symptoms (American Psychiatric Association, 2013; Faraone, 2009; Faraone & Buitelaar, 2010). Other approved indications for stimulant medications include the treatment of sleep disorders (e.g., narcolepsy) and eating disorders (Centers for Medicare & Medicaid Services, 2017). Lastly, stimulant medications are used off-label for various conditions, such as treatment-resistant major depressive disorder (American Psychiatric Association, 2010). It is important to keep in mind that clinical efficacy associated with the stimulant medications must always be balanced with the risks for medical and nonmedical misuse and diversion, which have resulted in their Schedule II designation by the Drug Enforcement Administration (DEA; Drug Enforcement Administration 2012). The abuse potential of these medications is discussed in greater detail below, following a description of their pharmacodynamic and pharmacokinetic properties.

Although the most commonly used stimulant medications fall into either the methylphenidate or amphetamine pharmacological classes, there are numerous stimulant formulations available for therapeutic use. Table 3.1 lists the currently available psychostimulant medication formulations along with their Food and Drug Administration–approved indication(s). As the table demonstrates, there are now a great number of specific stimulant formulations available for appropriate therapeutic use; however, these medications have found their way to medical misuse (e.g., a prescribed patient uses the stimulant in ways the provider did not intend, whether for the prescribed condition, but at higher doses, or for euphoric purposes) and nonmedical use (e.g., prescription stimulant use without a prescription, often following diversion of the stimulant from an individual with a valid stimulant prescription).

The prescription stimulant landscape continuously changes, and clinicians and researchers must be vigilant and follow the literature on a regular basis to remain current. For example, as this chapter was being written, Mydayis (mixed salts single-entity amphetamine) began being marketed for use, with evidence of improved ADHD control at 16 hours postdose (Food and Drug Administration, 2017). As this example illustrates, the prescription stimulant armamentarium is constantly changing, and Table 3.1 is meant to serve as an overview at the time of this writing.

Pharmacodynamics and Pharmacokinetics

Psychostimulant medications are sympathomimetic in that they stimulate the sympathetic nervous system and typically increase dopaminergic and noradrenergic neurotransmission to various degrees (Prince et al., 2017; Westfall & Westfall, 2011). They often have structural similarities to naturally occurring catecholamines (Westfall & Westfall, 2011).

For example, Figure 3.1 compares amphetamine structures to the structures of naturally occurring catecholamine neurotransmitters in the central nervous system (CNS), such as norepinephrine and dopamine (Heal, Smith, Gosden, & Nutt, 2013). As shown in the figure, amphetamines and the catecholamine neurotransmitters all share the phenethylamine core structure, which is made of the benzene ring connected to an ethylamine side chain (Westfall & Westfall, 2011). Variations made to this phenethylamine structure result in various substances with sympathomimetic effects. For an

Table 3.1 Central Nervous System Psychostimulant Medications

Pharmacologic Class	Stimulant Formulations	Approved Indication(s)
Methylphenidate (MPH) Medications		
Short/Intermediate Acting *(duration of action 3–8 hours)*	Generic MPH; Ritalin; Methylin MPH SR (wax matrix); Ritalin SR (wax matrix); Metadate ER (wax matrix); Methylin ER; QuilliChewER [MPH]	ADHD Narcolepsy
	Focalin [dexmethylphenidate]	
Long Acting *(duration of action >8 hours)*	Ritalin LA (50%IR/50%ER beads); Metadate CD (30%IR/70%ER beads);	ADHD
	Concerta (OROS);	
	Daytrana (transdermal);	
	Aptensio XR (40%IR/60%ER);	
	Quillivant [MPH] XR Suspension (20%IR/80%ER)	
	Focalin XR [dexmethylphenidate] (50%IR/50%ER beads)	
Amphetamine (AMPH) Medications		
Short/Immediate Acting *(duration of action 3–8 hours)*	Mixed amphetamine salts (75% d-AMPH + 25% l-AMPH); Adderall	ADHD Narcolepsy
	Dextroamphetamine; Dexedrine; Dextrostat; Dexedrine Spansule	
Long Acting *(duration of action >8 hours)*	Adderall XR (dextro/levo 3:1 ratio)—in addition to 50%IR/50%ER	ADHD Narcolepsy [1]Exogenous Obesity [2]Moderate to severe binge-eating disorder
	Adzenys XR-ODT (dextro/levo in 3:1 ratio) - microparticles	
	Dyanavel XR Suspension (dextro/levo in 3.2:1 ratio)—ion exchange tech.	
	Evekeo[1] (dextro/levo 1:1 ratio)—up to 10 hours	
	Vyvanse[2] [lisdexamfetamine] (prodrug converted to dextroamphetamine)	

(continued)

Table 3.1 *(continued)*

Pharmacologic Class	Stimulant Formulations	Approved Indication(s)
Miscellaneous Stimulant Medications		
Short/Immediate Acting *(duration of action 3–8 hours)*	Provigil [Modafinil] Nuvigil [Armodafinil]	Sleep Disorders (e.g., adjunct for obstructive sleep apnea)
Long Acting *(duration of action >8 hours)*	Phentermine (in combination with other agents)	Weight Loss

Table adapted from the following sources: CMS.gov, 2017; Dopheide & Pliszka, 2017; and Prince et al., 2017.

Abbreviations: ER & XR = extended release; IR = immediate release; ODT = orally disintegrating tablets; LA= long acting

extensive listing of phenethylamine derivatives (i.e., compounds with stimulant activity), including a visual representation of their chemical structures, the reader is referred to Westfall & Westfall (2011).

Pharmacology

Stimulants block reuptake of monoamine neurotransmitters via the monoamine transporters and, in some cases (e.g., amphetamines), stimulate monoamine release from the neuron via displacement of neurotransmitters from presynaptic vesicles (Westfall & Westfall, 2011). For example, methylphenidate blocks the reuptake of dopamine and norepinephrine back into the nerve terminal, and amphetamine-based medications have this mechanism in addition to stimulating monoamine neurotransmitter release from the nerve terminal (Biaggioni & Robertson, 2015).

Taken together, these pharmacological effects result in CNS activation, with observable increases in both behavioral and motor activity in the individual using them (Schatzberg & Nemeroff, 2017). In some cases, this activation is used for therapeutic purposes or can lead to side effects. In other cases, these stimulant properties may be used for recreational or self-treatment purposes. For example, it is thought that dopaminergic and noradrenergic modulation in the prefrontal cortex caused by stimulant medication could treat ADHD symptoms (Stahl, 2010; Swanson, Baler, & Volkow, 2011), which is often referred to as enhanced "top-down" executive control. In contrast, increases in stereotyped behavior (e.g., rocking back and forth) following stimulant ingestion are likely due to striatal dopaminergic increases and could be considered a side effect, depending on severity. Lastly, we know (as discussed in "Pharmacokinetic Contribution") that individuals misuse these stimulant medications for their dopaminergic effects in the reward pathway and possibly for their activating noradrenergic effects throughout the CNS.

Methylphenidate and amphetamine consist of multiple isomers (Prince et al., 2017). However, these stimulants are also available as pure isomers. In the case of methylphenidate, d-methylphenidate is more pharmacologically active and is available in medication form as dexmethylphenidate. The same is true of amphetamines, with d-amphetamine being more potent and available in medication form as dextroamphetamine. Currently, the relative contribution of each isomer to clinical advantages (or disadvantages) remains to be determined with certainty. However, it is possible that pure isomer medications may offer advantages over their racemic mixture counterparts, and this represents

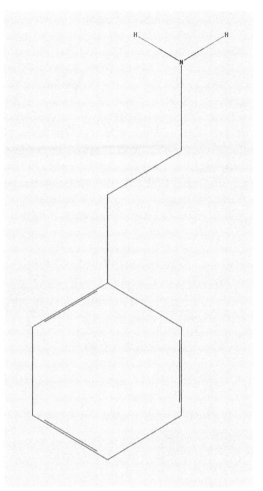

Figure 3.1   National Center for Biotechnology Information: PubChem Compound Database; CID=1001, https://pubchem.ncbi.nlm.nih.gov/compound/1001 (accessed Nov. 20, 2017; NCBI, 2017)

an area for future research and medication development efforts.

Modafinil (Provigil) and armodafinil are relatively new stimulant medications and possess a unique, and not currently well-understood, mechanism of action compared to the methylphenidate and amphetamine medications discussed above. Given their relatively low prevalence of use, medical misuse, and nonmedical misuse, they are not the focus of this chapter. However, their place in the stimulant medication toolkit needs further study, as do both their abuse liability and any other potentially adverse effects.

Physiologic and Adverse Effects

Many of the effects (both desired and adverse) that stimulant medications exert on the body can be reliably predicted based on their sympathomimetic mechanism of action. For example, an increase in alertness and vigilance is consistent with a sympathomimetic response. However, too much sympathetic stimulation may result in anxiety, restlessness, and irritability. Table 3.2 provides common examples of both normal physiologic and adverse effects that may occur as a result of stimulant medication ingestion.

In regard to the overlap that exists between the desired therapeutic efficacy and adverse effects of stimulant medications, consider a patient case in which the wakefulness-promoting effects of stimulant medications may be desired (e.g., excessive sleepiness resulting from sleep apnea); in another

Table 3.2   Physiologic Effects (including Adverse Effects) of Stimulant Medications

	Physiologic Effect	**Adverse Effect**
Cardiac/vascular Effects	Increased heart rate	Tachycardia
	Increased blood pressure	Cardiac arrhythmias
		Cerebrovascular accidents
		Peripheral vasculopathy (e.g., Raynaud's phenomenon)
Central nervous system effects *(likely dependent on baseline status of individual, i.e., whether the individual has a preexisting condition, such as ADHD)*	Increased wakefulness	Restlessness/anxiety
	Increase in psychomotor activity	Tremor
		Headache
	Increased vigilance	Insomnia
	Improved attention	Long-term neurotoxicity *(particularly following frequent or high stimulant doses, which may damage nerve terminals)*
	Appetite suppression	Malnutrition/undesired weight loss *(although adherence to nutritional diet can reduce the unwanted weight loss when using these medications long-term for ADHD)*
Ocular *(i.e., relating to the eyes)*	Pupil dilation	Mydriasis *(common observable sign of recent stimulant ingestion)*

Table adapted from following sources: Dopheide & Pliszka, 2017; Westfall & Westfall, 2011.

patient, the sleep-interfering effects of stimulant use may be undesired and might be considered side effects (e.g., an adolescent with ADHD who stops taking her medication because of stimulant-induced insomnia). Thus, whether a particular physiologic effect is considered efficacious versus an adverse effect depends on the unique situation.

Other effects are not as reliably predicted as those shown in Table 3.2. For example, given the potent dopaminergic effects of stimulants, someone using a stimulant may rapidly develop manic or psychotic behaviors, which are typically listed as warnings or precautions for stimulant medications in their prescribing information (i.e., package inserts). In fact, antipsychotic medications that possess potent dopaminergic blockade are used clinically to treat stimulant intoxication, especially when other approaches (e.g., benzodiazepines) are nonefficacious.

Stimulant Intoxication

Table 3.2 is meant to highlight examples of sympathomimetic adverse effects that can occur at even typical stimulant dosages. However, beyond these typical stimulant doses, individuals often use excessive amounts of stimulants, which can and often do result in stimulant intoxication. The signs and symptoms of stimulant intoxication generally fall into two broad categories:

- *mood/behavioral effects:* elated mood, hypervigilance, anxiety/panic, impaired judgment, violent behavior, delusional thinking, hallucinations
- *neurologic/neuromuscular effects:* mydriasis (i.e., pupil dilation); headache; tremor; increased motor activity; compulsive/stereotyped movements (e.g., skin picking, grinding teeth); hyperthermia; rhabdomyolysis (i.e., severe muscle breakdown, with potentially deleterious effects on the kidneys); seizure activity

Some of these above signs and symptoms can result in medical emergencies, which is a key reason that medical misuse and nonmedical misuse of prescription stimulants can be a very dangerous form of substance use. In other words, prescription stimulant misuse is not always a benign substance use behavior.

Acute versus Chronic Effects

As with any substance, adverse effects can generally be thought of as acute versus chronic. For example, an acute stimulatory cardiac effect following stimulant use might be a concerning elevation in heart rate and blood pressure or possibly even sudden death due to cardiovascular complications.

In contrast, following years of long-term (i.e., chronic) stimulant use, especially in high or frequent doses, cardiomyopathy can occur despite any life-threatening acute complications. The issue of acute side effect versus chronic toxicity is particularly relevant to the central nervous system, as the long-term impact of stimulants on the brain have been (and continue to be) debated among the clinical and scientific community, given their widespread use for ADHD and other disorders.

Pharmacokinetics

Pharmaceutical delivery systems for stimulant medications have greatly expanded over the years, which, in turn, has amplified the variation of their pharmacokinetic profiles. However, despite the numerous formulations currently available in the United States, stimulant medications are often classified into two clinically relevant and useful categories: short/intermediate-acting and long-acting. These categories are related to their pharmaceutical delivery system and the half-life of the active pharmacologic substance. This simplified approach helps clinicians choose appropriate stimulant medication therapy based on patient needs (e.g., choosing a long-acting medication for a student who needs a full day of stimulant coverage for ADHD symptoms compared to another student with ADHD who prefers to take a short-acting medication in the morning to avoid insomnia in the evening).

Broadly speaking, clinical pharmacokinetics are generally concerned with absorption, distribution, metabolism, and elimination (ADME). In regard to the issues being discussed in this chapter, the most relevant pharmacokinetic parameters of stimulant medications are how quickly they are absorbed and distributed throughout the body—and the brain in particular—and how quickly they are metabolized and eliminated from the body. Again, these pharmacokinetic parameters are manipulated by various delivery systems. For example, the Focalin XR delivery system produces a bimodal plasma concentration over time curve that occurs via the use of a proprietary spheroidal oral drug absorption system (SODAS; Novartis Pharmaceuticals Corporation, 2007). Thus, it is as important to understand the pharmaceutical delivery system as the pharmacokinetics of the active pharmacological substance (e.g., dexmethylphenidate). See Prince et al. (2017) for a concise review of the pharmacokinetic differences among the stimulant medications.

Abuse Potential

Stimulant medications possess abuse potential (Kollins, 2007), which is clearly reflected in their DEA Schedule II classification (American Psychiatric Association, 2013; Drug Enforcement Administration, 2012); the black box warning of abuse and dependence present in the prescribing information for amphetamine- and methylphenidate-based psychostimulants; and the fact that stimulant use disorders (including disorders from prescription stimulant use) are present in the *Diagnostic and Statistical Manual of Mental Disorders* (DSM-5; American Psychiatric Association, 2013). According to the DSM-5, there are three unique stimulant-related disorders: (1) stimulant intoxication, (2) stimulant withdrawal, and (3) stimulant use disorder, any of which can result from prescription stimulant use. It should be noted that physical dependence and tolerance to stimulant medications are often normal consequences of long-term therapeutic stimulant use, compared to the process of "addiction" to stimulants, which is an entirely distinct phenomenon and is covered under the third DSM-5 category of "stimulant use disorder." Lastly, there have been a great deal of reports describing the medical misuse, nonmedical misuse, and illicit use of prescription stimulants over recent years and among various populations (McCabe et al., 2005; Wilens et al., 2008).

Pharmacokinetic Contribution

The abuse potential associated with a stimulant medication can be directly traced to its mechanism of action and pharmacokinetic parameters. Similar to most substances that are misused by humans, psychostimulants increase extracellular dopamine concentrations in the brain's reward pathway (Volkow, 2006). Furthermore, stimulants that result in a more rapid rise in drug concentrations in the brain tend to produce more positive reinforcement and hence drug likability (Volkow, 2006). These are the clinical pharmacokinetic parameters of absorption and distribution referred to above. A rapid rise in CNS drug concentration is accompanied by a rapid increase in dopamine levels in the reward pathway from the ventral tegmental area to the nucleus accumbens. This reward pathway in the midbrain is often referred to as the "least common denominator" associated with all pleasurable substances that are misused by humans.

Likewise, medications that are eliminated quickly from the body often produce a greater withdrawal presentation and hence result in negative reinforcement, which, in simple terms, implies the use of the medication or other substance to alleviate adverse withdrawal symptoms or craving. This process can occur following ingestion of most, if not all, psychoactive stimulant substances. For example, although not the focus of this chapter, cocaine is a classic example of a stimulant that causes significant withdrawal symptoms given how quickly it is eliminated from the body. The same concept applies to stimulant medications, as rapid elimination from the body and brain could result in greater withdrawal symptoms and hence use of the substance to eliminate those withdrawal symptoms, which can include craving for the substance. This process is a portion of the *addiction cycle* that is often referred to when speaking of substance use disorders.

Abuse-Deterrent Formulations

To lessen the abuse potential of stimulant medications, abuse-deterrent formulations have been and continue to be developed to deliver medication concentrations into the body at a consistent rate to slow the rate of rise of dopamine in the brain. For example, Spencer et al. (2006) demonstrated that a methylphenidate formulation with a longer time to maximum concentrations (known as the T_{max}) was associated with slower rates of dopamine transporter occupancy and less "likeability." Table 3.1 provides examples of many abuse-deterrent formulations, such as transdermal patches and oral delivery systems that deliver continuous or bolus doses of medication. Perhaps the most novel of these orally delivered abuse-deterrent delivery systems is the commercially available Vyvanse (lisdexamfetamine), which consists of a stimulant bound to an amino acid. In the stomach, the stimulant separates from the amino acid and becomes a pharmacologically active substance. It is important to note, though, that once the stimulant is freed from the amino acid, it is an active amphetamine with similar sympathomimetic characteristics to other stimulant medications.

Individual Characteristics

In addition to the inherent pharmacodynamic and pharmacokinetic principles of the stimulant medications, other nonmedication factors are involved in the overall abuse potential of these medications.

Performance Enhancement Motives

Motives have been linked to the abuse potential of the stimulant medications (Drazdowski, 2016; Teter, McCabe, LaGrange, Cranford, & Boyd, 2006). This line of research illustrates that, in addition to typical substance use behaviors (e.g., using stimulants for their positive reinforcing effects), motives consistent with performance enhancement explain at least some prescription stimulant misuse. For example, because stimulants increase alertness, individuals with and without diagnosed disorders, such as ADHD, may take higher or more frequent doses to stay awake for longer durations of time and to promote concentration. This pattern of use can lead to, or exacerbate, aberrant drug-taking behaviors (e.g., medical misuse or nonmedical misuse), in which an individual's stimulant use becomes compulsive and maladaptive (American Psychiatric Association, 2013). Those who misuse stimulants while endorsing performance-enhancement motives may require unique intervention or prevention efforts as compared to those engaged in recreational stimulant misuse, who typically misuse these medications primarily for their dopaminergic effects (e.g., euphoria, high) described in "Pharmacokinetic Contribution."

Pharmacologic Cognitive Enhancement

Recent evidence further suggests that in addition to using these stimulant medications to help study and increase mental concentration (Teter et al., 2006), students perceive stimulant medications as efficacious for improving their cognitive abilities (Arria et al., 2017). While this may be true among individuals with ADHD (Lu et al., 2017), there are extremely mixed findings in the literature among normal healthy (e.g., non-ADHD) individuals (Bagot & Kaminer, 2014; Repantis, Schlattmann, Laisney, & Heuser, 2010; Smith & Farah, 2011). Although this literature describes the occasional positive finding for specific memory tasks and describes the possibility of benefits in "specific cognitive domains," the real-world (i.e., natural setting) significance of these relatively isolated laboratory-based findings cannot be determined at this time. For instance, there are no concrete findings that students without ADHD who engage in prescription stimulant use for cognitive-enhancement purposes demonstrate fewer problem behaviors and superior academic performance compared to their peers; indeed, the bulk of the evidence suggests poorer academic performance in those misusing stimulants (Arria et al., 2013; Garnier-Dykstra, Caldeira, Vincent, O'Grady, & Arria, 2012), though causality cannot be inferred from the study designs used.

This lack of real-world efficacy may be due to the isolated laboratory findings that have demonstrated pharmacologic cognitive enhancement reveal very modest effect sizes (Ilieva, Hook, & Farah, 2015; Marraccini, Weyandt, Rossi, & Gudmundsdottir, 2016). In any case, given both that stimulant medications are commonly theorized to help with top-down cognitive abilities via their ability to enhance tonic dopamine (DA) and norepinephrine (NE) activity in the prefrontal cortex (Stahl, 2013) and that there is likely an optimal balance between too little and too much CNS neurotransmitter activity (Stahl, 2013), the distinction between cognitive-enhancement efficacy among individuals with disorders such as ADHD and normal healthy individuals needs a great deal of clarification.

Pharmacologic Motivational Enhancement

An explanation for the perceived efficacy of pharmacologic cognitive enhancement that has been put forth in the literature is that prescription stimulants simply increase an individual's motivation toward a task (Ilieva & Farah, in press). For example, findings from a sample of college students indicate that stimulants increased their interest in academic work (DeSantis,

Webb, & Noar, 2008). This finding has been supported using laboratory techniques; for example, methylphenidate was associated with increased ratings of tasks being "interesting," "exciting," and "motivating," which correlated to dopaminergic increases in the CNS (Volkow et al., 2004). The authors postulated that methylphenidate may increase the saliency and motivation to complete a task, which could, in turn, result in improved ability; of note, performance on tasks was not reported (Volkow et al., 2004). This motivation-centered explanation is certainly credible given that dopamine is essential to both learning and motivation (Blum et al., 2014). A related mechanism for engaging in stimulant misuse might be explained by research that demonstrates subjective arousal with mere expectation of receiving methylphenidate during cognitive batteries. Evidence for cognitive enhancement was not identified in this "placebo effect" study, although findings suggest that the experience of subjective arousal could propagate stimulant use, despite lack of proven efficacy (Looby & Earleywine, 2011).

Pharmacological cognitive or motivational enhancement is a topic of ongoing and intense debate and, while not the focus of this chapter, certainly impacts the discussion of prescription stimulant medication misuse. That said, it is important to note that the risks of stimulant misuse appear to outweigh any perceived cognitive benefits among normal healthy individuals (Weyandt et al., 2016). Further research should help clarify these important public health issues.

Summary

Stimulants are highly effective medications, particularly for ADHD symptoms and sleep disorders such as narcolepsy; yet, use imparts the significant risks of medical misuse and nonmedical use. A stimulant's abuse potential is partly dictated by its pharmacodynamics and pharmacokinetic properties, the latter of which is manipulated by its delivery system. Thus, one must understand the pharmacokinetics and pharmacodynamics of a particular psychostimulant, in addition to its delivery system, to fully predict the possible outcomes associated with that stimulant medication. Of course, the characteristics of those using stimulants must be considered in addition to the stimulant being used or misused. The interaction between the stimulant and the characteristics of those engaged in use or misuse can help predict the potential misuse of these important therapeutic medications.

It is important to remember that stimulant medications used in a dose and timing schedule that deliver consistent drug concentrations to the brain typically produce a therapeutic benefit, but rapid stimulant delivery to the brain could produce euphoria, a higher abuse potential, and, ultimately, stimulant use disorders. While the risk for misuse of stimulant medications exists, they remain highly effective medications that can help many individuals suffering from CNS disorders.

References

American Psychiatric Association. (2010). *Practice Guideline for the Treatment of Patients with Major Depressive Disorder* (3rd ed.). Arlington, VA: American Psychiatric Association.

American Psychiatric Association. (2013). *Diagnostic and Statistical Manual of Mental Disorders* (5th ed.). Arlington, VA: American Psychiatric Association.

Arria, A. M., Geisner, I. M., Cimini, M. D., Kilmer, J. R., Caldeira, K. M., Barrall, A. L., . . . Larimer, M. E. (2017). Perceived academic benefit is associated with nonmedical prescription stimulant use among college students. *Addictive Behaviors, 76*, 27–33. doi:10.1016/j.addbeh.2017.07.013.

Arria, A. M., Wilcox, H. C., Caldeira, K. M., Vincent, K. B., Garnier-Dykstra, L. M., & O'Grady, K. E. (2013). Dispelling the myth of "smart drugs": Cannabis and alcohol use problems predict nonmedical use of prescription stimulants for studying. *Addictive Behaviors, 38*(3), 1643–1650. doi:10.1016/j.addbeh.2012.10.002.

Bagot, K. S., & Kaminer, Y. (2014). Efficacy of stimulants for cognitive enhancement in non-attention deficit hyperactivity disorder youth: A systematic review. *Addiction, 109*(4), 547–557.

Biaggioni, I., & Robertson, D. (2015). Adrenoceptor agonists & sympathomimetic drugs. In B. G. Katzung & A. J. Trevor (Eds.), *Basic & Clinical Pharmacology* (13th ed.), 133–151. New York: McGraw-Hill Medical.

Blum, K., Febo, M., McLaughlin, T., Cronjé, F. J., Han, D., & Gold, S. M. (2014). Hatching the behavioral addiction egg: Reward Deficiency Solution System (RDSS)™ as a function of dopaminergic neurogenetics and brain functional connectivity linking all addictions under a common rubric. *Journal of Behavioral Addictions, 3*(3), 149–156. doi:10.1556/JBA.3.2014.019.

Centers for Medicare & Medicaid Services. (2017). Program integrity: Pharmacy education toolkit. https://www.cms.gov/Medicare-Medicaid-Coordination/Fraud-Prevention/Medicaid-Integrity-Education/Pharmacy-Education-Materials/pharmacy-ed-materials.html.

Chai, G., Governale, L., McMahon, A. W., Trinidad, J. P., Staffa, J., & Murphy, D. (2012). Trends of outpatient prescription drug utilization in US children, 2002–2010. *Pediatrics, 130*(1), 23–31. doi:10.1542/peds.2011-2879.

DeSantis, A. D., Webb, E. M., & Noar, S. M. (2008). Illicit use of prescription ADHD medications on a college campus: A multimethodological approach. *Journal of American College Health, 57*(3), 315–324. doi:10.3200/JACH.57.3.315-324.

Dopheide, J. A., & Pliszka, S. R. (2017). Attention deficit/hyperactivity disorder. In J. T. DiPiro, R. L. Talbert, G. C. Yee, G. R. Matzke, B. G. Wells, & L. M. Posey (Eds.), *Pharmacotherapy: A Pathophysiologic Approach, 10e*, 945–958. New York: McGraw-Hill Education.

Drazdowski, T. K. (2016). A systematic review of the motivations for the nonmedical use of prescription drugs in young adults. *Drug and Alcohol Dependence, 162*, 3–25. doi:10.1016/j.drugalcdep.2016.01.011.

Drug Enforcement Administration. (2012). Title 21 United States Code (USC) Controlled Substances Act. https://www.deadiversion.usdoj.gov/21cfr/21usc/index.html.

Faraone, S. V. (2009). Using meta-analysis to compare the efficacy of medications for attention-deficit/hyperactivity disorder in youths. *Pharmacy and Therapeutics, 34*(12), 678–694.

Faraone, S. V., & Buitelaar, J. (2010). Comparing the efficacy of stimulants for ADHD in children and adolescents using meta-analysis. *European Child and Adolescent Psychiatry, 19*(4), 353–364. doi:10.1007/s00787-009-0054-3.

Food and Drug Administration. (2017). Mydayis: Highlights of prescribing information. https://www.accessdata.fda.gov/drugsatfda_docs/label/2017/022063s000lbl.pdf.

Fortuna, R. J., Robbins, B. W., Caiola, E., Joynt, M., & Halterman, J. S. (2010). Prescribing of controlled medications to adolescents and young adults in the United States. *Pediatrics, 126*(6), 1108–1116. doi:10.1542/peds.2010-0791.

Garnier-Dykstra, L. M., Caldeira, K. M., Vincent, K. B., O'Grady, K. E., & Arria, A. M. (2012). Nonmedical use of prescription stimulants during college: Four-year trends in exposure opportunity, use, motives, and sources. *Journal of American College Health, 60*(3), 226–234. doi:10.1080/07448481.2011.589876.

Heal, D. J., Smith, S. L., Gosden, J., & Nutt, D. J. (2013). Amphetamine, past and present—A pharmacological and clinical perspective. *Journal of Psychopharmacology, 27*(6), 479–496. doi:10.1177/0269881113482532.

Ilieva, I. P., & Farah, M. J. (in press). Attention, motivation, and study habits in users of unprescribed ADHD medication. *Journal of Attention Disorders.* doi:10.1177/1087054715591849.

Ilieva, I. P., Hook, C. J., & Farah, M. J. (2015). Prescription stimulants' effects on healthy inhibitory control, working memory, and episodic memory: A meta-analysis. *Journal of Cognitive Neuroscience, 27*(6), 1069–1089. doi:10.1162/jocn_a_00776.

Kollins, S. H. (2007). Abuse liability of medications used to treat attention-deficit/hyperactivity disorder (ADHD). *American Journal on Addictions, 16 Suppl 1*, 35–42. doi:10.1080/10550490601082775.

Looby, A., & Earleywine, M. (2011). Expectation to receive methylphenidate enhances subjective arousal but not cognitive performance. *Experimental and Clinical Psychopharmacology, 19*(6), 433–444. doi:10.1037/a0025252.

Lu, Y., Sjölander, A., Cederlöf, M., D'Onofrio, B. M., Almqvist, C., Larsson, H., & Liechtenstein, P. (2017). Association between medication use and performance on higher education entrance tests in individuals with attention-deficit/hyperactivity disorder. *JAMA Psychiatry, 74*(8), 815–822. doi:10.1001/jamapsychiatry.2017.1472.

Marraccini, M. E., Weyandt, L. L., Rossi, J. S., & Gudmundsdottir, B. G. (2016). Neurocognitive enhancement or impairment? A systematic meta-analysis of prescription stimulant effects on processing speed, decision-making, planning, and cognitive perseveration. *Experimental and Clinical Psycho-pharmacology, 24*(4), 269–284. doi:10.1037/pha0000079.

McCabe, S. E., Knight, J. R., Teter, C. J., & Wechsler, H. (2005). Non-medical use of prescription stimulants among US college students: Prevalence and correlates from a national survey. *Addiction, 100*(1), 96–106. doi:10.1111 /j.1360-0443.2005.00944.x.

McCabe, S. E., Veliz, P., Wilens, T. E., & Schulenberg, J. E. (2017). Adolescents' prescription stimulant use and adult functional outcomes: A national prospective study. *Journal of the American Academy of Child and Adolescent Psychiatry, 56*(3), 226–233 e224. doi:10.1016/j.jaac.2016.12.008.

National Center for Biotechnology Information. (2017). PubChem identifier: CID 1001. https://pubchem.ncbi.nlm.nih.gov/compound/1001.

Novartis Pharmaceuticals Corporation. (2007). Focalin XR: Dexmethylphenidate hydrochloride. https://www.pharma.us.novartis.com/sites/www.pharma .us.novartis.com/files/focalinXR.pdf.

Prince, J. B., Wilens, T. E., Spencer, T. J., & Biederman, J. (2017). Stimulants and other medications for ADHD. In T. A. Stern, M. Fava, T. E. Wilens, & J. F. Rosenbaum (Eds.), *Massachusetts General Hospital Psychopharmacology and Neurotherapeutics*, 99–112. New York: Elsevier.

Repantis, D., Schlattmann, P., Laisney, O., & Heuser, I. (2010). Modafinil and methylphenidate for neuroenhancement in healthy individuals: A systematic review. *Pharmacology Research, 62*(3), 187–206. doi:10.1016/j.phrs .2010.04.002.

Safer, D. J. (2016). Recent trends in stimulant usage. *Journal of Attention Disorders, 20*(6), 471–477. doi:10.1177/1087054715605915.

Schatzberg, A. F., & Nemeroff, C. B. (Eds.). (2017). *Textbook of Psychopharmacology* (5th ed.). Arlington, MA: American Psychiatric Association Publishing.

Smith, M. E., & Farah, M. J. (2011). Are prescription stimulants "smart pills"? The epidemiology and cognitive neuroscience of prescription stimulant use by normal healthy individuals. *Psychological Bulletin, 137*(5), 717–741. doi:10.1037/a0023825.

Spencer, T. J., Biederman, J., Ciccone, P. E., Madras, B. K., Dougherty, D. D., Bonab, A. A., . . . Fischman, A. J. (2006). PET study examining pharmacokinetics, detection and likeability, and dopamine transporter receptor occupancy of short- and long-acting oral methylphenidate. *American Journal of Psychiatry, 163*(3), 387–395. doi:10.1176/appi.ajp.163.3.387.

Stahl, S. M. (2010). Mechanism of action of stimulants in attention-deficit/ hyperactivity disorder. *Journal of Clinical Psychiatry, 71*(1), 12–13. doi:10 .4088/JCP.09bs05890pur.

Stahl, S. M. (2013). *Stahl's Essential Psychopharmacology: Neuroscientific Basis and Practical Application* (4th ed.). Cambridge, UK: Cambridge University Press.

Swanson, J., Baler, R. D., & Volkow, N. D. (2011). Understanding the effects of stimulant medications on cognition in individuals with attention-deficit hyperactivity disorder: A decade of progress. *Neuropsychopharmacology,* *36*(1), 207–226. doi:10.1038/npp.2010.160.

Teter, C. J., McCabe, S. E., LaGrange, K., Cranford, J. A., & Boyd, C. J. (2006). Illicit use of specific prescription stimulants among college students: prevalence, motives, and routes of administration. *Pharmacotherapy,* *26*(10), 1501–1510. doi:10.1592/phco.26.10.1501.

Volkow, N. D. (2006). Stimulant medications: How to minimize their reinforcing effects? *American Journal of Psychiatry, 163*(3), 359–361. doi:10.1176/appi .ajp.163.3.359.

Volkow, N. D., Wang, G. J., Fowler, J. S., Telang, F., Maynard, L., Logan, J., . . . Swanson, J. M. (2004). Evidence that methylphenidate enhances the saliency of a mathematical task by increasing dopamine in the human brain. *American Journal of Psychiatry, 161*(7), 1173–1180.

Westfall, T. C., & Westfall, D. P. (2011). Adrenergic agonists and antagonists. In L. L. Brunton, B. A. Chabner, & B. C. Knollmann (Eds.), *Goodman & Gilman's: The Pharmacological Basis of Therapeutics* (12th ed.), 277–334. New York: McGraw-Hill Education.

Weyandt, L. L., Oster, D. R., Marraccini, M. E., Gudmundsdottir, B. G., Munro, B. A., Rathkey, E. S., & McCallum, A. (2016). Prescription stimulant medication misuse: Where are we and where do we go from here? *Experimental and Clinical Psychopharmacology, 24*(5), 400–414. doi:10.1037/pha 0000093.

Wilens, T. E., Adler, L. A., Adams, J., Sgambati, S., Rotrosen, J., Sawtelle, R., . . . Fusillo, S. (2008). Misuse and diversion of stimulants prescribed for ADHD: A systematic review of the literature. *Journal of the American Academy of Child and Adolescent Psychiatry, 47*(1), 21–31. doi:10.1097/chi.0b013e 31815a56f1.

Wolraich, M., Brown, L., Brown, R. T., DuPaul, G., Earls, M., Feldman, H. M., . . . Visser, S. (2011). ADHD: Clinical practice guideline for the diagnosis, evaluation, and treatment of attention-deficit/hyperactivity disorder in children and adolescents. *Pediatrics, 128*(5), 1007–1022. doi:10.1542/peds .2011-2654.

CHAPTER FOUR

Benzodiazepines[1]

Michael Weaver

Benzodiazepines are sedative medications that are widely used for the treatment of insomnia and anxiety, but they have the potential for misuse and abuse by patients. It is important to address problematic patient behaviors regarding benzodiazepines for reasons of patient safety (e.g., to prevent morbidity and mortality from overdose or withdrawal) and ethical issues, such as appropriate treatment of sedative use disorder (SUD) and prevention of drug diversion.

Sedative drugs include benzodiazepines, barbiturates, and other sleeping pills. These are commonly prescribed for insomnia and other sleep problems and are also used for anxiety, either generalized anxiety or for panic attacks (Ciraulo & Knapp, 2014). Benzodiazepines are similar to alcohol in that they facilitate the inhibitory effects of gamma-aminobutyric acid (GABA) at the GABA-A receptor complex, primarily by binding nonselectively to the benzodiazepine subtype 1 (BZ1) and 2 (BZ2) receptors. Some benzodiazepines (e.g., oxazepam, lorazepam, temazepam) are directly conjugated via glucuronyl transferase and then excreted, while others (e.g., alprazolam, diazepam) are first metabolized by the cytochrome P-450 isozyme 3A4 or 3A5 (Altamura et al., 2013). Many different benzodiazepines are prescribed, with different durations of action, rates of onset, and intensities of euphoria (see Table 4.1).

---

[1]Portions of the chapter have been adapted from Weaver, M. F. (2015). Prescription sedative misuse and abuse. *Yale Journal of Biology and Medicine, 88*(3), 247–256. Used by permission of the *Yale Journal of Biology and Medicine.*

Table 4.1   Benzodiazepines

Generic Name	Brand Name	Slang Name(s)	Typical Oral Dose (mg)	Typical Dosing Interval (hours)
Alprazolam	Xanax	Gold bars, school bus, X	1	6
Chlordiazepoxide	Librium	Lobbies	25	6
Clonazepam	Klonopin	Clozzies, k-pins, Klondike bars	2	8
Clorazepate	Tranxene	Tranx	7.5	8
Diazepam	Valium	Valley girls, Vs	10	6
Flunitrazepam	Rohypnol	Roofies, rope, Mexican Valium	1	
Flurazepam	Dalmane		15	12
Lorazepam	Ativan	Dots, lozzies, pam	2	8
Oxazepam	Serax		10	6
Temazepam	Restoril	Beans, temmies	15	6
Triazolam	Halcion		0.25	2

There are also other agonists that bind to the same binding site as benzo-diazepines at the GABA-A receptor but only act on the BZ1 subtype receptor (Richardson & Roth, 2001) and thus are similar to typical benzodiazepines (i.e., diazepam, alprazolam, and others), even though they are more selective receptor subtype agonists. These sedatives are zolpidem (Ambien), zaleplon (Sonata), and eszopiclone (Lunesta) (Dang, Garg, & Rataboli, 2011) and are often called "z-drugs." Increasing reports of bizarre and complex behavioral effects from z-drugs have prompted regulatory agencies such as the Food and Drug Administration (FDA) to issue warnings and restrictions on the pre-scribing, dispensing, and use of z-drugs (Dolder & Nelson, 2008).

Use and Misuse

Uses

Benzodiazepines as a group are one of the most widely used drugs in the world (Lader, 2011). They have a variety of recognized therapeutic uses, including the treatment of insomnia, reduction of anxiety, acute treatment and prevention of panic attacks, acute treatment and prevention of seizures, muscle relaxation, induction of anesthesia, amnesia for procedural memory loss, and acute treatment of alcohol withdrawal syndrome. They are most commonly prescribed in outpatient settings for the treatment of anxiety or insomnia. According to some surveys, up to 33 percent of elderly North American patients are prescribed either a benzodiazepine or other sedative for a sleep problem (Glass, Lanctot, Herrmann, Sproule, & Busto, 2005). Patients who are elderly, women, and those who have poor perceived health and poor actual physical health are more likely to engage in the long-term use of sedatives, especially benzodiazepines (Lader, 2014). Half of the patients who receive a prescription for benzodiazepines obtain it from a primary care physician (Kroll, Nieva, Barsky, & Linder, 2016).

Even though there are multiple accepted and appropriate medical purposes for prescribing benzodiazepines, their use is associated with higher mortality (Weich et al., 2014). This may be due in part to the higher rates of medical comorbidity among patients who are prescribed benzodiazepines reflected in higher rates of health care utilization (Kroll et al., 2016). Benzodiazepine use is linked to higher rates of respiratory depression in patients with chronic obstructive pulmonary disease (Ekström, Bornefalk-Hermansson, Abernethy, & Currow, 2014) and worsening of obstructive sleep apnea (Lavie, 2007). There is also an increased risk of falls and injury (Finkle et al., 2011), which is particularly concerning for older patients. Furthermore, this mortality risk is magnified in patients who take benzodiazepines for nontherapeutic purposes. Among patients who regularly inject opioids, benzodiazepine use was more strongly associated with mortality than any other substance of misuse (Walton et al., 2016).

In addition to taking benzodiazepines for personal use, at least one has a history of being given surreptitiously to unsuspecting others for its ability to cause amnesia, or memory loss. Flunitrazepam (Rohypnol) is a short-acting benzodiazepine that is available by prescription in South America and Europe, but not in the United States, and its potency is about 10 times that of diazepam (Gahlinger, 2004). It has achieved notoriety as a date-rape drug because it is colorless, odorless, and miscible with alcohol (which enhances the sedative and amnestic effects). These properties have made it popular among sexual predators, as they can add it to the drink of a potential victim. The expected effects of a high-potency benzodiazepine can incapacitate the unsuspecting recipient and facilitate the perpetrator in committing a crime (often rape) against the victim.

Self-Medication

Some patients take controlled substances that have been prescribed for specific conditions, such as benzodiazepines for panic disorder, to obtain other benefits: to induce sleep, to reduce anxiety from acute stressful life circumstances, or to elevate their mood when depressed. This behavior is a form of self-medication and has also been termed "chemical coping" (Weaver, 2015). Patients who engage in self-medication may develop tolerance to these other effects of benzodiazepines more rapidly than to the therapeutic effect for which it was prescribed, leading to dose escalation. Increases in emotional stress (e.g., disputes with family or friends, professional pressures, financial worries) can heighten a patient's sensitivity to discomfort from anxiety symptoms, leading to increased consumption of benzodiazepines (Weaver, 2009). However, such self-medication is not the same as intentional malingering to obtain benzodiazepines. Presentations of intentional malingering may include exaggerating symptoms of anxiety or insomnia; resisting access to outside medical records; exacerbation of symptoms or clinical deterioration when the benzodiazepine dose is due to be reduced; a significant number of tests, consults, and treatments have been performed with little success; noncompliance with diagnostic or treatment recommendations; or evidence from tests that disputes information provided by the patient.

Self-medication can have several features in common with a substance use disorder (SUD), but they are not the same disorder. SUD is an addiction in which patients are focused on the euphoric effects of benzodiazepines, even in the face of adverse consequences resulting from inappropriate use of benzodiazepines. In contrast, self-medication is prompted by a search for relief from intolerable symptoms of anxiety or depression, not euphoria. A short-acting benzodiazepine is not an appropriate treatment of depression, especially when the patient is escalating the dose to attempt to achieve some symptom relief despite increasing tolerance to the medication.

Self-medication behavior is challenging for clinicians to address. Somatization of psychological distress into physical symptoms is pervasive in medical practice (Katon, Sullivan, & Walker, 2001), and the boundary between physical and mental distress is not clear and distinct for many patients. Use of prescribed benzodiazepines becomes a reliable coping skill for the patient, but it is maladaptive. The challenge for the treating clinician is to help patients identify the underlying (often nonconscious) reasons for reliance on other inappropriate effects of the medication and then to help the patient begin the process of developing new coping skills for dealing with symptoms of anxiety and depression. Utilization of specific antidepressant medications can be a very effective way to shift the focus away from inappropriate use of benzodiazepines and toward treatment of the underlying condition. The selective serotonin reuptake inhibitors and the serotonin-norepinephrine reuptake inhibitors are safe and not prone to misuse and can be accompanied by cognitive-behavioral therapy for long-term treatment of comorbid psychiatric diagnoses such as depression and anxiety.

Sedative Use Disorder

In addition to reducing anxiety and inducing sleep, benzodiazepines can cause euphoria, so they are subject to misuse as recreational drugs. Tolerance, dependence, and withdrawal are all reported with benzodiazepines (Hajak, Muller, Wittchen, Pittrow, & Kirch, 2003). The high from benzodiazepines is described as being very similar to alcohol intoxication. Sedative use disorder is a type of SUD involving sedative, hypnotic, and anxiolytic substances, which includes benzodiazepines (American Psychiatric Association, 2013). Specific criteria have been established to diagnose SUD (see Table 4.2). This diagnosis takes into account social and psychiatric consequences resulting from ongoing use of benzodiazepines and other sedatives as well as physiologic manifestations, such as tolerance and withdrawal. Patients with SUD are not solely taking increasing doses of benzodiazepines. They also demonstrate other problematic behaviors, such as mixing different benzodiazepines or other sedatives, escalating the doses, engaging in recreational as well as specific therapeutic use, or obtaining benzodiazepines illegally (Ashton, 2005).

Some patients with SUD receive benzodiazepine prescriptions from a prescriber, albeit with an indication that may not be clear or appropriate (Voyer, Cappeliez, Pérodeau, & Préville, 2005). These patients maintain contact with the health care system as their primary means of obtaining benzodiazepines. They often have underlying anxiety or other psychiatric diagnoses for which they are taking benzodiazepines, but self-medication leads to problematic use. Other patients primarily obtain benzodiazepines illegally for recreational use, often from friends or family members but also on the black market. These patients do not usually come into contact with the health care system until they experience significant health consequences from benzodiazepine use, such as an overdose or severe withdrawal. These patients are usually younger and do not have significant psychiatric comorbidities, but they have more severe SUD when they do come in for medical attention.

Developed countries show rates of long-term benzodiazepine use in 2–17.5 percent of the population, and 3–4 percent demonstrate clear SUD (Lader, 2011). Not surprisingly, the highest rates of recreational benzodiazepine use in the United States are among young adults (aged 18–29 years), which is the population with the highest rates of use of all illicit substances and recreational use of prescription medications such as opioids (Kurtz, Buttram, & Surratt, 2017). Even though flunitrazepam is the only benzodiazepine classified as a club drug by the National Institute on Drug Abuse, illicit use of a variety of benzodiazepines is prevalent among those using club drugs. Rates of problems related to benzodiazepines among those who use club drugs are as high as 24 percent, and SUD is associated with younger

Table 4.2 Sedative Use Disorder Criteria

Over a 12-month time frame, meeting at least two of these criteria, which causes the individual to experience distress or impaired function that is clinically significant and directly related to use of sedatives:

1. Using higher quantities or for a longer time frame than the initial intent.

2. Unable to reduce or control use, or experiencing sustained thoughts about using.

3. Spending significant time on seeking, consuming, and resuming other activities after effects have worn off.

4. Cravings.

5. Repeated use causes significant problems related to occupation, educational activities, or domestic roles.

Experiencing intense or persistent impulses to use

Examples:

Occupation:

1. Frequent time away from job.

2. Problems accomplishing job tasks and responsibilities.

Educational activities:

1. Tardiness or delinquency.

2. Lower grades or academic suspension.

3. Dismissal or discontinuation in school facility.

Domestic roles:

1. Child neglect or abandonment.

2. Problems accomplishing chores or family responsibilities.

Examples:

1. Marital discord, including disagreements about effects of sedative use.

2. Violent altercations.

6. Ongoing use even though it causes or worsens issues with relationships, either domestic or other.

7. Intentionally choosing sedative use over other life roles, including interpersonal interactions, work-related activities, sports, or relaxation.

8. Repeated use when or where it may be physically dangerous or result in injury or property damage.

Examples:
1. Operating a motor vehicle while intoxicated.
2. Using other machinery while intoxicated.

9. Persistent use even though there is awareness that it has resulted in or worsened medical or mental health issues.

10. Tolerance.

Defined by either:
a. Larger quantities must be consumed to obtain the same level of effects.
b. Using the same quantity results in a reduction in the effects being sought.

11. Withdrawal syndrome.

Characterized by:
a. Symptom constellation that is specific to reduction in sedative quantity used.
b. To prevent or ameliorate the effects of dose reduction, sedatives or other similar cross-dependent substances are used.

Severity Classification:

1. Mild: 2–3 criteria are met within the 12-month time frame.

2. Moderate: 4–5 criteria are met within the 12-month time frame.

3. Severe: 6 or more criteria are met within the 12-month time frame.

Remission Classification:

1. Early: After meeting at least 2 criteria, no criteria at all are clinically significant for a period of not less than 3 months, but not more than 12 months (except for criterion #4, cravings).

2. Sustained: After meeting at least 2 criteria, no criteria at all are clinically significant for a period of more than 12 months (except for criterion #4, cravings).

Specifier (in a controlled environment). The individual currently resides in an environment with no ability to obtain or consume sedatives, such as a correctional facility, a treatment program, or an inpatient hospital setting.

Source: American Psychiatric Association (APA). Diagnostic and Statistical Manual of Mental Disorders, 5th Edition. Washington, D.C.: American Psychiatric Association, 2013.

age, psychiatric comorbidity, and use of other drugs, especially cannabis or opioids (Kurtz et al., 2017). Problems from benzodiazepine use have continued to grow with time. Admissions for treatment of SUD due to benzodiazepines nearly tripled from 22,400 admissions in 1998 to 60,200 in 2008 (Substance Abuse and Mental Health Services Administration, 2011).

Long-Term Effects

There are few indications for long-term use of benzodiazepines, and even these can be controversial (Lader, 2011). Chronic use of benzodiazepines can worsen underlying depression and anxiety (Rickels, Lucki, Schweizer, Garcia-Espana, & Case, 1999). Unfortunately, few data are available about long-term physiological and psychological consequences of intermittent high-dose use of sedatives in the setting of use of multiple substances of abuse.

Studies of those using high doses of benzodiazepines have shown very significant changes in all neuropsychological domains, even in those who are relatively young and who did not have significant comorbid psychiatric diagnoses or SUDs (Federico et al., 2017). Multiple studies have shown an association between long-term use of benzodiazepines and development of dementia (Zhong, Wang, Zhang, & Zhao, 2015); benzodiazepine use may double the risk for dementia (Billioti de Gage, Pariente, & Begaud, 2015), but the mechanism for this is not yet known. Discussing this information with patients may help motivate them to consider stopping chronic or inappropriate benzodiazepine use.

Safe Prescribing

Risk Factors for Misuse

A thorough history is very important for safe prescribing of controlled prescription medications, especially benzodiazepines. This includes gathering information about past medications, vitamins and herbal supplements, illicit substance use history, and any problems with medication management (e.g., running out early, going to the emergency department for medication refills). Screening instruments to assess risks related to benzodiazepine and other sedative use are not readily available. Records from previous treatment providers and information from significant others can help to corroborate the patient's history.

Some patient characteristics have been identified in research studies as risk factors for a higher likelihood of aberrant medication-taking behaviors (AMTB) due to SUD. A history of previous SUD, especially multiple substances used, is the strongest predictor of problems with management or misuse of controlled prescription medications. A history of cocaine or current tobacco use are each significant single substances of abuse that indicate a higher risk for AMTB (Turk, Swanson, & Gatchel, 2008). Use of nicotine in any form, including tobacco cigarette smoking, smokeless tobacco use (chew, snuff), or vaping electronic cigarettes, is an often overlooked but important predictor of possible SUD because the patient has already established a specific SUD (nicotine), usually from an early age. Other characteristics indicating higher risk for medication misuse are younger age (Ives et al., 2006); a history of childhood sexual abuse (Turk et al., 2008); legal problems (especially charges for drug possession or driving under the influence; Ives et al., 2006); a history of lost or stolen controlled medication prescriptions (Michna et al., 2004); or obtaining controlled substance prescriptions from sources other than the primary prescriber, such as taking from a friend or family member, "doctor shopping," or buying on the street/black market (Turk et al., 2008). A history of any of these indicators does not mean that the patient will certainly demonstrate serious AMTB or develop a SUD, so they should not be used to deny care to patients. The presence of risk factors such as these indicates a need for caution with the prescribing of long-term controlled prescription medications, including benzodiazepines.

Prescription Drug Monitoring Programs

A prescription drug monitoring program (PDMP) is a statewide electronic database that collects information on selected medications dispensed in the state. PDMPs are covered extensively in chapter 12, but a brief overview and discussion of their utility is warranted here. The purpose of a PDMP is to promote the appropriate use of controlled medications for legitimate medical purposes while also deterring misuse and diversion (Morgan, Weaver, Sayeed, & Orr, 2013). The availability of PDMP data can provide clinicians with additional information to refute or corroborate what a patient tells a prescriber. This allows clinicians to make better decisions about prescribing for a given patient.

Data from a PDMP helps determine the rate at which a patient is using a medication, based on dates of filling, refilling, or partial filling in relation to the original prescription date. Information from the PDMP can verify that patients are only obtaining controlled substance prescriptions from a single provider and a single pharmacy, with use of multiple providers or multiple pharmacies signaling AMTB (Weaver, 2009). PDMP information is better used by the prescriber as a deterrent to prevent problem behaviors by the patient instead of being an attempt to catch the patient in the act. As with other indicators described above, data from a PDMP should not be used to deny care to patients at high risk but to raise awareness of a need for caution when prescribing benzodiazepines. If a PDMP inquiry results in information that is concerning to the prescriber, this should be addressed directly with the patient. Informing the patient about the prescriber's concerns regarding specific AMTB and asking direct questions can help clarify any misunderstanding. This provides an opportunity to enhance patient-prescriber communication, and specific examples can be provided for expected versus inappropriate behaviors.

It is important to recognize that there are clear limitations in using PDMP data for clinical decision making, many of which are covered in chapter 12. Different states update data at different intervals, often up to seven days after filling, so the most recent prescription data may not be available. Also, PDMPs are statewide only; therefore, providers may need to register for access to PDMPs in several states. Finally, PDMP data does not cover illegally obtained prescription medications. For clinical decision making, PDMP data is best used in combination with other medication-monitoring strategies, such as those described below.

Urine Drug Screening

Urine drug screening (UDS) is another important component of medication monitoring. It verifies the presence of prescribed medications and identifies substances that should not be present in the patient's urine. This enhances the prescriber-patient relationship by providing documentation of adherence to the treatment plan. Problematic results should be discussed with the patient in a supportive fashion with the goal of encouraging appropriate patient behavior.

Unfortunately, no individual immunoassay test can recognize all benzodiazepines at clinically relevant concentrations (Glover & Allen, 2010). Point-of-care immunoassays for benzodiazepines are usually optimized to detect alprazolam and diazepam and often yield false-negative results for benzodiazepines of other types, particularly lorazepam and clonazepam. If warranted by significant clinical concern, confirmatory testing for specific benzodiazepine metabolites can be requested from the testing laboratory. Most benzodiazepines can be detected in urine for two to four days after use, but some may be detected for longer if they have multiple metabolites. Short-acting benzodiazepines are usually detectable for only 24 hours; in contrast, long-acting benzodiazepines, such as chlordiazepoxide or diazepam, may be detectable for more than seven days after the last dose, especially with specific confirmatory testing. An unexpected positive UDS result for benzodiazepines may occur when the patient is legitimately and appropriately receiving the medication from another doctor and does not realize that the medications are similar. This situation can offer a teaching opportunity to help the patient to recognize potential problems.

Some patients may attempt to mask the presence of unauthorized benzodiazepines (or other substances) in their urine sample. The simplest way to do this is by "water loading," which involves ingesting a large amount of water just prior to giving a urine sample to dilute the urine and lower the amount of unauthorized benzodiazepine to below the threshold of detection by the UDS immunoassay. Another way to mask unauthorized benzodiazepines is by adding an adulterant to the urine. Sodium hypochlorite is found in laundry detergent and other household products, such as Drano, and will effectively mask the presence of a benzodiazepine (as well as some other drugs) by interfering with the screening immunoassay when added to the urine sample. Another adulterant is tetrahydrozoline, which is found in over-the-counter Visine eye drops; this compound can be difficult to detect when added directly to the urine sample. Glutaraldehyde is an adulterant that is commercially available through the Internet under the brand name Urinaid, but because it has been fairly widely used to interfere with UDS (for marijuana as well as benzodiazepines), some labs test for it specifically to determine adulteration of a urine sample. If a patient does adulterate a urine sample, this is clearly an inappropriate behavior that should be addressed with the patient and prompt closer monitoring by the prescriber.

Medication Monitoring

Benzodiazepine medication compliance can be monitored by having patients bring the original medication containers from the pharmacy to each visit so that the prescriber can count any unused medication, allowing for determination of the rate at which the patient is taking the prescription (Weaver & Schnoll, 2002a). Pill counts can also be performed between visits by calling the patient on short notice (up to 24 hours before) to bring the medication containers to the office.

Basic monitoring of patients being prescribed controlled prescription medications requires some effort by the prescribing physician. This includes regular inquiries to a PDMP, only issuing prescriptions in person at scheduled office visits, pill counts, and random UDS (Weaver & Schnoll, 2002b). A patient without significant risk factors for medication misuse may initially have only basic monitoring activities. This may consist of one or two random UDS per year, a query to the PDMP once a year, and pill counts randomly at some office visits. Ongoing assessment and documentation of successfully met clinical goals (e.g., improved function, no AMTB) supports continuation of therapy. A failure to meet goals requires reevaluation and a change in the treatment plan (Gourlay, Heit, & Almahrezi, 2005).

A thorough history and records from previous physicians can assist with determining in advance which patients are likely to need enhanced monitoring or whether basic monitoring activities are adequate when prescribing or continuing benzodiazepines (Weaver, 2009). For example, a history of illicit substance use and previous documentation of rapidly escalating medication doses are signs that should prompt closer monitoring of ongoing benzodiazepine use. Such a patient may have UDS at nearly every visit initially, pill counts and UDS on short notice between visits, and queries to the PDMP every few weeks (if available and updated that frequently in the state of residence). Such enhanced monitoring aims to deter AMTB from occurring and assist the patient in achieving adequate medication management, leading to better treatment outcomes. The clinician may utilize counseling strategies such as motivational interviewing to assist patients with medication management or refer the patient to a behavioral therapist for additional assistance. As patients demonstrate an ability to manage their benzodiazepine prescriptions appropriately, the enhanced monitoring can be gradually reduced by the prescriber to just basic monitoring efforts.

Any patient may display AMTB at some point during treatment. For less serious problems, it is reasonable to initiate enhanced monitoring that includes more frequent visits and tighter limits on the amount of benzodiazepine prescribed at a time. For example, an isolated UDS positive for an illicit drug or unauthorized medication results in closer monitoring with more frequent UDS; recurrent positive results may prompt referral to an addiction medicine specialist for further evaluation and possible treatment of a SUD. Repeated AMTB or patient refusal to adhere to all aspects of an appropriate treatment program should result in loss of the privilege to receive prescriptions for benzodiazepines, but this does not necessarily indicate that the patient should be completely discharged from treatment with the practitioner (Weaver & Schnoll, 2002b). The prescriber may choose to continue to see the patient and provide other forms of treatment that do not include benzodiazepines (Weaver, Heit, Savage, & Gourlay, 2007). This may take the form of alternative medications or individual counseling for anxiety or insomnia. However, if benzodiazepines are to be discontinued, this should be done carefully and cautiously to prevent development of sedative withdrawal syndrome. Patients can be slowly tapered off or referred for inpatient detoxification.

Intoxication

The clinical features of acute benzodiazepine intoxication are similar to alcohol intoxication. Psychiatric manifestations include impaired attention, inappropriate behavior, labile mood, and impaired judgment. Physical signs include nystagmus, decreased reflexes, and unsteady gait. As the amount consumed increases, especially beyond the established tolerance of an individual, progressively more impairment occurs in judgment and neurobehavioral functioning. Initial signs include slurred speech, followed by nystagmus (repetitive and uncontrolled eye movements), incoordination (especially in complex tasks such as driving), ataxia (unsteadiness), and memory impairment (Weaver, Jewell, & Tomlinson, 2009). At high doses, sedatives can cause anterograde amnesia, which means the individual using stops encoding memories despite being awake and alert, so there is no memory of events during the time of the sedative effect. Similar to heavy alcohol use, this is known as a "blackout," but it is not the same thing as "passing out" (oversedation). Patients who misuse sedatives may not realize they have experienced a blackout until someone informs them of things they said or did during an amnesic period. Severe overdose may lead to stupor, and high levels result in suppression of the autonomic respiratory drive and may result in coma or death from anoxic brain injury (Weaver, 2010a). One study showed that benzodiazepines accounted for nearly 30 percent of deaths from pharmaceutical agents, and 75 percent of overdose deaths overall were unintentional (Jones, Mack, & Paulozzi, 2013).

Initial management of intoxication and overdose involves general supportive care, as for any clinically significant intoxication, including maintenance of an adequate airway, ventilation, and cardiovascular function. Attention to airway patency and supportive management of ventilation and hemodynamics are usually sufficient. Following stabilization of respiratory and cardiac function, activated charcoal should be given (Jones & Volans, 1999). A competitive benzodiazepine antagonist, flumazenil (Romazicon), is available for the treatment of acute benzodiazepine intoxication. However, it may not completely reverse respiratory depression, and it can provoke withdrawal seizures in patients with physical dependence on benzodiazepines (Weinbroum, Flaishon, Sorkine, Szold, & Rudick, 1997). Its most common side effects are nausea and vomiting. Flumazenil should be withheld in patients with current seizures or a history of seizures and in patients who have concurrently ingested other drugs that lower the seizure threshold, such as antipsychotics or stimulants. Flumazenil should not be routinely administered to comatose patients when the identity of ingested drug(s) is uncertain. Flumazenil is short-acting, and sedation may recur after an initial awakening, which can be treated by repeating doses at 20-minute intervals as needed. Repeat doses should be administered slowly in patients who are physically dependent on benzodiazepines.

Treatment of an acute overdose is not sufficient treatment for SUD in itself, and long-term specialty SUD treatment can lead to recovery with less disability (Hasin, Stinson, Ogburn, & Grant, 2007). Referral for counseling in a group or individual format should be offered to the patient. This can help prevent worsening medical and psychiatric consequences of SUD.

Withdrawal

Presentation

Patients who chronically take benzodiazepines, whether prescribed by a physician or bought illegally on the black market, are at risk for an acute withdrawal syndrome that is clinically indistinguishable from alcohol withdrawal. Risk factors for severe withdrawal include larger amounts of sedatives taken chronically, longer time of use, older age, and comorbid medical or psychiatric problems. The severity of withdrawal is worsened by concurrent medical or psychiatric illness (Saitz, 1995), and up to 20 percent of patients develop severe withdrawal if left untreated (Cross & Hennessey, 1993). Recognition and effective treatment of benzodiazepine withdrawal is important to prevent excess mortality due to complications. There is individual variability in the threshold at which a patient may develop withdrawal, so it is difficult to predict who will and who will not enter withdrawal. The best predictor of whether a patient will develop acute withdrawal is a previous history of benzodiazepine withdrawal.

The clinical features of the acute withdrawal syndrome are identical for all sedatives, including alcohol, which may be considered a short-acting sedative. Abrupt reduction or cessation of benzodiazepine use results in a characteristic set of signs and symptoms, including tremor; anxiety; agitation; hyperreflexia; autonomic hyperactivity (i.e., elevated heart rate, blood pressure, body temperature, and sweating); hallucinations; and seizures (American Psychiatric Association, 2013). Withdrawal symptoms are generally the opposite of the symptoms of acute benzodiazepine intoxication. The initial indication of withdrawal is an elevation of vital signs (e.g., heart rate, blood pressure, temperature). Tremors develop next, first a fine tremor of the hands and fasciculation of the tongue that is sometimes followed by gross tremors of the extremities. Disorientation and mild hallucinations (often auditory, occasionally visual) may develop as the withdrawal syndrome progresses, accompanied by diaphoresis. Seizures can be an early sign of withdrawal, and they may be the presenting symptom for those seeking medical care. The symptoms may appear as soon as 4 to 8 hours after the last dose, and withdrawal symptoms usually manifest within 48 hours. For benzodiazepines with long-acting metabolites, however, the patient may not show signs of withdrawal for up to 7 to 10 days after stopping chronic use.

Withdrawal symptoms usually peak at around five days (Blondell, Powell, Dodds, Looney, & Lukan, 2004). Some patients do not progress to severe withdrawal, and their symptoms simply subside after a few days, with or without treatment. Still, it is impossible to predict which patients will progress or not. The signs of severe withdrawal consist of worsening diaphoresis, nausea, and vomiting (which may result in aspiration pneumonia); delirium with frank hallucinations; and rapid, severe fluctuation in vital signs (Monte Secades et al., 2008). Sudden changes in blood pressure and heart rate may result in complications, such as myocardial infarction (heart attack) or a cerebrovascular event (stroke), and increased variability in the QT segment on electrocardiogram demonstrates elevated risk for serious cardiac arrhythmias (Bar et al., 2007). Progression to severe withdrawal results in significant morbidity and even death (Monte Secades et al., 2008), but adequate treatment early in the clinical course can help prevent the progression of withdrawal.

Pharmacologic Treatment

Chronic benzodiazepine use can result in a withdrawal syndrome that requires detoxification with medical monitoring. However, there is little consistency in the treatment of benzodiazepine withdrawal, and there are no standard protocols for withdrawal management in widespread use (Weaver & Schnoll, 1996). Pharmacotherapy is indicated for management of moderate to severe withdrawal.

Acute withdrawal is most safely managed in an inpatient setting if the patient has been using high doses of benzodiazepines, has a history of seizures or severe withdrawal, or has unstable comorbid medical or psychiatric problems (Saitz, 1998). This allows for close medical monitoring during benzodiazepine withdrawal treatment to prevent complications from progression to severe withdrawal, which can be life-threatening. Stable patients on low to moderate doses of a benzodiazepine may be tapered off in the outpatient setting. This may be accomplished by gradually reducing the dose over several weeks, and at least 10 weeks is recommended to be successful for achieving long-term abstinence from benzodiazepines (Denis, Fatseas, Lavie, & Auriacombe, 2006). It is usually better to reduce the dose rather than the time between doses to avoid development of benzodiazepine withdrawal symptoms between doses. For patients tapering off short-acting benzodiazepines, it is preferable to substitute a long-acting benzodiazepine.

For pharmacologic prevention and management of benzodiazepine withdrawal syndrome, the choice of medication depends on such characteristics as duration of action, metabolism, and speed of onset of effects. Both benzodiazepines and barbiturates have been effectively used to treat benzodiazepine withdrawal syndrome. Clonazepam is a long-acting benzodiazepine with generally less euphoria than other benzodiazepines, such as diazepam or chlordiazepoxide, so it is more suitable for detoxification. However, for patients who have been abusing benzodiazepines, a different type of sedative may be appropriate to use for treatment of withdrawal symptoms. Barbiturates have been used successfully to treat acute sedative withdrawal syndrome in a variety of clinical settings, and phenobarbital (Luminal) is a long-acting barbiturate that may be preferable to other sedatives for treatment of acute sedative withdrawal syndrome (Weaver et al., 2009). It has a long half-life of up to 100 hours (Wiehl, Hayner, & Galloway, 1994); dosing is very flexible (it can be given orally as tablets or elixir or administered parenterally); it is inexpensive; and there is almost no street market for it, in contrast to the benzodiazepines.

A specific type of prolonged benzodiazepine withdrawal syndrome, symptom rebound, may be seen following long-term use of benzodiazepines (Weaver, Jarvis, & Schnoll, 1999). This can manifest after a relatively short tapering off of the benzodiazepine. Associated symptoms of insomnia and anxiety may last for several months. Although not life-threatening, this prolonged abstinence syndrome may be sufficiently uncomfortable that it may trigger a relapse to benzodiazepine use or misuse. To avoid this, it may be useful to taper the original benzodiazepine, or a long-acting substitute such as clonazepam or phenobarbital, over an extended period of at least two to three months (Higgitt, Fonagy, Toone, & Shine, 1990).

Rates of long-term abstinence from benzodiazepines vary significantly. Older adults who were prescribed benzodiazepines in a general practice setting have shown abstinence rates of up to 80 percent (Curran et al., 2003). However, patients who use high doses of benzodiazepines or have comorbid psychiatric diagnoses, especially alcohol use disorder, are likely to have lower rates of abstinence, only around 25 percent at one year (Vorma, Naukkarinen, Sarna, & Kuoppasalmi, 2003). This helps demonstrate the importance of providing additional treatment resources for patients with SUD, including referral for specialty treatment. Support for the patient and specialty treatment of the SUD can help to improve rates of long-term abstinence from benzodiazepines.

Treatment of Sedative Use Disorder

Acute and long-term treatment is necessary once the diagnosis of SUD is made (McLellan, Lewis, O'Brien, & Kleber, 2000). Addressing overdose or withdrawal is only the initial step in overall treatment of SUD. Recovery from SUD is possible, and those who are treated have less disability than those who remain untreated (Hasin et al., 2007). Patients identified with SUD should be provided with information linking them to local community treatment resources. In the United States, physicians certified in treatment of SUDs can be found through the American Society of Addiction Medicine (www.asam.org) or the American Academy of Addiction Psychiatry (www.aaap.org). At times, it may be more expedient and cost-effective to refer the patient to a nonphysician counselor (Weaver, 2010b), which can be found through the National Association for Alcohol and Drug Abuse Counselors (www.naadac.org). The Substance Abuse and Mental Health Services Administration provides a treatment finder guide on its website that can help providers or patients and their families locate various treatment resources for SUD in their geographic area. This is available at the findtreatment.samhsa.gov website.

There are several types of formal counseling available for treatment of problems due to SUD. Motivational interviewing is a counseling style that seeks to motivate the patient to reduce or stop drug use or to seek further treatment (Miller & Rollnick, 2013). Cognitive-behavioral treatment helps patients identify life stressors, high-risk situations for benzodiazepine use, and coping skills deficits; it then uses modeling and rehearsal to address these. Relapse prevention therapy (Marlatt & Donovan, 2005) helps identify triggers for benzodiazepine use (as well as for other substances), provides practice avoiding them through rehearsal with a trained therapist, and emphasizes responsibility for recovery.

Conclusions

There are many different types of sedatives, and they are widely prescribed for insomnia and anxiety. Benzodiazepines are very popular, especially alprazolam and diazepam. Patients may misuse benzodiazepines to self-medicate symptoms of underlying depression or anxiety, a condition sometimes known as *chemical coping*. Benzodiazepines may be used recreationally for euphoria, either obtained from prescribers under false pretenses directly for this purpose or diverted to the black market and sold on the street. The number of admissions to treatment programs for sedative SUD has continued to grow. To help prevent misuse and diversion of benzodiazepines, prescribers can use appropriate precautions similar to those used when prescribing other controlled substances, such as opioids. This includes obtaining previous medical records, utilizing the state PDMP, performing pill counts and UDS, and promptly addressing any AMTB with the patient.

Misuse of benzodiazepines may lead to overdose or a withdrawal syndrome, either of which may be fatal. Fortunately, overdose with benzodiazepines responds to an antagonist, flumazenil, although it has its limitations and potential adverse effects. Sedative withdrawal syndrome can be avoided by slowly tapering down the dose of the benzodiazepine over several weeks to months. More serious withdrawal is treated by substitution with a long-acting sedative and requires close medical supervision in the outpatient or inpatient setting. After treatment of these consequences, the SUD should be addressed with long-term treatment that involves individual or group counseling with the help of a SUD treatment professional.

References

Altamura, A. C., Moliterno, D., Paletta, S., Maffini, M., Mauri, M. C., & Bareggi, S. (2013). Understanding the pharmacokinetics of anxiolytic drugs. *Expert Opinion on Drug Metabolism & Toxicology, 9*(4), 423–440. doi:10.1517/1742 5255.2013.759209.

American Psychiatric Association. (2013). *Diagnostic and Statistical Manual of Mental Disorders* (5th ed). Washington, D.C.: American Psychiatric Association.

Ashton, H. (2005). The diagnosis and management of benzodiazepine dependence. *Current Opinion in Psychiatry, 18*(3), 249–255. doi:10.1097/01.yco
.0000165594.60434.84.

Bar, K. J., Boettger, M. K., Koschke, M., Boettger, S., Groteluschen, M., Voss, A.,
& Yeragani, V. K. (2007). Increased QT interval variability index in acute
alcohol withdrawal. *Drug and Alcohol Dependence, 89*(2-3), 259–266.
doi:10.1016/j.drugalcdep.2007.01.010.

Billioti de Gage, S., Pariente, A., & Begaud, B. (2015). Is there really a link
between benzodiazepine use and the risk of dementia? *Expert Opinion on
Drug Safety, 14*(5), 733–747. doi:10.1517/14740338.2015.1014796.

Blondell, R. D., Powell, G. E., Dodds, H. N., Looney, S. W., & Lukan, J. K. (2004).
Admission characteristics of trauma patients in whom delirium develops.
American Journal of Surgery, 187(3), 332–337. doi:10.1016/j.amjsurg.2003
.12.027.

Ciraulo, D., & Knapp, C. (2014). The pharmacology of nonalcohol sedative hypnotics. In R. Ries, D. Fiellin, S. Miller, & R. Saitz (Eds.), *The ASAM Principles of Addiction Medicine* (5th ed.), 117–134. Chevy Chase, MD: Lippincott
Williams & Wilkins.

Cross, G. M., & Hennessey, P. T. (1993). Principles and practice of detoxification. *Primary Care, 20*(1), 81–93.

Curran, H. V., Collins, R., Fletcher, S., Kee, S. C., Woods, B., & Iliffe, S. (2003).
Older adults and withdrawal from benzodiazepine hypnotics in general
practice: Effects on cognitive function, sleep, mood and quality of life.
Psychological Medicine, 33(7), 1223–1237.

Dang, A., Garg, A., & Rataboli, P. V. (2011). Role of zolpidem in the management
of insomnia. *CNS Neuroscience & Therapeutics, 17*(5), 387–397. doi:10.1111
/j.1755-5949.2010.00158.x.

Denis, C., Fatseas, M., Lavie, E., & Auriacombe, M. (2006). Pharmacological
interventions for benzodiazepine mono-dependence management in outpatient settings. *Cochrane Database of Systematic Reviews* (3), CD005194.
doi:10.1002/14651858.CD005194.pub2.

Dolder, C. R., & Nelson, M. H. (2008). Hypnosedative-induced complex behaviours: Incidence, mechanisms and management. *CNS Drugs, 22*(12), 1021–
1036. doi:10.2165/0023210-200822120-00005.

Ekström, M. P., Bornefalk-Hermansson, A., Abernethy, A. P., & Currow, D. C.
(2014). Safety of benzodiazepines and opioids in very severe respiratory
disease: National prospective study. *BMJ: British Medical Journal, 348*,
g445. doi:10.1136/bmj.g445.

Federico, A., Tamburin, S., Maier, A., Faccini, M., Casari, R., Morbioli, L., &
Lugoboni, F. (2017). Multifocal cognitive dysfunction in high-dose benzodiazepine users: A cross-sectional study. *Neurological Sciences, 38*(1),
137–142. doi:10.1007/s10072-016-2732-5.

Finkle, W. D., Der, J. S., Greenland, S., Adams, J. L., Ridgeway, G., Blaschke, T., . . .
VanRiper, K. B. (2011). Risk of fractures requiring hospitalization after an
initial prescription for zolpidem, alprazolam, lorazepam, or diazepam in

older adults. *Journal of the American Geriatric Society, 59*(10), 1883–1890. doi:10.1111/j.1532-5415.2011.03591.x.

Gahlinger, P. M. (2004). Club drugs: MDMA, gamma-hydroxybutyrate (GHB), Rohypnol, and ketamine. *American Family Physician, 69*(11), 2619–2626.

Glass, J., Lanctot, K. L., Herrmann, N., Sproule, B. A., & Busto, U. E. (2005). Sedative hypnotics in older people with insomnia: Meta-analysis of risks and benefits. *BMJ: British Medical Journal, 331*(7526), 1169. doi:10.1136 /bmj.38623.768588.47.

Glover, S. J., & Allen, K. R. (2010). Measurement of benzodiazepines in urine by liquid chromatography-tandem mass spectrometry: Confirmation of samples screened by immunoassay. *Annals of Clinical Biochemistry, 47*(Pt 2), 111–117. doi:10.1258/acb.2009.009172.

Gourlay, D. L., Heit, H. A., & Almahrezi, A. (2005). Universal precautions in pain medicine: A rational approach to the treatment of chronic pain. *Pain Medicine, 6*(2), 107–112. doi:10.1111/j.1526-4637.2005.05031.x.

Hajak, G., Muller, W. E., Wittchen, H. U., Pittrow, D., & Kirch, W. (2003). Abuse and dependence potential for the non-benzodiazepine hypnotics zolpidem and zopiclone: A review of case reports and epidemiological data. *Addiction, 98*(10), 1371–1378.

Hasin, D. S., Stinson, F. S., Ogburn, E., & Grant, B. F. (2007). Prevalence, correlates, disability, and comorbidity of DSM-IV alcohol abuse and dependence in the United States: Results from the National Epidemiologic Survey on Alcohol and Related Conditions. *Archives of General Psychiatry, 64*(7), 830–842. doi:10.1001/archpsyc.64.7.830.

Higgitt, A., Fonagy, P., Toone, B., & Shine, P. (1990). The prolonged benzodiazepine withdrawal syndrome: anxiety or hysteria? *Acta Psychiatrica Scandinavica, 82*(2), 165–168.

Ives, T. J., Chelminski, P. R., Hammett-Stabler, C. A., Malone, R. M., Perhac, J. S., Potisek, N. M., . . . Pignone, M. P. (2006). Predictors of opioid misuse in patients with chronic pain: A prospective cohort study. *BMC Health Services Research, 6*, 46. doi:10.1186/1472-6963-6-46.

Jones, A. L., & Volans, G. (1999). Management of self poisoning. *BMJ: British Medical Journal, 319*(7222), 1414–1417. doi:10.1136/bmj.319.7222.1414.

Jones, C. M., Mack, K. A., & Paulozzi, L. J. (2013). Pharmaceutical overdose deaths, United States, 2010. *JAMA, 309*(7), 657–659. doi:10.1001/jama.2013.272.

Katon, W., Sullivan, M., & Walker, E. (2001). Medical symptoms without identified pathology: Relationship to psychiatric disorders, childhood and adult trauma, and personality traits. *Annals of Internal Medicine, 134*(9 Pt 2), 917–925.

Kroll, D. S., Nieva, H. R., Barsky, A. J., & Linder, J. A. (2016). Benzodiazepines are prescribed more frequently to patients already at risk for benzodiazepine-related adverse events in primary care. *Journal of General Internal Medicine, 31*(9), 1027–1034. doi:10.1007/s11606-016-3740-0.

Kurtz, S. P., Buttram, M. E., & Surratt, H. L. (2017). Benzodiazepine dependence among young adult participants in the club scene who use drugs. *Journal of Psychoactive Drugs, 49*(1), 39–46. doi:10.1080/02791072.2016.1269978.

Lader, M. (2011). Benzodiazepines revisited—Will we ever learn? *Addiction,* *106*(12), 2086–2109. doi:10.1111/j.1360-0443.2011.03563.x

Lader, M. (2014). Benzodiazepine harm: How can it be reduced? *British Journal of Clinical Pharmacology, 77*(2), 295–301. doi:10.1111/j.1365-2125.2012 .04418.x.

Lavie, P. (2007). Insomnia and sleep-disordered breathing. *Sleep Medicine, 8 Suppl 4,* S21–25. doi:10.1016/s1389-9457(08)70005-4.

Marlatt, G. A., & Donovan, D. M. (Eds.). (2005). *Relapse Prevention: Maintenance Strategies in the Treatment of Addictive Behaviors* (2nd ed.). New York: The Guilford Press.

McLellan, A. T., Lewis, D. C., O'Brien, C. P., & Kleber, H. D. (2000). Drug dependence, a chronic medical illness: Implications for treatment, insurance, and outcomes evaluation. *JAMA, 284*(13), 1689–1695.

Michna, E., Ross, E. L., Hynes, W. L., Nedeljkovic, S. S., Soumekh, S., Janfaza, D., . . . Jamison, R. N. (2004). Predicting aberrant drug behavior in patients treated for chronic pain: Importance of abuse history. *Journal of Pain and Symptom Management, 28*(3), 250–258. doi:10.1016/j.jpainsymman .2004.04.007.

Miller, W. R., & Rollnick, S. (2013). *Motivational Interviewing: Helping People Change* (3rd ed.). New York: The Guilford Press.

Monte Secades, R., Casariego Vales, E., Pertega Diaz, S., Rabunal Rey, R., Pena Zemsch, M., & Pita Fernandez, S. (2008). [Clinical course and features of the alcohol withdrawal syndrome in a general hospital]. *Revista Clínica Española, 208*(10), 506–512.

Morgan, L., Weaver, M., Sayeed, Z., & Orr, R. (2013). The use of prescription monitoring programs to reduce opioid diversion and improve patient safety. *Journal of Pain & Palliative Care Pharmacotherapy, 27*(1), 4–9. doi:10 .3109/15360288.2012.738288.

Richardson, G. S., & Roth, T. (2001). Future directions in the management of insomnia. *Journal of Clinical Psychiatry, 62 Suppl 10,* 39–45.

Rickels, K., Lucki, I., Schweizer, E., Garcia-Espana, F., & Case, W. G. (1999). Psychomotor performance of long-term benzodiazepine users before, during, and after benzodiazepine discontinuation. *Journal of Clinical Psychopharmacology, 19*(2), 107–113.

Saitz, R. (1995). Recognition and management of occult alcohol withdrawal. *Hosp Pract (1995), 30*(6), 49–54, 56–48.

Saitz, R. (1998). Introduction to alcohol withdrawal. *Alcohol Health Res World, 22*(1), 5–12.

Substance Abuse and Mental Health Services Administration. (2011). *The TEDS Report: Substance Abuse Treatment Admissions for Abuse of Benzodiazepines.* Rockville, MD: Center for Behavioral Health Statistics and Quality.

Turk, D. C., Swanson, K. S., & Gatchel, R. J. (2008). Predicting opioid misuse by chronic pain patients: A systematic review and literature synthesis. *Clinical Journal of Pain, 24*(6), 497–508. doi:10.1097/AJP.0b013e31816b1070.

Vorma, H., Naukkarinen, H., Sarna, S., & Kuoppasalmi, K. (2003). Long-term outcome after benzodiazepine withdrawal treatment in subjects with complicated dependence. *Drug and Alcohol Dependence, 70*(3), 309–314.

Voyer, P., Cappeliez, P., Pérodeau, G., & Préville, M. (2005). Mental health for older adults and benzodiazepine use. *Journal of Community Health Nursing, 22*(4), 213–229.

Walton, G. R., Hayashi, K., Bach, P., Dong, H., Kerr, T., Ahamad, K., . . . Wood, E. (2016). The impact of benzodiazepine use on mortality among polysubstance users in Vancouver, Canada. *Public Health Reports, 131*(3), 491–499. doi:10.1177/0033354916131003315.

Weaver, M. F. (2009). Prescribing medications with potential for abuse. *Journal of Clinical Outcomes Management, 16*(4), 171–179.

Weaver, M. F. (2010a). Medical sequelae of addiction. In D. Brizer & R. Castaneda (Eds.), *Clinical Addiction Psychiatry*, 24–36). New York: Cambridge University Press.

Weaver, M. F. (2010b). Substance-related disorders. In J. L. Levenson (Ed.), *Textbook of Psychosomatic Medicine* (2nd ed.), 381–403. Washington, D.C.: American Psychiatric Press.

Weaver, M. F. (2015). Prescription sedative misuse and abuse. *Yale Journal of Biology and Medicine, 88*(3), 247–256.

Weaver, M. F., Heit, H., Savage, S., & Gourlay, D. (2007). Clinical case discussion: Chronic pain management. *Journal of Addiction Medicine, 1*(1), 11–14. doi:10.1097/ADM.0b013e3180442ee8.

Weaver, M. F., Jarvis, M. A., & Schnoll, S. H. (1999). Role of the primary care physician in problems of substance abuse. *Archives of Internal Medicine, 159*(9), 913–924.

Weaver, M. F., Jewell, C., & Tomlinson, J. (2009). Phenobarbital for treatment of alcohol withdrawal. *Journal of Addictions Nursing, 20*(1), 1–5. doi:10.1080/10884600802693066.

Weaver, M. F., & Schnoll, S. H. (1996). Drug overdose and withdrawal syndromes. *Current Opinion in Critical Care, 2*(3), 242–247.

Weaver, M. F., & Schnoll, S. H. (2002a). Abuse liability in opioid therapy for pain treatment in patients with an addiction history. *Clinical Journal of Pain, 18*(4 Suppl), S61–69.

Weaver, M. F., & Schnoll, S. H. (2002b). Opioid treatment of chronic pain in patients with addiction. *Journal of Pain & Palliative Care Pharmacotherapy, 16*(3), 5–26.

Weich, S., Pearce, H. L., Croft, P., Singh, S., Crome, I., Bashford, J., & Frisher, M. (2014). Effect of anxiolytic and hypnotic drug prescriptions on mortality hazards: Retrospective cohort study. *BMJ: British Medical Journal, 348*, g1996. doi:10.1136/bmj.g1996.

Weinbroum, A. A., Flaishon, R., Sorkine, P., Szold, O., & Rudick, V. (1997). A risk-benefit assessment of flumazenil in the management of benzodiazepine overdose. *Drug Safety, 17*(3), 181–196.

Wiehl, W. O., Hayner, G., & Galloway, G. (1994). Haight Ashbury Free Clinics' drug detoxification protocols—Part 4: Alcohol. *Journal of Psychoactive Drugs, 26*(1), 57–59. doi:10.1080/02791072.1994.10472601.

Zhong, G., Wang, Y., Zhang, Y., & Zhao, Y. (2015). Association between benzo-diazepine use and dementia: A meta-analysis. *PLoS One, 10*(5), e0127836. doi:10.1371/journal.pone.0127836.

CHAPTER FIVE

Misuse and Abuse of Over-the-Counter Medicines

Richard Cooper

Introduction

An important group of medicines are those that are available for purchase without prescription in many countries. Such nonprescription, or over-the-counter (OTC), medicines are primarily available from sources such as pharmacies. They may also be obtained from general retail stores and the Internet. Such medicines are important because they offer members of the public the opportunity to self-manage many conditions and symptoms and to avoid the need to have a medical consultation, which may have related issues of time and cost. OTC medicines range considerably in terms of therapeutic groups and span treatments for pain, allergy, viral infections and infestations, gastrointestinal, skin, and ophthalmic conditions. In the United Kingdom, oral adult analgesics, cough and cold remedies, and skin treatments account for 23.2 percent, 18.7 percent, and 17.8 percent, respectively, of all OTC medicines sold, with increases of 2.5 percent in 2015 (Connelly, 2016). Globally, OTC sales represent a considerable and increasing economic market, which has been estimated to amount to $162 billion by 2020 (Technavio, 2016). The OTC market may provide a further benefit by not burdening health care systems through medical appointments and medicine costs (Bond & Bradley, 1996).

Despite these benefits and the tendency to view nonprescription medicine as being safer (Bissell, Ward, & Noyce, 2001), there are potential problems

Table 5.1 Summary of the Different Characteristics of Misuse, Abuse, Dependence, and Substitution

	Misuse	Abuse	Substitution
Legitimate	Yes	No	No
Intentional	No	Yes	Yes
Inappropriate	Yes	Yes	Yes
OTC medicines implicated	All	Opioids, sedatives, decongestants, dissociative substances, laxatives, nicotine replacement	Opioids, decongestants
Examples	Incorrect dose, indication or duration	Intention to exploit side effect to experience high or lose weight	Using OTC opioid when illicit opioid cannot be obtained

associated with the OTC medicine supply. These can be broadly divided into issues relating to their misuse and abuse (Akram, 2000). Although these terms are somewhat ambiguous, contested, and, in some cases, synonymous (Cooper, 2013b), the misuse of OTC medicines relates to their legitimate but inappropriate use, whereas abuse involves intentional and illegitimate use (see Table 5.1). Also recognized in the literature is substitution, which involves OTC medicines being used when illicit drugs or medicines cannot be obtained. A final definition related to OTC medicines concerns dependence. Research in this area has often used *dependence*, which again has been defined differently by various commentators but relates to the continued desire to use an OTC medicine, to signify difficulty in trying to stop and change medication use (World Health Organization, 1994).

This chapter is mainly concerned with the misuse, abuse, and dependence potential of OTC medicines and will explore in further detail the implicated medicines and resulting harms, the scale of the problem and who is affected, and strategies for prevention and treatment. It should be noted however, that this chapter relates to OTC medicines that are legal and licensed for supply through the sources mentioned above. This must be contrasted with the illegal or unregulated supply of prescription medicines through pharmacies and other nonmedical routes that is the focus of much of this volume.

Key Categories of OTC Medicines of Abuse and Misuse

As Table 5.1 indicates, all OTC medicines can be associated with unintentional misuse, as this occurs for benign reasons, such as low levels of health literacy or incorrect advice. Abuse, though, occurs only with certain groups of medicines. These comprise opioid medicines, sedative antihistamines, stimulants such as decongestants, dissociative substances that are often contained in cough and cold remedies, and laxatives (Cooper, 2013b; Lessenger & Feinberg, 2008). These medications are covered in more detail below.

Opioids and Compound Analgesics

Arguably the most widely recognized medicines of OTC misuse and abuse are opioids, particularly compound analgesics. Although these are not available without prescription in the United States and several other countries, they are of concern in many countries globally. Opioid medicines are used as strong analgesics due to their effect on opioid receptors in nerve cells and can be distinguished from weaker analgesics, such as paracetamol/acetaminophen, aspirin, and ibuprofen (see chapters 2 and 9 for more on opioids). They are also used to treat cough and diarrhea due to their more complex pharmacological action on different sites. As a class of medicines, opioids include naturally occurring alkaloids, such as morphine and codeine, and synthetic ones, such as diamorphine and tramadol.

Abuse occurs through exploiting the side effect of euphoria, through the pleasurable effect caused by dopamine release via the central reward pathway. However, in relation to OTC supply, only less potent opioids are licensed for supply, and this typically involves only codeine and dihydrocodeine. Furthermore, the quantity and strength of opioids available OTC are often less than that permitted on prescription. In relation to codeine availability in Europe, for example, only one country allowed the supply of the same 30mg tablet strength as prescription formulations, and many countries limited these to between 8mg and 12.8mg (Foley et al., 2015). Of note is that OTC opioid analgesics are formulated as compound preparations, usually with nonopioid analgesics such as paracetamol or ibuprofen, and sometimes include caffeine. In some countries, codeine is available for the treatment of cough in liquid formulation, either alone or with other cough and cold medicines. As noted, a more conservative stance exists in the United States and around half of European countries, where opioids are only available via prescription, reflecting public health policy concerns about potential harms. Australia, too, recently up-scheduled codeine to prescription-only supply following abuse concerns. As such, the distribution of those affected by OTC opioid abuse is dependent on where it is available, but such availability is a recognized problem in many countries (Cooper, 2013b).

Opioid harms arise primarily through their potential to cause dependence and for side effects such as euphoria to be exploited or, as noted in Table 5.1, where they may be sought when illicit opioids are not available (i.e., substitution). In relation to dependence, this may result in additional morbidity, or harm, if withdrawal is attempted. There are a range of other recognized problems associated with dependence more generally, such as increased risks of accidents, adverse effects on social and work environments, and even criminal activity (Cooper, 2013b; Lessenger & Feinberg, 2008). There are also particular concerns associated with compound opioid analgesic preparations and where, in combination with the previously mentioned harms, increased doses of analgesics are consumed and the harm occurs due to the compound analgesic (Frei, Nielsen, Dobbin, & Tobin, 2010; Robinson, Robinson, McCarthy, & Cameron, 2010). In the case of paracetamol (acetaminophen) combinations, where formulations are typically 500mg per dose, harm relates to hepatotoxicity (Cooper, 2013b; Lessenger & Feinberg, 2008), and for ibuprofen compound products, gastrointestinal hemorrhage (bleeding), renal impairment, and hypokalemia (low blood potassium levels) represent significant concerns. Reported abuse can involve very significant amounts, and in Australia, for example, "doses of up to 100 tablets daily, the equivalent of 16 times the recommended OTC maximum daily dose of ibuprofen have been reported" from individuals (Tobin, Dobbin, & McAvoy, 2013, p. 484). OTC opioid abuse also leads to mortality, and in England, deaths where paracetamol and codeine compound analgesics were the primary cause increased by 21 percent in 2014, although this figure includes prescription formulations as well as OTC (Office for National Statistics, 2015). In Australia, 40 percent of reported deaths involving codeine between 2000 and 2008 involved OTC medicines (Tobin et al., 2013).

Stimulants

The second key group of OTC medicines of abuse involve those that have a centrally acting stimulant effect. The most common type of medicines in this group are sympathomimetics, which include ephedrine, pseudoephedrine, and phenylpropanolamine. These are indicated OTC not for their stimulant effect, but as decongestants, due to their vasoconstrictive properties and action on sites such as the nasal sinuses. They are found in a range of cough and cold remedies, either alone in strengths that are comparable to those on prescription or in compound preparations with analgesics, antihistamines, and antitussives. Abuse occurs when a nonmedical stimulant side effect is exploited, often at higher doses, but other nonmedical effects such as priapism and enhanced sexual performance have also been reported (Lessenger & Feinberg, 2008). Stimulants are also recognized as appetite suppressants, and further concerns have emerged in relation to stimulant abuse to promote weight loss. As well as sympathomimetic decongestants, a further class of medicine with stimulant properties is caffeine. While caffeine is well recognized as a beverage, it is also licensed as an OTC medicine to prevent tiredness and is included in compound formulations. Stimulants are available in many countries as OTC medicines, and abuse appears to be widespread (Cooper, 2013b).

In relation to harms, stimulants can lead to a variety of adverse effects. Psychoactive effects include changes in mood and the potential for agitation, anxiety, and even psychotic behavior (Pentel, 1984). Also, there are recognized cardiovascular complications, such as tachycardia (Lessenger & Feinberg, 2008) and hypertension (Berman, Setty, Steiner, Kaufman, & Skotzko, 2006). In some cases, even more severe complications can arise, such as hypertensive encephalopathy or intracerebral hemorrhage with decongestants and, for caffeine, seizures and tachyarrhythmia (Pentel, 1984).

Sedative Antihistamines

Antihistamines are primarily used in OTC formulations as treatments for allergies and conditions such as hay fever and urticarial (allergic skin rash). Recent medicines have relatively few side effects, but older antihistamines are still available that have significant sedating side effects related to their central action. These include medicines such as chlorphenamine, diphenhydramine, promethazine, and cyclizine, and due to additional anticholinergic activity, some are also licensed for use in preventing motion sickness and treating symptoms of nausea. In some countries, licensing of such medicines actually exploits the pronounced nature of the sedative side effect for the short-term treatment of insomnia. However, it is chiefly this sedative side effect that is the cause of misuse and abuse. Issues of concern relate to the development of rebound insomnia due to overuse of sedative antihistamines, and there have been isolated cases of more severe side effects, such as acidosis and convulsions (Murao, Manabe, Yamashita, & Sekikawa, 2008).

Dextromethorphan

Particular concerns have emerged about OTC medicines that have the potential to cause a dissociative effect in the brain, with the cough suppressant dextromethorphan chiefly implicated. Dextromethorphan, or DXM, as it is known colloquially, is available in a wide range of cough and cold remedies in many countries, in tablet, capsule, and liquid formulation, often with additional ingredients. At low doses, it is mainly used to suppress cough, but at higher doses (potentially up to 30 times the recommended dose), it can cause euphoria and a dissociative effect. Less commonly, such high doses can cause hallucinations and effects similar to ketamine (Martinak, Bolis, Black, Fargason, & Birur, 2017). Unlike other categories of OTC medicines that are liable to abuse, dextromethorphan is more selectively abused, and evidence suggests that it is more common among U.S. teenagers and males (Cooper, 2013b; Steinman, 2006). Recreational use often aims to exploit a series of dose-dependent "plateaus." Unlike other medicines considered in this chapter, dextromethorphan has established a cultural significance, with use often referred to as "Robotripping" based on one of the popular cough medicine brands. Of further public health concern, however, are more severe psychotic psychiatric outcomes associated with dextromethorphan, including delusional thoughts, paranoia, and reports of assaults, suicide, and homicide (Logan et al., 2012). This has led to restrictions on sales to adolescents in several U.S. states and increased educational awareness campaigns (Wilson, Ferguson, Mazer, & Litovitz, 2011).

Nicotine Replacement Therapy

Introduced in the 1990s, different formulations of nicotine are available without prescription to assist in smoking cessation. These were offered as various strengths of gums, patches, or inhaled preparations with the aim of helping individuals who were nicotine dependent via tobacco to reduce their nicotine dose over time. Concerns emerged, however, that such OTC medicines may cause agitation (Lessenger & Feinberg, 2008) and may be misused or abused in three scenarios: by never-smokers, for noncessation reasons, or when combined with cigarettes (Hughes, Pillitteri, Callas, Callahan, & Kenny, 2004). Empirical studies, however, have suggested that the incidence of such scenarios was relatively low among a sample of the U.S. public (Hughes et al., 2004) and was identified only in a minority of participants in a U.K. study (Fingleton, Watson, Duncan, & Matheson, 2016).

Laxatives

In contrast to the medicines considered so far, there is further group of OTC medicines that are recognized as causing misuse and abuse but which do not have a centrally acting, psychoactive effect. These involve laxatives, which increase the frequency of bowel movements and are used to treat constipation. Laxatives vary considering in their mode of action, including those with stimulant effects, such as senna and bisacodyl; osmotic laxatives; and stool softeners. Misuse can occur through prolonged use of such medicines and particularly with stimulant laxatives, which can exacerbate constipation in the longer term. Of more concern, though, is that some individuals abuse laxatives because they are thought to assist in weight reduction. Laxative abuse is a well-recognized problem and is associated with a range of eating disorders (Austin, Penfold, Johnson, Haines, & Forman, 2013; Bryant-Waugh, Turner, & East, 2005). Harms can result due to gastrointestinal disturbances and may lead to a worsening of eating disorder symptoms and the development of other psychopathology (Tozzi et al., 2006).

Who and How Many Are Affected by OTC Medicine Abuse?

Various attempts have been made to quantify the extent of OTC medicine abuse across several countries. Unfortunately, no clear trend is apparent in the available evidence, as estimates of abuse range from around 1 percent in the United Kingdom to nearly a quarter of a public sample in Nigeria (see Table 5.2). Different emphases and definitions of misuse, abuse, and dependence (Cooper, 2013b), together with different populations and medicine groups, make comparisons between studies difficult. They do however reveal that problematic OTC medicine use occurs in a range of settings and in different types of individuals. As noted above and in the next section, different licensing and policies may also be important factors in explaining the variance observed.

Those most likely to be affected by problematic OTC use have been identified as younger people (Fingleton et al., 2016; Nielsen, Cameron, & Pahoki, 2010; Wazaify, Shields, Hughes, & McElnay, 2005); those with long-standing illnesses (Fingleton et al., 2016); previous illicit substance use (Fingleton et al., 2016; Nielsen et al., 2010); lower educational attainment; and poorer employment history (Nielsen et al., 2010). Sex appeared to be a factor for OTC medicine abuse in only some studies, with females suspected of abusing laxatives more frequently (Pates, McBride, Li, & Ramadan, 2002; Sweileh, Arafat, Al-Khyat, Al-Masri, & Jaradat, 2004) and among high school students engaged in misuse (Steinman, 2006).

Preventing Harm and Providing Support

Various attempts have been made to address the issue of OTC medicine misuse and abuse, and these can be summarized in terms of prevention strategies at the level of policy and regulation, practitioner and public awareness and pharmacy level, and treatment approaches of either formal or informal types. A key aspect of OTC medicine supply that may make prevention difficult is the transactional nature of OTC medicine purchases and the ability for individuals to visit multiple pharmacies to obtain supplies without records being kept (Cooper, 2013a, 2013b, 2013c).

As noted earlier, perhaps the most obvious preventative strategy is to prohibit OTC sales completely, as has been done in several countries, including Australia, where recent up-scheduling occurred (Tobin et al., 2013), and suggested in others, such as Canada (MacKinnon, 2016). This would require medicines to be obtained via prescription only and require a medical consultation. While this would not prevent abuse and dependence of products such as opioids and codeine completely (Office for National Statistics, 2015; Roxburgh et al., 2015), it could significantly reduce opportunities to obtain them (MacKinnon, 2016; Tobin et al., 2013). However, increased regulation of

Table 5.2 Summary of Evidence of the Scale of OTC Medicine, Misuse, Abuse and Dependence

Country	OTC Medicines	Sample	Misuse	Abuse	Dependence
Region of France (Orriols, Gaillard, Lapeyre-Mestre, & Roussin, 2009)	Opioids, sedative antihistamines, pseudoephedrine, dextromethorphan	Pharmacy customers	15.1%	7.5%	7.5%
France (Roussin, Bouyssi, Pouché, Pourcel, & Lapeyre-Mestre, 2013)	Codeine and paracetamol	Pharmacy customers	6.8%	0.85%	17.8%
Northern Ireland (Wazaify et al., 2005)	Any	Public	–	29.8%*	–
South Yorkshire, England (Cooper & Gavens, 2015)	Opioids, sedative antihistamines, pseudoephedrine, laxatives	Pharmacy customers	1.2%	1.2%	0%
Australia (Nielsen et al., 2010)	Opioids	Public	–	–	17.3%
United Kingdom (Fingleton et al., 2016)	Any	Public	19.3%	4.1%	2.0%
Jos, Nigeria (Agaba, Agaba, & Wigwe, 2004)	Analgesics	Public	–	–	22.6%
Ohio, USA (Steinman, 2006)	Any	High school students	4.7%	–	–
Ohio, USA (Le et al., 2017)	Any	University students	21.4%	–	–

* Self-reported awareness of OTC abuse (by self or other).

supply has also been argued not to have an influence on overall sales. Using the sale of OTC codeine in Iceland as an example, work suggests that increasing access was not responsible for the increasing sales of codeine between 1993 and 1998 (Almarsdóttir & Grímsson, 2000).

Other policy approaches have been to alter the licensing of medicines and, as in the United Kingdom for example, to set a three-day limit for the recommended use of codeine-based analgesics, reduce maximum pack sizes (from 100 previously to 32), and adding addiction warning labels (Medicines and Healthcare Products Regulatory Agency, 2009). Other approaches include preventing direct advertising to the public, providing mandatory customer advice, setting age restrictions, and requiring pharmacist-supervised sales (Foley et al., 2015; McBride, Pates, Ramadan, & McGowan, 2003). Increasing awareness about the harm potential of some OTC medicines has been advocated through providing training (Fleming, McElnay, & Hughes, 2004; Wazaify, Hughes, & McElnay, 2006) and offering guidance on how to identify those affected and recognition of the different medicines involved (Royal College of General Practitioners, 2014a).

Several basic pharmacy-specific strategies have been reported, including hiding medicines from the sight of customers, refusing sales, signposting to other health professionals, limiting amounts sold, claiming medicines were not available, and limited forms of monitoring and surveillance (Albsoul-Younes, Wazaify, Yousef, & Tahaineh, 2010; Cooper, 2013c; Matheson, Bond, & Pitcairn, 2002; Pates et al., 2002). In relation to treatment, formal services include the use of specialist drug treatment clinics (Cooper, 2013a; Mattoo, Basu, Sharma, Balaji, & Malhotra, 1997; Myers, Siegfried, & Parry, 2003) and general practitioners or family physicians, with the latter being argued to be more suited, given the different profiles of those abusing OTC medicines compared to illicit substances (Cooper, 2013b; Royal College of General Practitioners, 2014b). A range of pharmacological therapies, such as the use of opioid-substitution therapy, particularly buprenorphine for opioid dependence, and psychological approaches are available (Royal College of General Practitioners, 2014b). Research has also suggested that those affected by OTC medicine abuse may represent a hard to reach group (Reay, 2009) who may also not want to present to any formal health services due to concerns about being identified and their addiction being recorded (Cooper, 2013a). This may explain the diversity of several informal treatment and support services, which include use of Narcotics Anonymous, use of online support groups, and other attempts to self-manage the problem (Cooper, 2013a).

Relationship between OTC and Prescription Medicine Use and Abuse

It is not uncommon for OTC and prescription medicine misuse and abuse to be considered together as a single issue or for evidence and reporting to combine the two, but while there are arguably many similarities, it is important to consider them as distinct but related issues. In a recent study, U.S. university students' self-reported use of OTC and prescription medicines suggested that those misusing OTC cough medicines, stimulants, and sleeping aids were more likely to also use equivalent prescription medicines, although use of prescription medicines was around half that of OTC medicines: 11.2 percent compared to 21.4 percent, respectively (Le et al., 2017). In another study, a complex interrelationship was identified between OTC and prescription medicines with four different types of co-use being identified (Cooper, 2013a):

- Switching from prescription to OTC use once the former had stopped being prescribed was a common initial introduction to OTC medicines.
- Using OTC medicines to cover gaps when a prescription medicine had run out.
- "Topping-up" prescription medicines with OTC medicines to increase the total amount taken.
- Controlling the dose taken to enable lower doses than of prescription medication to be taken when the symptoms were less severe.

Such relationships are important when considering how OTC abuse can be identified and treated.

Summary

This chapter has introduced a number of distinct types of OTC medicines that, while potentially not being as potent as prescription medicines, are potentially problematic. These include opioids and compound analgesics, stimulants, sedative antihistamines, dextromethorphan, nicotine replacement therapies, and laxatives. Evidence exists as to their causing significant morbidity and even mortality, with opioid compound analgesic (paracetamol/acetaminophen or ibuprofen) products a particular concern due to hepatotoxicity and gastric bleeding. Such problems have been identified in several countries, although further research is needed to compare the scale of the problem effectively, given all the implicated OTC medicine types and different populations. Several individual characteristics have been identified that may be associated with OTC abuse that can be used to potentially identify and predict problematic use; those using may be younger, have a long-term condition, and have a previous history of problematic substance use. A range of prevention, treatment, and support options exist, but OTC medicine abuse represents a potentially difficult issue to control due to the transactional nature of customer-pharmacy relationships and the ability to purchase from multiple pharmacies. Overall, OTC medicines remain an important way for the public to access treatment and reduce the workload of other health services, but use needs to be balanced with public health concerns over the risks posed by the medicines described in this chapter.

References

Agaba, E. I., Agaba, P. A., & Wigwe, C. M. (2004). Use and abuse of analgesics in Nigeria: A community survey. *Nigerian Journal of Medicine, 13*(4), 379–382.

Akram, G. (2000). Over-the-counter medication: An emerging and neglected drug abuse? *Journal of Substance Use, 5*(2), 136–142. doi:10.3109/146598 90009053078.

Albsoul-Younes, A., Wazaify, M., Yousef, A. M., & Tahaineh, L. (2010). Abuse and misuse of prescription and nonprescription drugs sold in community pharmacies in Jordan. *Substance Use & Misuse, 45*(9), 1319–1329. doi:10.3109/10826080802490683.

Almarsdóttir, A. B., & Grímsson, A. (2000). Over-the-counter codeine use in Iceland: The impact of increased access. *Scandinavian Journal of Public Health, 28*(4), 270–274. doi:10.1177/14034948000280041001.

Austin, S. B., Penfold, R. B., Johnson, R. L., Haines, J., & Forman, S. (2013). Clinician identification of youth abusing over-the-counter products for weight control in a large U.S. integrated health system. *Journal of Eating Disorders, 1*(1), 40. doi:10.1186/2050-2974-1-40.

Berman, J. A., Setty, A., Steiner, M. J., Kaufman, K. R., & Skotzko, C. (2006). Complicated hypertension related to the abuse of ephedrine and caffeine alkaloids. *Journal of Addictive Diseases, 25*(3), 45–48. doi:10.1300/J069v25 n03_06.

Bissell, P., Ward, P. R., & Noyce, P. R. (2001). The dependent consumer: Reflections on accounts of the risks of non-prescription medicines. *Health, 5*(1), 5–30. doi:10.1177/136345930100500101.

Bond, C. M., & Bradley, C. (1996). Over the counter drugs: The interface between the community pharmacist and patients. *BMJ: British Medical Journal, 312*(7033), 758–760. doi:10.1136/bmj.312.7033.758.

Bryant-Waugh, R., Turner, H., & East, P. (2005). Over-the-counter laxatives and eating disorders: A survey of pharmacists' and other retailers' views and practice. *Pharmaceutical Journal, 275*, 87–91.

Connelly, D. (2016). The OTC market in Britain in 2015. *Pharmaceutical Journal, 296*, 154–155.

Cooper, R. J. (2013a). "I can't be an addict. I am." Over-the-counter medicine abuse: A qualitative study. *BMJ Open, 3*(6). doi:10.1136/bmjopen-2013-002913.

Cooper, R. J. (2013b). Over-the-counter medicine abuse—A review of the literature. *Journal of Substance Use, 18*(2), 82–107. doi:10.3109/14659891.2011. 615002.

Cooper, R. J. (2013c). Surveillance and uncertainty: Community pharmacy responses to over the counter medicine abuse. *Health & Social Care in the Community, 21*(3), 254–262. doi:10.1111/hsc.12012.

Cooper, R. J., & Gavens, J. (2015). *OTC medicine misuse, abuse and dependence in the UK: A pilot survey study.* University of Sheffield. Unpublished Study.

Fingleton, N. A., Watson, M. C., Duncan, E. M., & Matheson, C. (2016). Non-prescription medicine misuse, abuse and dependence: A cross-sectional survey of the UK general population. *Journal of Public Health, 38*(4), 722–730. doi:10.1093/pubmed/fdv204.

Fleming, G. F., McElnay, J. C., & Hughes, C. M. (2004). Development of a community pharmacy-based model to identify and treat OTC drug abuse/misuse: A pilot study. *Pharmacy World and Science, 26*(5), 282–288. doi:10.1023/b:phar.0000042891.66983.60.

Foley, M., Harris, R., Rich, E., Rapca, A., Bergin, M., Norman, I., & Van Hout, M. C. (2015). The availability of over-the-counter codeine medicines across the European Union. *Public Health, 129*(11), 1465–1470. doi:10.1016/j.puhe .2015.06.014.

Frei, M. Y., Nielsen, S., Dobbin, M. D., & Tobin, C. L. (2010). Serious morbidity associated with misuse of over-the-counter codeine-ibuprofen analgesics: A series of 27 cases. *Medical Journal of Australia, 193*(5), 294–296.

Hughes, J. R., Pillitteri, J. L., Callas, P. W., Callahan, R., & Kenny, M. (2004). Misuse of and dependence on over-the-counter nicotine gum in a volunteer sample. *Nicotine & Tobacco Research, 6*(1), 79–84. doi:10.1080/14622 200310001656894.

Le, V. T., Norris Turner, A., McDaniel, A., Hale, K. M., Athas, C., & Kwiek, N. C. (2017). Nonmedical use of over-the-counter medications is significantly associated with nonmedical use of prescription drugs among university students. *Journal of American College Health*, 1–8. doi:10.1080/07448481. 2017.1356312.

Lessenger, J. E., & Feinberg, S. D. (2008). Abuse of prescription and over-the-counter medications. *Journal of the American Board of Family Medicine, 21*(1), 45–54. doi:10.3122/jabfm.2008.01.070071.

Logan, B. K., Yeakel, J. K., Goldfogel, G., Frost, M. P., Sandstrom, G., & Wickham, D. J. (2012). Dextromethorphan abuse leading to assault, suicide, or homicide. *Journal of Forensic Sciences, 57*(5), 1388–1394. doi:10.1111/j.1556 -4029.2012.02133.x.

MacKinnon, J. I. J. (2016). Tighter regulations needed for over-the-counter codeine in Canada. *Canadian Pharmacists Journal/Revue des Pharmaciens du Canada, 149*(6), 322–324. doi:10.1177/1715163516660572.

Martinak, B., Bolis, R. A., Black, J. R., Fargason, R. E., & Birur, B. (2017). Dextro-methorphan in cough syrup: The poor man's psychosis. *Psychopharmacology Bulletin, 47*(4), 59–63.

Matheson, C., Bond, C. M., & Pitcairn, J. (2002). Misuse of over-the-counter medicines from community pharmacies: A population survey of Scottish pharmacies. *Pharmaceutical Journal, 269*, 66–68.

Mattoo, S. K., Basu, D., Sharma, A., Balaji, M., & Malhotra, A. (1997). Abuse of codeine-containing cough syrups: A report from India. *Addiction, 92*(12), 1783–1787. doi:10.1111/j.1360-0443.1997.tb02898.x.

McBride, A. J., Pates, R., Ramadan, R., & McGowan, C. (2003). Delphi survey of experts' opinions on strategies used by community pharmacists to reduce over-the-counter drug misuse. *Addiction, 98*(4), 487–497. doi:10.1046/j.1360-0443.2003.00345.x.

Medicines and Healthcare Products Regulatory Agency. (2009). *MHRA Public Assessment Report: Codeine and Dihydrocodeine-containing Medicines: Minimising the Risk of Addiction.* London, England: MHRA.

Murao, S., Manabe, H., Yamashita, T., & Sekikawa, T. (2008). Intoxication with over-the-counter antitussive medication containing dihydrocodeine and chlorpheniramine causes generalized convulsion and mixed acidosis. *Internal Medicine, 47*(11), 1013–1015.

Myers, B., Siegfried, N., & Parry, C. D. (2003). Over-the-counter and prescription medicine misuse in Cape Town—Findings from specialist treatment centres. *South African Medical Journal, 93*(5), 367–370.

Nielsen, S., Cameron, J., & Pahoki, S. (2010). *Over the Counter Codeine Dependence Final Report 2010.* Fitzroy, Victoria, Australia: Turning Point Alcohol and Drug Centre.

Office for National Statistics. (2015). *Deaths Related to Drug Poisoning in England and Wales: 2014 Registrations.* Newport, UK: Office for National Statistics.

Orriols, L., Gaillard, J., Lapeyre-Mestre, M., & Roussin, A. (2009). Evaluation of abuse and dependence on drugs used for self-medication. *Drug Safety, 32*(10), 859–873. doi:10.2165/11316590-000000000-00000.

Pates, R., McBride, A. J., Li, S., & Ramadan, R. (2002). Misuse of over-the-counter medicines: A survey of community pharmacies in the South Wales health authority. *Pharmaceutical Journal, 268*, 179–182.

Pentel, P. (1984). Toxicity of over-the-counter stimulants. *JAMA, 252*(14), 1898–1903.

Reay, G. (2009). *An Inquiry into Physical Dependence and Addiction to Prescription and Over-the-Counter Medication.* London, England: All-Party Parliamentary Drugs Misuse Group.

Robinson, G. M., Robinson, S., McCarthy, P., & Cameron, C. (2010). Misuse of over-the-counter codeine-containing analgesics: Dependence and other adverse effects. *New Zealand Medical Journal, 123*(1317), 59–64.

Roussin, A., Bouyssi, A., Pouché, L., Pourcel, L., & Lapeyre-Mestre, M. (2013). Misuse and dependence on non-prescription codeine analgesics or sedative H1 antihistamines by adults: A cross-sectional investigation in France. *PLoS One, 8*(10), e76499. doi:10.1371/journal.pone.0076499.

Roxburgh, A., Hall, W. D., Burns, L., Pilgrim, J., Saar, E., Nielsen, S., & Degenhardt, L. (2015). Trends and characteristics of accidental and intentional codeine overdose deaths in Australia. *Medical Journal of Australia, 203*(7), 299.

Royal College of General Practitioners. (2014a). *Prescription and Over-the-Counter Medicines Misuse and Dependence. Fact Sheet 3. Identification. How Are Patients Who Are Misusing or Dependent on Prescription-only or Over-the-Counter Medicines Identified?* London, England: RCGP.

Royal College of General Practitioners. (2014b). *Prescription and Over-the-Counter Medicines Misuse and Dependence. Fact Sheet 4. Treatment. How Are Patients Who Misuse and/or Become Dependent on Prescription-only or Over-the-Counter Medicines Treated?* London, England: RCGP.

Steinman, K. J. (2006). High school students' misuse of over-the-counter drugs: A population-based study in an urban county. *Journal of Adolescent Health, 38*(4), 445–447. doi:10.1016/j.jadohealth.2005.08.010.

Sweileh, W. M., Arafat, R. T., Al-Khyat, L. S., Al-Masri, D. M., & Jaradat, N. A. (2004). A pilot study to investigate over-the-counter drug abuse and misuse in Palestine. *Saudi Medical Journal, 25*(12), 2029–2032.

Technavio. (2016). *Global Over-the-Counter Drug Market 2016–2020.* Toronto, Canada: Infiniti Research, Ltd.

Tobin, C. L., Dobbin, M., & McAvoy, B. (2013). Regulatory responses to over-the-counter codeine analgesic misuse in Australia, New Zealand and the United Kingdom. *Australian and New Zealand Journal of Public Health, 37*(5), 483–488. doi:10.1111/1753-6405.12099.

Tozzi, F., Thornton, L. M., Mitchell, J., Fichter, M. M., Klump, K. L., Lilenfeld, L. R., . . . Price Foundation Collaborative Group. (2006). Features associated with laxative abuse in individuals with eating disorders. *Psychosomatic Medicine, 68*(3), 470–477. doi:10.1097/01.psy.0000221359.35034.e7.

Wazaify, M., Hughes, C. M., & McElnay, J. C. (2006). The implementation of a harm minimisation model for the identification and treatment of over-the-counter drug misuse and abuse in community pharmacies in Northern Ireland. *Patient Education and Counseling, 64*(1), 136–141. doi:https://doi.org/10.1016/j.pec.2005.12.008.

Wazaify, M., Shields, E., Hughes, C. M., & McElnay, J. C. (2005). Societal perspectives on over-the-counter (OTC) medicines. *Family Practice, 22*(2), 170–176. doi:10.1093/fampra/cmh723.

Wilson, M. D., Ferguson, R. W., Mazer, M. E., & Litovitz, T. L. (2011). Monitoring trends in dextromethorphan abuse using the National Poison Data System: 2000–2010. *Clinical Toxicology (Philadelphia, PA), 49*(5), 409–415. doi:10.3109/15563650.2011.585429.

World Health Organization. (1994). *Lexicon of Alcohol and Drug Terms.* Geneva, Switzerland: WHO.

CHAPTER SIX

Nonmedical Prescription Drug Use in Adolescents and Young Adults

*Lian-Yu Chen, Alexander S. Perlmutter, Luis Segura,
Julian Santaella-Tenorio, Julia P. Schleimer,
Mariel Mendez, Lilian Ghandour,
Magdalena Cerdá, and Silvia S. Martins*

Nonmedical use of prescription drugs (NMPD) is defined as the use of prescription drugs for reasons other than prescribed, for a time period longer than prescribed or simply without a doctor's prescription. NMPD use has become a worldwide concern in the past few decades, with multiple surveys from Europe, South Asia, Latin America, and the Middle East illustrating its rising prevalence (Center for Behavioral Health Statistics and Quality, 2016b; Martins & Ghandour, 2017; Novak et al., 2016; United Nations Office on Drugs and Crime, 2011a, 2011b). NMPD use in the United States has received special attention because it is considered a rising epidemic (Martins & Ghandour, 2017), with NMPD use ranking as the second most prevalent form of illicit drug use, following only marijuana use (Center for Behavioral Health Statistics and Quality, 2016a). In fact, NMPD in the United States is considered a major public health issue, with the past-year prevalence estimated at 7.1 percent based on results from 2015 National Survey on Drug Use and Health (NSDUH; Center for Behavioral Health Statistics and Quality, 2016a).

However, the scale of the problem of NMPD is probably underestimated, given the difficulty in capturing the population that uses these legally pre-scribed drugs for nonmedical reasons through epidemiologic surveys. NMPD has been associated with numerous health consequences as well as potential adverse effects on adolescents and young adults, including a higher likeli-hood of other risky behaviors, psychiatric comorbidities, and other sub-stance use problems (Chen, Crum, Strain, Martins, & Mojtabai, 2015; Johnston, O'Malley, Bachman, Schulenberg, & Miech, 2016; McCabe, West, & Wechsler, 2007).

The most commonly nonmedically used prescription drugs in the United States are opioids, followed by tranquilizers, stimulants, and sedatives, and young adults aged 18–25 years old constitute the largest group of those engaged in nonmedical prescription opioid (NMPO) use (Hughes et al., 2016). Prescription opioids are usually taken nonmedically to elicit a feeling of euphoria, though they are indicated for the treatment of chronic and can-cer pain. Prescription opioids have received the highest level of public atten-tion due to the soaring numbers of opioid overdose deaths. Nonmedical prescription stimulant (NMPS) use, like nonmedical prescription opioid use, has also increased in the past two decades, particularly among adolescents and young adults (Chen et al., 2015; McCabe, 2005; McCabe, Teter, & Boyd, 2004). Prescription stimulants mainly refer to medications prescribed for treatment of attention-deficit hyperactivity disorder (ADHD), including methylphenidate and mixed-salts amphetamines. They are typically used nonmedically for cognitive enhancement or getting high (Teter, McCabe, LaGrange, Cranford, & Boyd, 2006). NMPS use among adolescents and young adults is also a public health issue noted mostly in the United States and Canada.

Research on nonmedical use of tranquilizers (primarily composed of ben-zodiazepines) and sedatives has mostly been conducted among older popula-tions; hence, worldwide data describing the situation among adolescents and young adults is relatively scarce. Promoting sleep onset is a leading reason for nonmedical sedative use, while promotion of relaxation and sleep are leading motivations for nonmedical tranquilizer use (Center for Behavioral Health Statistics and Quality, 2016b). Prescription tranquilizers and sedatives deliver a feeling of calm to those taking them, but nonmedical use may result in respiratory depression, apnea, and even death if used in large quantities (Nattala, Murthy, Thennarasu, & Cottler, 2014). The problem of nonmedical use of sedatives and tranquilizers is particularly prominent in East and Southeast Asia, particularly in Brunei, Indonesia, Malaysia, the Philippines, and Singapore (United Nations Office on Drugs and Crime, 2011b), though the exact extent of this problem is largely unknown. In the United States, literature on nonmedical tranquilizer and sedative use is relatively limited despite the growing problem within the past decade (Treatment Episode

Data Set, 2011). Data on these drug classes in the United States have been measured by the NSDUH and the Monitoring the Future (MTF) study, while in Eastern European countries, the European School Survey on Alcohol and Other Drugs (ESPAD) has recently documented high a prevalence of nonmedical use.

In the following sections, we will summarize (1) the health burden nonmedical prescription drug use imposes in the United States and (2) each drug class's historical perspective and public health significance, separately for adolescents and young adults. While we try to draw on the global data, most evidence originates where it was published, mainly the United States and Canada.

Health Burden of Nonmedical Prescription Drug Use in the United States

Over the last two decades, NMPD, particularly among young adults (aged 18–25 years old), has increasingly become a public health concern in the United States. Increasingly relaxed prescription regulations and policies and surges in pharmaceutical production and marketing of medications for pain management were the primary changes leading to the current NMPD epidemic in the United States. From 1996, the sales of one of those opioid medications, OxyContin (oxycodone), grew from $48 million to $1.1 billion in 2000 in the United States alone (Van Zee, 2009). As of 2009, the United States has been the world's leading opioid prescriber and consumer, consuming 99 percent of the world's hydrocodone and 81 percent of the world's oxycodone (Manchikanti & Singh, 2008). These ecological changes have led to serious public health issues, including an increase in opioid overdose-related deaths. Between 1999 and 2015, more than 183,000 people died in the United States from overdoses involving prescription opioids (Centers for Disease Control and Prevention, 2016). The rising number of fatalities related to prescription opioid misuse triggered the president's Prescription Drug Abuse Prevention Plan aimed at curbing prescription drug misuse nationwide (White House, 2011).

Canadians and Europeans have also reported that NMPO use is a rising epidemic (United Nations Office on Drugs and Crime, 2011b). Aside from increasing overdose and hospitalization prevalences, prescription opioid consumption can lead to substance use disorder symptoms. Prescription rates for another drug class, stimulants, have increased for children, adolescents, and adults, with more than 2.6 million people using them nonmedically in 2009 (Substance Abuse and Mental Health Services Administration, 2010). Prescription stimulants are mainly used nonmedically for cognitive enhancement and for euphoric reasons (i.e., "to get high"). Stimulant nonmedical use is associated with suicide in adolescents and eating disorders in young adults, and between 2005 and 2010, emergency room visits involving these medications tripled from 13,379 to 31,244 (Substance Abuse and Mental Health Services Administration, 2013).

Nonmedical prescription sedative and tranquilizer use is both a related problem to the opioid epidemic in the United States and an independent one elsewhere. Prescription sedatives are often found in those who have died from a prescription opioid overdose in the United States (Centers for Disease Control and Prevention, 2017). The psychiatric illnesses associated with nonmedical sedative and tranquilizer use are somewhat similar to those associated with nonmedical prescription opioid use. While not as physiologically addicting, those nonmedically using tranquilizers and sedatives have elevated odds of depression and risky behaviors regarding other substance use. Evidently, nonmedical prescription drug use, across medication classes, has significant negative health determinants and consequences.

Nonmedical Prescription Opioid Use (NMPO)

Historical Trends among Adolescents

NMPO among adolescents has not been historically significant as a form of substance use in the United States. In fact, between 1975 and 1992, its prevalence among high school seniors fell from near 6 percent to just below 4 percent (Johnston, O'Malley, Miech, Bachman, & Schulenberg, 2016). However, since 1992 (3.3%), the prevalence of NMPO use has increased dramatically, plateauing between 2003 and 2009 with a prevalence of 9 percent to 10 percent before slowly decreasing to 5.4 percent in 2015 (Johnston, O'Malley, Miech et al., 2016). NSDUH reports and studies using local samples of adolescents aged 12–17 years old suggest that the prevalence of past-year NMPO is about 3.5 percent to 4 percent (Boyd, Young, & McCabe, 2014; Hughes et al., 2016), while MTF data from 2010–2011 reported NMPO use as 5.5 percent (Veliz, Boyd, & McCabe, 2013). The MTF report shows drops in 8th, 10th, and 12th graders' NMPO, whose combined prevalence was above 8 percent from 2001 to 2009. Both Wu and colleagues and Zullig and colleagues found NMPO use to be about 7 percent among 12- to 17-year-olds using 2005 and 2006 NSDUH data (Wu, Ringwalt, Mannelli, & Patkar, 2008) and among high school students in five U.S. cities (Zullig, Divin, Weiler, Haddox, & Pealer, 2015).

In Wu and colleagues' analysis of adolescents using 2005 and 2006 NSDUH data, more than one-third of those who reported NMPO further reported one or more symptoms of DSM-IV substance abuse or dependence; specifically, 6.7 percent reported abuse, 19.6 percent were at the threshold for dependence, and 9.1 percent were found to be dependent regardless of abuse (Wu et al., 2008). It is worth noting that prevalence of prescription opioid use disorder among 12- to 17-year-olds in 2002 was 1 percent, compared to 0.6 percent in 2012, 0.5 percent in 2013, and 0.7 percent in 2014, illustrating a relatively stable trend for opioid use disorder in adolescents (Center for Behavioral Health Statistics and Quality, 2015a). Martins and colleagues' analysis of 12- to 17-year-olds with NMPO use disorder or heroin use among those engaged in NMPO found no change from 2002 to 2014 for either case, although 2004, 2005, and 2011 had significant peaks during that time frame (Martins et al., 2017). Regarding overdose, data from Centers for Disease Control and Prevention (CDC) does not differentiate between adolescents and emerging adults aged 18–25 years old. Though the 2014 and 2015 NMPO overdose death rates for the older age groups were higher, overdose death rates among 15- to 24-year-olds in 2014 and 2015 nearly doubled in only one year from 1.2 to 2.3 per 100,000, a 91.7 percent increase (Rudd, 2016). Overall, NMPO overdose rates increased every year from 2002 until 2011 (Center for Behavioral Health Statistics and Quality, 2015), and benzodiazepines (sedatives) were involved in most opioid-related overdose deaths (Centers for Disease Control and Prevention, 2017).

Public Health Significance and Correlates of NMPO among Adolescents

Adolescents rarely have any of the indications for which opioids are prescribed, yet they use opioids nonmedically at higher rates than stimulants, which are typically prescribed to adolescents with ADHD (Hughes et al., 2016). Adolescents may directly receive opioid prescriptions for conditions for which opioids are not indicated, such as sports injuries and headaches (Dowell, Haegerich, & Chou, 2016) and indirectly through diversion from friends or family.

Initiation of NMPO among adolescents has recently become a new threat in combating the opioid epidemic. In the 2015 NSDUH report on drug initiation, 415,000 12- to 17-year-olds initiated NMPO in the past year, compared to 276,000 who initiated NMPS (Lipari, Williams, Copello, & Pemberton, 2016). The 2009 to 2012 Secondary Student Life Survey data shows the age of first opioid medical use initially rising between ages 9 and 10, with larger rises and smaller falls up to age 13, when onset prevalence reaches 4 percent. From ages 13–16, onset prevalence reaches 10 percent, falling slightly at age 17. This contrasts with the onset prevalence of NMPO in another study, where it rose from near zero at age 11 to 3 percent by age 16 (Austic, McCabe, Stoddard, Ngo, & Boyd, 2015). The 2015 MTF report backs this finding as nonmedical OxyContin and Vicodin use rose with increasing age among American 8th (0.8% and 0.9%, respectively), 10th (2.6% and 2.5%), and 12th graders (3.7% and 4.4%). Vaughn and colleagues show that among non-Hispanic/Latino Whites, 15- to 17-year-olds were 32 percent more likely to use opioids nonmedically than 12- to 14-year-olds (Vaughn, Nelson, Salas-Wright, Qian, & Schootman, 2016).

NMPO also varies by demographic characteristics among youth. Vaughn and colleagues combined 2004 to 2013 NSDUH data, showing that non-Hispanic/Latino White, non-Hispanic/Latino Black, and Hispanic females were all between 1.3 to 1.4 times more likely to use opioids nonmedically than male counterparts (Vaughn et al., 2016). MTF data shows that 12th grade males and females in 2015 had a NMPO prevalence rate slightly above and below 5 percent, respectively (Johnston, O'Malley, Miech, Bachman, & Schulenberg, 2017). Since 2004, racial and ethnic differences in NMPO have attenuated; non-Hispanic/Latino White NMPO prevalence was 8 percent during 2004–2005, but it has more recently dropped to 5 percent, near minority NMPO levels (Vaughn et al., 2016). This trend can be seen in 12th grade MTF participants as well (Johnston et al., 2017). Non-Hispanic/Latino White children from families annually earning less than $20,000, $20,000–$49,999 or $50,000–$74,999 were 64 percent, 34 percent, and 23 percent more likely to use opioids nonmedically than those with household incomes greater than $75,000 (Vaughn et al., 2016). Non-Hispanic/Latino Blacks from families in the lowest two income categories were 37 percent to 38 percent more likely to use opioids nonmedically than youth from the highest-earning non-Hispanic/Latino Black families (Vaughn et al., 2016).

Adolescents engaged in NMPO may encounter grave health concerns related to their opioid use, including overdose, psychiatric disorders, and other substance use and problematic use. Adolescents using opioids both medically (i.e., appropriately) and nonmedically face a higher risk of adverse health associations because overdoses have been observed in this population, which have not been observed among those uniquely using other prescription drug classes nonmedically (Zosel, Bartelson, Bailey, Lowenstein, & Dart, 2013). Data on 13- to 19-year-olds from 2007 to 2009, during a relative peak in adolescent NMPO, found that poison center calls (i.e., events) related to intentional opioid (i.e., purposeful medical or nonmedical) exposures found that, of 8,866 events, 22 percent, 51 percent, 22 percent, and 5 percent had no, minor, moderate, and major effects, with 0.2 percent (or 20 events) resulting in death (Zosel et al., 2013). Martins and colleagues (2017) revealed that 12- to 17-year-olds engaged in NMPO had high levels of opioid use disorder and heroin use. From 2002 to 2014, opioid use disorder among those engaged in NMPO never dropped below 10 percent and was close to 20 percent in 2004 (Martins et al., 2017). While still problematic, heroin use among those who use opioids was much less common, at about 2 percent for most of the period and near 4 percent in 2011 (Martins et al., 2017). Adolescent NMPO is also associated with increased rates of psychiatric illness, as a Michigan high school study found that affective, anxiety, attention-deficit hyperactivity, and conduct disorders were more prevalent in those who are nonmedically using opioids for recreational purposes than those not using, those using appropriately, and those self-treating pain (Boyd et al., 2014).

Contributing to the diffusion of opioids in American society is the common practice of opioid diversion to friends and family as well as reselling pills for profit. Combined 2005–2006 NSDUH data revealed that adolescents engaged in NMPO most commonly received their opioid from friends or relatives (Schepis & Krishnan-Sarin, 2009). These adolescents had 2.03, 2.25, and 2.29 greater odds of binge drinking alcohol, smoking cigarettes daily, and using marijuana monthly, respectively, than those who obtained their opioids from physicians (Schepis & Krishnan-Sarin, 2009). However, those who stole opioids or wrote fake prescriptions to obtain opioids were 1.5 and 3 times less likely to have 10 or more prescriptions and have a past-year major depressive episode (MDE), respectively, than those who received their opioids from physicians (Schepis & Krishnan-Sarin, 2009). In fact, those who received opioids from friends or relatives for free, purchased their opioids, or obtained opioids from other nonphysician sources were at least two times less likely to have a past-year MDE, but they were more likely to have aforementioned concomitant alcohol, cigarette, and marijuana use (Schepis & Krishnan-Sarin, 2009).

Historical Trends among Young Adults

NMPO prevalence on college campuses was 3.1 percent, 3.8 percent, 4.5 percent, and 7.3 percent in 1993, 1997, 1999 and 2001, respectively (McCabe et al., 2007). By 1994, NMPO prevalence among college students had gradually declined to 2.4 percent, which was under half (5.1%) of the 1980 prevalence rate (Johnston, O'Malley, Bachman et al., 2016); this decline mirrored the same trend for those not attending college. By 2006, the prevalence of college students' past-year NMPO had increased to 8.8 percent (Johnston, O'Malley, Bachman et al., 2016). Prevalence of NMPO use among college students was lower (3.3%) compared to non-college-attending emerging adults (5.9%), who compose 65 percent of 18- to 24-year-olds cohort (Johnston, O'Malley, Bachman et al., 2016). A study on educational attainment among college-aged (i.e., 18–22 years old) emerging adults found that prescription opioid use decreased from 2008 (12.4%) to 2010 (11.8%), but this decline was not significant (Martins et al., 2015).

While the prevalence of NMPO may be a marker for the extent of the epidemic over several years, rates of DSM-IV opioid abuse and dependence are clear indicators of the severity of the epidemic. The prevalence of NMPO is currently on the decline, with the peak levels among young adults having occurred from 2003 to 2006. Martins and colleagues' analysis of 2002–2014 NSDUH data found that opioid use disorder (12.0% to 15.1%) and heroin use (2.1% to 7.4%) among 18- to 25-year-olds engaged in NMPO both increased significantly (Martins et al., 2017). Between 1999 and 2008, there was a 122 percent increase in hospitalizations due to drug overdoses of prescription opioid pain medications among 18- to 24-year-olds (White, Hingson, Pan, & Yi, 2011).

Public Health Significance and Correlates of NMPO among Young Adults

College years are a period during which students are introduced to opioids and NMPO. In 1,253 incoming first-year college students, Arria and colleagues estimated an 85.7 percent increase in lifetime prevalence of NMPO from precollege to sophomore year (Arria, Caldeira et al., 2008). Moreover, the increase in NMPO started at age 16, and by age 18, 50 percent of students had tried NMPO (Arria, Caldeira et al., 2008). At least one-third of 18-year-old students who experimented with NMPO continued to do so beyond age 18 (McCabe, Schulenberg, O'Malley, Patrick, & Kloska, 2014).

Those who remain engaged in NMPO vary demographically. Among college students, NMPO is more likely to occur among students who are White (Ford & Arrastia, 2008; McCabe, Teter, Boyd, Knight, & Wechsler, 2005); Hispanic (Ford & Arrastia, 2008); residents of fraternity and sorority houses; those who attended more competitive colleges (McCabe et al., 2005); those who were sexually active; and those less involved in college activities (e.g., student organizations, sports activities, volunteer work, etc.; Ford & Arrastia, 2008). Evidence on the sex and sexual orientation differences in NMPO among college students remains unclear; however, some studies suggest a higher rate of NMPO among males (Jones, Paulozzi, & Mack, 2014; Martins & Ghandour, 2017); young females (Lieb, Pfister, & Wittchen, 1998); and lesbian and bisexual women (Kelly & Parsons, 2007).

NMPO negatively affects academic performance and academic behaviors (Arria, O'Grady, Caldeira, Vincent, & Wish, 2008; Ford & Arrastia, 2008). In a prospective study, Arria and colleagues found that college-attending students engaged in NMPO had lower grade point averages than those who did not nonmedically use, spent less time studying during weekdays and weekends, studied for fewer hours per day, and socialized more during weekdays (Arria, O'Grady et al., 2008). The authors attributed the adverse effect of NMPO on academic performance to skipping classes. Not attending college is also associated with NMPO. Martins and colleagues found that non-college-attending adults with a high school degree or less were 25 percent more likely to use opioids nonmedically than college-attending young adults (Martins, Kim et al., 2015). Among young adults engaged in NMPO who were not in college, the prevalence of opioid use disorder secondary to NMPO was higher (19.1% vs. 11.7%) than those in college (Martins, Kim et al., 2015). The relationship between educational attainment and past-year opioid use disorder secondary to NMUPO seems to be moderated by ethnicity and gender, particularly non-Hispanic/Latino Whites and females; females not enrolled in college had the highest rates of opioid use disorder compared to both male and female college students and males who did not attend college (Martins, Kim et al., 2015).

The use of other substances in combination with opioids among young adults attending college is of particular concern. Alcohol use is more common in college students engaged in NMPO than in college students not engaged in NMPO (Garnier et al., 2009; Ghandour, El Sayed, & Martins, 2013). Evidence from prospective studies suggests that 58 percent of college students engaged in NMPO are concurrent users of alcohol (Garnier et al., 2009). Those engaged in NMPO who also consume alcohol have more drinks per day—an average of 7.5 per day—than those using alcohol only (Garnier et al., 2009). Other studies had similar findings where those engaged in NMPO were more likely than those who were not engaged in NMPO to binge drink (Ford & Arrastia, 2008); drive after binge drinking; be a passenger with a drunk driver (McCabe et al., 2005; Whiteside et al., 2013); report marijuana use (Ford & Arrastia, 2008; Ghandour et al., 2013); and use cocaine (McCabe et al., 2005). Young adults engaged in NMPO perceive opioids as safer and less addictive than other illegal drugs (Mateu-Gelabert, Guarino, Jessell, & Teper, 2015). Additional risky behaviors have been reported among young adults engaged in NMPO, including needle sharing, unprotected sex with casual partners, exchange sex, group sex, and sexual violence (Mateu-Gelabert et al., 2015; Whiteside et al., 2013). NMPO prevalence is higher among young college-aged females who reported recent violence by a partner and abused alcohol; NMPO prevalence was particularly high among those with cumulative (i.e., many subtypes of) violence exposure (Cole & Logan, 2010).

More recently, the possibility of transitioning from NMPO to heroin use has gained special attention, as heroin use prevalence has been increasing in the United States, particularly among those engaged in NMPO (Martins, Santaella-Tenorio, Marshall, Maldonado, & Cerda, 2015; Martins et al., 2017). Evidence from a 36-month follow-up cohort of 18- to 24-year-olds engaged in NMPO estimated a heroin initiation incidence rate of 2.8 percent per year (Carlson, Nahhas, Martins, & Daniulaityte, 2016). Moreover, those who transitioned from NMPO to heroin use were more likely to have had early initiation of opioid use, between 10 and 12 years of age (Cerda, Santaella, Marshall, Kim, & Martins, 2015), have reported lifetime opioid dependence; have used opioids to get high; have used nonoral opioid formulations (Carlson et al., 2016); have nonmedically used opioids more frequently; and were White or Hispanic/Latino (Martins, Santaella-Tenorio et al., 2015). NMPO in college-attending young adults has been linked to higher reporting of psychiatric symptoms, psychiatric disorders, and suicidal ideation (Kuramoto, Chilcoat, Ko, & Martins, 2012), while opioid abuse is linked to overdose, emergency department utilization, and death (Jones et al., 2014; Whiteside et al., 2013).

Nonmedical Prescription Stimulant Use (NMPS)

Historical Trends among Adolescents

Nonmedical prescription stimulant use (NMPS) was very prevalent during the late 1970s among high school seniors in the United States, with past-year NMPS prevalence peaking in 1981 at 26 percent. The prevalence then declined until 1992. Since 1992, the prevalence of NMPS has been steady at between 7 percent (in 2009) and 11 percent (in 2002) of adolescents (Johnston, O'Malley, Miech et al., 2016), with no significant gender differences (Johnston et al., 2017). NMPS prevalence among different cross sections of high school sophomores (starting in 1990) peaked in 1996 at 12.4 percent and was lowest in 2008 and 2011, at 6.4 percent and 6.6 percent, respectively (Johnston, O'Malley, Miech et al., 2016). NMPS prevalence among 8th graders, who are usually 13–14 years old, was 6.2 percent in 1991, peaked at 9.1 percent in 1996, and dropped steadily and linearly until 2012 to 2.9 percent (Johnston, O'Malley, Miech et al., 2016). Since then, a slight increase in prevalence has been observed (Johnston, O'Malley, Miech et al., 2016). Since 1991, when all three groups (i.e., 12th, 10th, and 8th graders) were asked whether it was easy to obtain prescription stimulants, 12th, 10th, and 8th graders evidence almost uninterrupted prevalence declines from 57 percent, 43 percent, and 32 percent, respectively, to 42 percent, 27 percent, and 11 percent (Johnston, O'Malley, Miech et al., 2016).

American adolescents have a higher prevalence rate of ADHD diagnoses and symptoms relative to young adults, who typically see symptoms reduce in severity or nearly disappear (National Institute on Drug Abuse, 2014). However, adolescents have a much smaller share of NMPS and other stimulant use (i.e., methamphetamine) than those of a college-attending age (Chen et al., 2014). For instance, combined 2006–2011 nationally representative data suggests that about 15 percent of those engaged in past month NMPS were 12- to 17-year-olds, while over half were 18–25 years old (Chen et al., 2016). More recent national data suggest that among those engaged in past-year NMPS, 7.3 percent were youth (Hughes et al., 2016). The same national data source revealed that only about 2 percent of those aged 12–17 years were engaged in past-year NMPS (Goldstein, 2008; Schepis & Krishnan-Sarin, 2009), which held through 2015 (Hughes et al., 2016). Other select samples (Boyd, Young, Grey, & McCabe, 2009; Guo et al., 2016; A. Young, Grey, Boyd, & McCabe, 2011) demonstrated higher prevalence rates of between 3 percent and 7 percent across time (Arria et al., 2008; Roy, Nolin, Traore, Leclerc, & Vasiliadis, 2015; Striley, Kelso-Chichetto, & Cottler, 2016; Zosel et al., 2013; Zullig et al., 2015).

Public Health Significance and Correlates of NMPS among Adolescents

NMPS usually begins at a young age, in part due to increased opportunities to try prescription stimulants. Wu and colleagues found that, in 2003,

15.2 percent and 42.5 percent of those engaged in NMPS initiated at or before age 14 and between ages 15 and 17, respectively (Wu, Pilowsky, Schlenger, & Galvin, 2007). More recent national data showed that 276,000 people aged 12–17 years old initiated NMPS (Lipari et al., 2016). Arria and colleagues' longitudinal study of 1,253 college students showed that 50 percent of all students ever had the opportunity to try stimulant medication, half of whom had the opportunity to initiate stimulant use before age 18 (Arria et al., 2008). The same study revealed NMPS prior to college to be 6 percent (Arria et al., 2008). A study using combined 2009–2012 data showed a nonlinear relationship of the prevalence distribution of age of first medical stimulant use (i.e., 5–17 years old), with a linear relationship of the prevalence distribution of first NMPS, but only from age 12 onward (Austic et al., 2015). From age 5 to age 12, the prevalence of first use was flat near zero, which increased for each additional year of age: age 13, 0.3 percent; age 14, 0.4 percent; age 15, 0.8 percent; age 16, 1.0 percent; and age 17, 1.5 percent (Austic et al., 2015). This finding supports Chen's concurrent analysis of adolescents engaged in past-year use, which saw 7.2 percent, 25.4 percent, and 62.4 percent of those engaged in NMPS to be 12–13, 14–15, and 16–17 years old, respectively; however, only 16- to 17-year-olds' use statistically differed from that of 12- to 13-year-olds (Chen et al., 2014). A Canadian study found a similar association (Pulver, Davison, & Pickett, 2015).

Current evidence suggests that the demographics of NMPS are no different than other NMPD. Adolescent Whites and other non-Hispanic/Latino racial/ethnic groups were 2.7 and 1.7 times more likely have used stimulants nonmedically in the past year compared to Blacks, respectively, while Hispanic/Latino NMPS was indistinguishable from that of Blacks (Striley et al., 2016). A suicide risk study of 4,148 adolescents in five public high schools in as many states found that females and male youths use stimulants at the same rates (Hughes et al., 2016; Zullig et al., 2015). Other drug use is common among adolescents who nonmedically use stimulants. An analysis of American adolescents using combined 2006–2011 data that 53.3 percent, 47.9 percent, and 23.4 percent of NMPS had concurrent alcohol, marijuana, and opioid use, respectively (Chen et al., 2015).

Adolescents face a risk of adverse, mostly psychosocial, health associations related to NMPS, even if otherwise prescribed stimulants. Risks include poisoning, which is associated with suicide. An analysis of the Researched Abuse Diversion and Addiction-Related Surveillance (RADARS) system data from 2007–2009 found that 4,582 of 16,209 intentional exposures were related to stimulants, 18 percent, 40 percent, 40 percent, and 3 percent of which had no, minor, moderate, and major effects, respectively (Zosel et al., 2013). The 2015 suicide risk study found that males and females reporting nonmedical stimulant use in the past year were 2.04 and 2.13 times (respectively) more likely to report feeling sad or hopeless every day for two or more weeks, seriously considering attempting suicide (2.37 and 2.48), and making a plan to commit suicide (2.24 and 2.65); suicide attempts were not elevated in those reporting NMPS (Zosel et al., 2013). Gambling, weight control behavior, depressed mood (Striley et al., 2016), problem behaviors (Boyd et al., 2009; Goldstein, 2008), and depression (Goldstein, 2008) have also been found among teen populations engaged in NMPS. Girls reporting NMPS aged 10–18 years old were 2.7, 1.9, 1.8, 4.4, and 5.1 times more likely to have depressed mood, gamble, have unhealthy weight control behaviors (WCB), have extreme WCB, and have both unhealthy and extreme WCB (Striley et al., 2016). Goldstein reported that 71 percent and 23 percent of youth engaged in past-year NMPS also took part in delinquent behaviors and experienced a major depressive episode, respectively, compared to 34 percent and 23 percent of youth not engaged in NMPS (Goldstein, 2008). An estimated 0.2 percent (38,000) of youths aged 12–17 years old had a stimulant use disorder, with 16,000 (not all necessarily with disorder) being treated for NMPS. Incoming and outgoing diversion of stimulants by adolescents may be related to NMPS and concurrent drug use (Lasopa, Striley, & Cottler, 2015; Schepis & Krishnan-Sarin, 2009).

Historical Trends among Young Adults

Among college students, past-year amphetamine use was estimated at 3.5 percent, 4.1 percent, and 3.7 percent in 1993, 1997, and 1999 (McCabe et al., 2007). Monitoring the Future (MTF) data from the last 15 years shows that 18-year-olds and 19- to 20-year-olds experienced declines in NMPS prevalence from 2002, at 11.1 percent and 9.1 percent, respectively, to 2014, at 7.7 percent and 7.6 percent (Johnston, O'Malley, Bachman et al., 2016). From 2002 to 2014, there was an increased prevalence (7.1% to 10.6%) in those aged 21–22 years old (Johnston, O'Malley, Bachman et al., 2016). NSDUH reports that 1.3 percent, 1.2 percent, and 2.5 percent of all people aged 18–22 years old nonmedically used stimulants in the past month in 2013, 2014, and 2015, respectively; please note that due to changes in methodology in 2015, NSDUH NMPD prevalence rates are not comparable to previous years. Among them, 1.7 percent (2013), 1.5 percent (2014), and 3.7 percent (2015) of full-time college students and 1.1 percent (2013), 1.0 percent (2014), and 1.8 percent (2015) of non-college-attending 18- to 25-year-olds nonmedically used stimulants in the past month (Center for Behavioral Health Statistics and Quality, 2016a). An analysis of combined 2009–2011 NSDUH data found that 18- to 25-year-olds made up 51 percent of those engaged in NMPS; however, they made up 8 percent of those using methamphetamine and 20 percent of individuals engaged in concurrent use, the least among all age groups (Chen et al., 2014).

Public Health Significance and Correlates of NMPS among Young Adults

Young adults aged 18–25 years old have a lower prevalence of ADHD than adolescents, yet a higher prevalence of past year NMPS. NSDUH data suggest that NMPS prevalence was constant at near 2 percent from 2000 to 2006 (Herman-Stahl, Krebs, Kroutil, & Heller, 2007; McCabe, Cranford, & Boyd, 2006). Local samples' prevalence corroborates that finding (McCabe, Boyd, & Teter, 2009; McCabe, Teter, & Boyd, 2006b), although some samples' prevalence rates were higher, near 5 percent (McCabe, Teter, & Boyd, 2006a; Teter, McCabe, Cranford, Boyd, & Guthrie, 2005; Teter et al., 2006) or even 10 percent (Carroll, McLaughlin, & Blake, 2006). Local samples from between 2007 and 2010 showed prevalence of NMPS use at between 6 percent and 8 percent (Teter, Falone, Cranford, Boyd, & McCabe, 2010; Weyandt et al., 2009). Combined 2005–2012 NSDUH data showed a weighted NMPS prevalence of between 2.7 percent and 3.2 percent (Wu, Swartz, Brady, Blazer, & Hoyle, 2014), depending on race/ethnicity. MTF data indicated that Adderall use prevalence is currently 7.7 percent and 10.7 percent among young adults and college students, respectively (Johnston, O'Malley, Bachman et al., 2016). While NMPS among college students was flat from 2009 to 2015, young adult prevalence is nearly two points higher (Johnston, O'Malley, Bachman et al., 2016). However, college students reported double the risk of using prescription stimulants nonmedically compared to their non-college-attending counterparts of the same age (Substance Abuse and Mental Health Services Administration, 2009), drawing significant mainstream media attention (Kraft, 2016).

As stated, access to stimulant medication in adolescent years is common. Half of all students aged 10–21 years old were presented with the opportunity to try a stimulant before age 18, with the other half having the opportunity during college-attending ages of 18–21 years old (Arria et al., 2008). The average age of initiation of NMPS is 22.3 (Lipari et al., 2016), which is an age after many four-year undergraduate students finish their bachelor's degrees. This could be potentially explained by MTF's finding that annual Adderall use prevalence spikes from 7.8 percent to 10.9 percent for ages 19–20 and 21–22, which then drops to 8.4 percent for 23- to 24-year-olds (Johnston, O'Malley, Bachman et al., 2016). During the same ages, Ritalin use prevalence is 2.6 percent, 1.2 percent, and 2.6 percent, respectively (Johnston, O'Malley, Bachman et al., 2016). Arria and colleagues' longitudinal study of 1,253 college students showed that lifetime use prevalence prior to college is 6 percent, doubling to 12 percent during the first year of college, and almost doubling again by sophomore year (Arria et al., 2008). College is unequivocally a time during which NMPS drastically increases through increased availability of prescription medication and experimentation and initiation of stimulant use and NMPS.

Demographic data on college attendees is more widely available and disparate than that of adolescents. The prevalence NMPS is similar between males and females (Wu et al., 2007), and both sexes' prevalence rates fall as age increases. In 2008–2010 NSDUH data, NMPS among males and females aged 18–22 years old was 4.1 percent and 3.9 percent, respectively (Martins, Kim et al., 2015). Martins and colleagues also showed that NMPS prevalence among 18- to 22-year-old non-Hispanic/Latino Whites, non-Hispanic/Latino Blacks, Native Americans/Hawaiians/Pacific Islanders, Asian Americans, and Hispanics was 5.4 percent, 0.7 percent, 4.6 percent, 1.9 percent, and 2.4 percent, respectively (Martins, Kim et al., 2015). Students belonging to families making more than $250,000 annually had 2.2 times greater odds of NMPS (McCabe, Teter et al., 2006a).

The NMPS use subtype that the largest proportion of college students endorse as the motive for use is to improve performance and enhance cognition (DeSantis, Webb, & Noar, 2008; Hartung et al., 2013; Stock, Litt, Arlt, Peterson, & Sommerville, 2013). Unlike NMPO, NMPS is positively associated with higher educational attainment. An analysis of 2002 18- to 25-year-old NSDUH participants found that NMPS prevalence was 2.1 percent and that those currently enrolled and formerly enrolled in college were 2.76 and 1.76 times more likely to have past-year NMPS than those who never enrolled, respectively (Herman-Stahl et al., 2007). This study and Martins and colleagues' study (Martins, Kim et al., 2015) span eight years and demonstrate that former college students have long had elevated NMPS prevalence. Like NMPO, NMPS is negatively associated with good academic performance (McCabe, Teter et al., 2006a), unlike the previous difference between NMPO and NMPS noted for educational attainment. A 2011 article (Gomes, Tavares, & de Azevedo, 2011) referenced in a systematic review (Nargiso, Ballard, & Skeer, 2015) provides evidence of high academic achievement among those endorsing NMPS, which conflicts with McCabe and colleagues or may be indicative of a more recent change in the NMPS-academic performance relationship (McCabe, Teter et al., 2006a).

Young adults reporting NMPS face numerous adverse health associations, many of them psychosocial. For instance, university students with frequent or nonoral NMPS use have more than double the odds of depressed mood than those who do not nonmedically use (Teter et al., 2010). Other studies shed light on university students' use of stimulants to promote weight control (Stock et al., 2013) and eating disorder behavior. Jeffers and Bentosch's study found that 3.5 percent and 6.7 percent of females and males used prescription stimulants for weight loss, respectively. Those nonmedically using stimulant medication for weight loss, versus those not reporting stimulant use for weight loss, reported greater binge eating (33.3% vs. 8.4%), vomiting (50.0% vs. 5.0%), and laxative/diet pill/diuretic use (46.4% vs. 5.8%) to control weight or shape (Jeffers & Benotsch, 2014). McCabe and Teter's 2005 survey of a college population found that those engaged in NMPS, intranasal NMPS, and those engaged in NMPS via nonoral routes were 4.6, 9, and 18 times more likely to endorse three or more items from a validated drug abuse screening test (DAST-10) instrument, respectively (McCabe & Teter, 2007). Some studies have shown that those endorsing NMPS were more likely to use other substances and engage in deviant behaviors (e.g., stealing or selling drugs) compared to those not engaged in NMPS (Chen, Strain, Alexandre et al., 2014; McCabe & West, 2013; McCabe et al., 2007; Teter et al., 2006).

Nonmedical Use of Prescription Tranquilizers and Sedatives

Historical Trends among Adolescents

Data from the U.S. MTF survey indicates that the past-year prevalence of tranquilizer, benzodiazepine, and non-benzodiazepine (e.g. Xanax, Valium) nonmedical use among 8th graders increased at the beginning of the 1990s (from 1.8% to 3.3%) and then remained in the range of 2.4 percent to 2.8 percent until it began to decrease again in 2011, reaching a prevalence of 1.7 percent in 2015. In 2001, past-year nonmedical use of tranquilizers and sedatives was 8.9 percent and 8.7 percent, respectively, among a national sample of high school students as per the MTF study (Johnston, O'Malley, Miech et al., 2016). Among 10th graders, there was a continuous increase in past-year tranquilizer use from 1991 to 2001 (3.6% to 7.7%), followed by a decrease starting in 2002 that continued through 2015 (3.9%; Johnston, O'Malley, Miech, Bachman, & Schulenberg, 2016).

Data from the NSDUH shows that among adolescents the prevalence of past month tranquilizer nonmedical use has been decreasing since 2002, from 0.8 percent to 0.4 percent in 2014, with the latter representing 103,000 adolescents. NSDUH data also shows that the prevalence of nonmedical sedative use was stable from 2002 to 2014, ranging from 0.1 to 0.2 percent, with the latter representing 41,000 adolescents (Center for Behavioral Health Statistics and Quality, 2015b). NSDUH data also shows that the prevalence of both past-year nonmedical tranquilizer and nonmedical sedative use was 1.9 percent in 2005 (Schepis & Krishnan-Sarin, 2008). Other studies, based on nationally representative U.S. data, have reported similar results for prevalence of past-year nonmedical tranquilizer (0.4% to 2.0%) and sedative (0.7% to 3.0%) use during the 2003–2005 period in adolescents (Young, Glover, & Havens, 2012). Boyd and colleagues showed that, among 7th to 12th grade students in southeastern Michigan in 2007, the annual prevalence of tranquilizer or sedative nonmedical use was 1.3 percent, and lifetime prevalence was 2.0 percent (Boyd et al., 2009). In terms of availability among both 8th and 10th graders, the proportion of those indicating is fairly or very easy to obtain tranquilizers has been declining since the beginning of the 1990s, per the MTF (Johnston, O'Malley et al., 2016). In Canada, the 2010–2011 Quebec Health Survey of High School Students (63,196 students in 2,651 secondary schools) showed that 1.1 percent nonmedically used sedatives, hypnotics, and other tranquilizers.

Much of the evidence on nonmedical prescription tranquilizer and sedative use among adolescents comes from outside of North America. A study of 85,000 16-year-old students from 31 European countries participating in the 2003 ESPAD showed that the lifetime prevalence of nonmedical tranquilizer or sedative use in all European countries was 5.6 percent, with the highest prevalence in Lithuania (13.6%) and the lowest in Ukraine (1.5%; Kokkevi, Fotiou, Arapaki, & Richardson, 2008). A more recent report shows that rates of lifetime tranquilizer or sedative nonmedical use have remained stable across 25 countries surveyed from 1995 to 2015, with only a slight reduction in 2015 (from 7% to 6%). Past-year prevalence was 2.5 percent in all countries, with higher prevalence among girls than boys, at 3 percent and 2 percent, respectively (European School Survey on Alcohol and Other Drugs, 2015). Medical use increased the odds of nonmedical use by 10.7 times in boys and 7.2 in girls. Nearly 21 percent of students endorsed that it is "fairly easy" or "very easy" to obtain tranquilizers or sedatives (Kokkevi et al., 2008). A study of all 27 Brazilian state capitals showed that the lifetime prevalence of tranquilizer or sedative nonmedical use is 5 percent, with a higher prevalence among females than males (6.6% vs. 3.1%) and in high versus low SES groups (9.3% vs. 3.7%). Having a previous medical prescription was associated with nonprescription use and with perceptions of low-risk perception for use, at 28.8 percent versus 3.6 percent (Opaleye et al., 2013). In China, a study including 3,273 students from schools in Guangzhou who were surveyed from 2009 to 2010 showed that 0.8 percent of students reported nonmedically using sedatives (Guo et al., 2016). A cross-sectional study of 986 high school students attending public and private high schools in Beirut, Lebanon, found that the lifetime and current prevalence of tranquilizer nonmedical use was 5.6 percent and 3.5 percent, respectively.

Public Health Significance and Correlates of Nonmedical Prescription Tranquilizer and Sedative Use among Adolescents

Results from the 2015 NSDUH indicated that approximately 210,000 adolescents aged 12–17 and 489,000 young adults aged 18–25 engaged in nonmedical prescription tranquilizer use for the first time in the past year, and 46,000 adolescents aged 12–17 and 86,000 young adults aged 18–25 reported nonmedical prescription sedative use for the first time in the past year (Lipari et al., 2016).

Different factors have been linked to prescription drug use. Data from the National Longitudinal Study of Adolescent Health (Add Health) showed that Black and Asian-American adolescents were less likely to report sedative/tranquilizer nonmedical use and that respondents whose highest-educated parent had completed some college were significantly more likely to engage in sedative/tranquilizer nonmedical use compared to respondents whose parents did not graduate from high school. Participants experiencing a financial hardship had significantly increased the odds (by 21%) of ever nonmedically using sedatives (Stewart & Reed, 2015). In a study by Ford and colleagues, using data from the 2005 NSDUH, low income was found to be associated with nonmedical use of tranquilizers, and school bond (e.g. enjoying going to school, belief of school work being meaningful) was negatively associated with tranquilizer and sedative nonmedical use (Ford, 2009). In another study using data from the 2005 NSDUH, the authors found that past-year major depressive episode, mental health treatment, being in jail or detention, and other substance use in the past year were factors associated with tranquilizer or sedative nonmedical use (Schepis & Krishnan-Sarin, 2008). Other factors associated with tranquilizer or sedative nonmedical use include living with one parent only (for tranquilizers), living in rural areas, and considering own health to be poor or fair (Simoni-Wastila, Yang, & Lawler, 2008).

Stabler and colleagues, using 2010 NSDUH data, showed that after controlling for demographic, interpersonal, and community factors, adolescents with low mobility (one to two moves in the past five years) and residential instability (three moves) were 16 percent and 25 percent more likely to report NMPD compared to nonmobile adolescents (zero moves), respectively (Stabler, Gurka, & Lander, 2015). Although low-mobile adolescents were 18 percent more likely to abuse opioids, no relationship was found between moving and tranquilizer, stimulant, or sedative nonmedical use. Moving in the past year was also found to be associated with tranquilizer and sedative nonmedical use among adolescents in NSDUH data (Schepis & Krishnan-Sarin, 2008).

In Canada, a survey on 44,344 7th to 12th graders, who responded to the 2008–2009 Youth Smoking Survey, showed that past-year nonmedical sedative or tranquilizer nonmedical use was reported by 2.1 percent of students, with the prevalence higher among females than males (2.4% vs. 1.9%). Students who identified as First Nations, Métis, or Inuit and those with lower school connectedness were more likely to have nonmedically used sedatives or tranquilizers in the past year (Currie & Wild, 2012). The authors suggested that ameliorating school connectedness may alleviate the problem among these populations (Currie & Wild, 2012).

The concomitant nonmedical use of prescription sedatives and opioids poses a public health risk due to the high prevalence of their concurrent use and the associated, and elevated, risk of morbidity and mortality (McCabe, 2005; Sun et al., 2017; Warner, Trinidad, Bastian, Minino, & Hedegaard, 2016). In a retrospective analysis of people with private health insurance in the United States from 2001–2013, researchers found that the concomitant use of these drugs significantly increased the odds of opioid-overdose hospitalization (emergency or inpatient visit) by 2.14 times compared to opioid use alone (Sun et al., 2017). Furthermore, 2014 data from the National Vital Statistics System showed that about 95 percent of sedative-overdose deaths in the United States involved another drug and that opioids were the most common concomitant drug involved in these deaths (Warner et al., 2016). Using 2003 NSDUH data, Simoni-Wastila and colleagues found that 30 percent of adolescents who engaged in NMPD reported using two to four prescription drug classes (Simoni-Wastila et al., 2008), indicating that poly-NMPD, with significant associated consequences, is common in adolescents.

Historical Trends among Young Adults

McCabe, West, and Wechsler reported that, in a nationally representative sample of U.S. college students, past-year and lifetime nonmedical sedative use increased from 1.3 percent and 4.8 percent in 1993 to 3.4 percent and 6.1 percent in 2001, respectively (McCabe et al., 2007). The authors reported similar trends for past-year and lifetime nonmedical tranquilizer use, such that percentages increased from 1.8 percent and 5.9 percent in 1993 to 4.6 percent and 8.1 percent in 2001, respectively (McCabe et al., 2007). Data from the 2001–2002 National Epidemiologic Survey on Alcohol and Related Conditions (NESARC) show that 18- to 24-year-olds reported higher levels of past-year nonmedical sedative and tranquilizer nonmedical use (2.76% and 2.59%, respectively) as compared to those aged 25 years and older (1.02% and 0.69%, respectively; McCabe, Cranford et al., 2006). Since the mid- to late-2000s, trends for the prevalence of nonmedical tranquilizer and sedative use have generally been declining. From 2003 to 2015, past-year nonmedical tranquilizer use among college students declined from about 7 percent to 5 percent, and nonmedical tranquilizer use among non-college-attending young adults declined from roughly 11 percent in 2002 to 7 percent in 2015; nonmedical sedative use among college students and non-college-attending young adults dropped from 4.0 percent in 2004 to 2.5 percent in 2015 and about 7.8 percent in 2008 to 4.0 percent in 2015, respectively (Johnston, O'Malley, Bachman et al., 2016). The 2015 NSDUH indicates that 1.7 percent and 0.2 percent of 18- to 25-year-olds engaged in nonmedical tranquilizer use and nonmedical sedative use in the past month, respectively (Center for Behavioral Health Statistics and Quality, 2016b).

Data from MTF provide further context to prevalence estimates by longitudinally comparing full-time U.S. college students with 12th graders and college-aged young adults who were not attending school. Since 1980, college students have had the lowest prevalence of annual sedative and tranquilizer nonmedical use, as compared to their non-college-attending peers and 12th graders (Johnston, O'Malley, Bachman et al., 2016). In 1980, annual nonmedical sedative use by college students was 2.9 percent, compared to roughly 6.4 percent and 6.5 percent for non-college-attending young adults and 12th graders, respectively (Johnston, O'Malley, Bachman et al., 2016). Nonmedical prescription sedative use declined in all three groups during the 1980s and early 1990s, with the gap between the three narrowing at this time (Johnston, O'Malley, Bachman et al., 2016). From the mid-1990s through much of the 2000s, annual nonmedical sedative use increased in all three groups, peaking at just over 4 percent in 2004 for college students, about 7.5 percent in 2005 for 12th graders, and almost 8 percent in 2008 for non-college-attending young adults (Johnston, O'Malley, Bachman et al., 2016). Prevalence declined from then on, with the exception of nonmedical use among college students, which increased again from 1.7 percent in 2011 to 3.1 percent in 2014 (Johnston, O'Malley, Bachman et al., 2016). Perceived availability of sedatives (measured by reporting sedatives would be "very easy" or "fairly easy" to get) among 19- to 22-year-olds slowly declined from 59.5 percent in 1980 to 35.3 percent in 2015 (Johnston, O'Malley, Bachman et al., 2016).

Similar to nonmedical sedative use, from 1980 to 2015, annual nonmedical prescription tranquilizer use among U.S. college students was less prevalent than such nonmedical use among 12th graders and college-aged young adults (Johnston, O'Malley, Bachman et al., 2016). In 1980, annual nonmedical tranquilizer use among college students was about 6.9 percent, whereas nonmedical use by college-aged young adults and 12th graders was roughly 10 percent and 8 percent, respectively (Johnston, O'Malley, Bachman et al., 2016). Rates of nonmedical tranquilizer use declined to their lowest rates by 1994 (below 4%), with no significant differences between the three groups (Johnston, O'Malley, Bachman et al., 2016). Starting in the mid-1990s, nonmedical tranquilizer use increased in all groups, with the steepest increase in non-college-attending young adults, reaching a peak of about 12 percent in 2002 (Johnston, O'Malley, Bachman et al., 2016). Since the early 2000s, nonmedical use has slowly declined; however, non-college-attending young adults still have higher rates than 12th graders and college students (Johnston, O'Malley, Bachman et al., 2016). Perceived availability of tranquilizers among 19- to 22-year-olds steadily decreased from 67.4 percent in 1980 to 19.7 percent in 2015 (Johnston, O'Malley, Bachman et al., 2016).

Public Health Significance and Correlates of Nonmedical Prescription Tranquilizer\ and Sedative Use among Young Adults

In the United States, a study of college students showed that the sophomore year of college was a time of increased nonmedical prescription tranquilizer use (Arria, Caldeira et al., 2008). McCabe found that more college students reported lifetime nonmedical benzodiazepine use; also, no gender differences were found for past-year benzodiazepine use (McCabe, 2005). Another study found that male college students were more likely to engage in sedative nonmedical use in the past year than females (McCabe, Boyd, & Teter, 2006). Other research has indicated that young adults are at increased risk for nonmedical benzodiazepine use if they are White, engage in other risky behavior, have higher rates of substance use, and are college students who have sex with both men and women (McCabe, 2005; McCabe et al., 2007; Tapscott & Schepis, 2013). In addition, McCabe, Cranford, and Boyd reported that, in 2001–2002, nonmedical tranquilizer and sedative use among 18- to 24-year-olds was positively correlated with alcohol use, with a dose-response relationship increasing from alcohol abstainers to those with DSM-IV alcohol dependence (McCabe, Cranford et al., 2006). Furthermore, according to the 2015 NSDUH, annual tranquilizer use disorder was reported by 0.7 percent of individuals aged 18–25 years old, representing 234,000 people (Center for Behavioral Health Statistics and Quality, 2016b). The average age of onset for tranquilizer and sedative use disorders in the United States are 21.9 and 21.2 years old, respectively, indicating the extent to which nonmedical use of these drugs affects young adults in the United States (Huang et al., 2006).

In a national sample of U.S. college students, McCabe found that schoolwide past-year nonmedical benzodiazepine use was significantly correlated with schoolwide past-year NMPO, NMPS, and marijuana use and binge drinking in the past two weeks (McCabe, 2005). Furthermore, young adults were significantly more likely to report more alcohol and drug use if they cited friends or peers (as opposed to family members) as the source for their prescription sedatives or tranquilizers (Tapscott & Schepis, 2013). Tapscott and Schepis also reported increased odds of nonmedical benzodiazepine use among females aged 18–25 years who reported feeling depressed, and Asian-American and Hispanic/Latino college students were less likely to nonmedically use benzodiazepines compared to Whites (Tapscott & Schepis, 2013). Similar results for Asian-American and Hispanic/Latino students were observed by McCabe in a 2001 sample of 119 colleges in 39 states; nonmedical benzodiazepine use was also less common among students at historically Black colleges and universities (McCabe, 2005).

Similar to adolescents, concomitant use of prescription opioids and sedatives significantly raises the risk of increased morbidity and mortality among college-aged young adults. McCabe and colleagues reported that, in 2001, 66 percent of college students in the United States who engaged in nonmedical use of prescription sedatives had also engaged in NMPO in the past year; the prevalence of NMPO in this group was 61 percent higher than students who did not engage in nonmedical use of prescription sedatives (McCabe, 2005).

As is the case among adolescents, nonmedical sedative and tranquilizer use among young adults is a greater problem outside of North America. In a study of 18- to 29-year-olds in Denmark, Germany, Great Britain, Spain, and Sweden, past-year nonmedical sedative use was 6.3 percent, and lifetime use in this age group was 10.2 percent; for those 12–17 years of age, past-year nonmedical sedative use was 1.2 percent, and lifetime nonmedical use was 1.7 percent (Novak et al., 2016). While the authors did not distinguish specific age groups, they found that among European Union countries in 2014, lifetime nonmedical sedative use was most common in Spain and Sweden and least common in Germany (Novak et al., 2016). In the European Union, students reported the lowest percentage of lifetime and past-year sedative nonmedical use compared to those who were working full-time, part-time, unemployed, or not in labor force (Novak et al., 2016). Regarding sedative use disorder in Germany, 0.7 percent of young adult males aged 18–24 years old endorsed sedative nonmedical use disorder, greater than the 0.2 percent of females endorsing such nonmedical use (Lieb et al., 1998).

In Canada, data from 40 universities surveyed in 2004 showed that 5.2 percent of undergraduate students nonmedically used tranquilizers in their lifetime, 2 percent in the past year and 1 percent in the past 30 days (Fischer, 2009). Barret and colleagues indicated that around 8.1 percent of Canadian university students reported lifetime nonmedical benzodiazepine use (Fischer, 2009). In Mexico, the United Nations Office on Drugs and Crime (UNODC) reported that tranquilizers are used nonmedically more often than other prescription medications, and men aged 26–34 years old and women aged 35 years and older nonmedically used them most often (United Nations Office on Drugs and Crime, 2011b). In the United States, geographical trends are not significant or consistent. Colleges with prevalence rates of nonmedical benzodiazepine use above 10 percent were primarily located in the South, and this risk was lower in the northern and central states (McCabe, 2005). However, analyses from the MTF found nonsignificant longitudinal regional differences in prevalence of nonmedical sedative and tranquilizer use in the United States (Johnston, O'Malley, Bachman et al., 2016). Among university students in Beirut in 2010, lifetime prevalence rates of medical and nonmedical use of anxiety medications were 8.3 percent and 4.6 percent, respectively, while they were 6.5 percent and 5.8 percent for sleeping medications (Ghandour, El Sayed, & Martins, 2012). In India, 5 percent of those treated for illicit drug use are treated specifically for sedative use (United Nations Office on Drugs and Crime, 2011a), and sedatives are one of the most common nonmedically used medications in Bangladesh (United Nations Office on Drugs and Crime, 2011a).

Novak and colleagues' EU analysis identified that, in 2014, certain characteristics, including male sex, having sexually transmitted diseases, having serious psychological problems, and having criminal involvement before age

15, were associated with higher odds and higher prevalence (specifically among those who were non-White, and unemployed) of past-year nonmedical sedative use; these characteristics were not moderated by age (Novak et al., 2016). Conversely, the authors found that those aged 18–29 years old had higher odds of nonmedical sedative use compared to those 12–17 years old (Novak et al., 2016).

Conclusion

To summarize, growing NMPD is a global health concern: past-year U.S. prevalence of NMPD was 7 percent for opioids, 2 percent for tranquilizers, and 1 percent for stimulants (Center for Behavioral Health Statistics and Quality, 2016b), and in Europe in 2014, it was reported to be 5 percent for opioids, nearly 6 percent for sedatives, and nearly 3 percent for stimulants (Novak et al., 2016). As limited data were available from many regions in the world (e.g., Asia, Africa, Latin America, the Middle East), tremendous work is still needed to fill the knowledge gap of the scale of NMPD use in these areas. China and India have large populations, so there is an urgent need to conduct national surveys on NMPD in these countries. For example, a school-based survey in Wuhan, China, showed up to 4 percent of middle school students had nonmedically used a benzodiazepine (Guo et al., 2016). In India, buprenorphine is the main drug of injection in most areas of the country, unlike many Western countries (United Nations Office on Drugs and Crime, 2011b). Similarly, there is an urgent need to conduct comprehensive national surveys on the topic in large Latin American countries, such as Brazil and Mexico. A more comprehensive study focusing on NMPD in countries in which only work on illicit drug use has been conducted is of high priority.

In this chapter, we reviewed the three most common types of NMPD context: opioids, stimulants, and tranquilizers/sedatives. NMPD and related phenomena are heterogeneous: different subpopulations reported NMPD of different substances, and regional- and country-level variations are prominent. Regardless of location or type of medication, NMPD was significantly associated with many adverse physical or psychological consequences (Assanangkornchai, Muekthong, Sam-Angsri, & Pattanasattayawong, 2007; Centers for Disease Control and Prevention, 2017; Chen et al., 2016; Martins & Ghandour, 2017; Mudur, 1999; Novak et al., 2016; United Nations Office on Drugs and Crime, 2011a, 2011b). Therefore, continued efforts to curb rising NMPD are crucial. Such efforts should also address misuse of over-the-counter (OTC) medication, which is a serious issue in many countries (Cooper, 2013), particularly in Asia (Assanangkornchai et al., 2007; Mudur, 1999). OTC misuse is addressed in this volume in chapter 5, and readers are referred there for further coverage of the issue.

As adolescents and young adults are at particular risk for substance use initiation due to the neurobehavioral developmental processes occurring at this time (Bava & Tapert, 2010), we found NMPD were prevalent in these groups, probably due to the relatively easy access of medications compared to illegal ones (Bartels, Binswanger, & Hopfer, 2016; Chen, Strain, Crum, Storr, & Mojtabai, 2014). Greater levels of medical consequences, deviant behaviors, and mortality were associated with these NMPD regardless of drug types or across counties (Centers for Disease Control and Prevention, 2017; Center for Behavioral Health Statistics and Quality, 2016b; Chen et al., 2016; Martins & Ghandour, 2017; McCabe et al., 2004; Novak et al., 2016; United Nations Office on Drugs and Crime, 2011a). Prevention programs, such as prescription drug monitoring programs (PDMPs; these are addressed in chapter 12 of this work), which adopt electronic databases to monitor controlled substances in the United States, have shown potential promising effects in curbing the increasing trends of prescription drug nonmedical use (Brady et al., 2014). Development of similar programs could be considered in countries where NMPD has become a threat to public health.

References

Arria, A. M., Caldeira, K. M., O'Grady, K. E., Vincent, K. B., Fitzelle, D. B., Johnson, E. P., & Wish, E. D. (2008). Drug exposure opportunities and use patterns among college students: Results of a longitudinal prospective cohort study. *Substance Abuse, 29*(4), 19–38. doi:10.1080/088970708024 18451.

Arria, A. M., O'Grady, K. E., Caldeira, K. M., Vincent, K. B., & Wish, E. D. (2008). Nonmedical use of prescription stimulants and analgesics: Associations with social and academic behaviors among college students. *Journal of Drug Issues, 38*(4), 1045–1060.

Assanangkornchai, S., Muekthong, A., Sam-Angsri, N., & Pattanasattayawong, U. (2007). The use of *Mitragynine speciosa* ("krathom"), an addictive plant, in Thailand. *Substance Use & Misuse, 42*(14), 2145–2157. doi:10.1080/108 26080701205869.

Austic, E., McCabe, S. E., Stoddard, S. A., Ngo, Q. E., & Boyd, C. (2015). Age and cohort patterns of medical and nonmedical use of controlled medication among adolescents. *Journal of Addiction Medicine, 9*(5), 376–382. doi:10.1097 /adm.0000000000000142.

Bartels, K., Binswanger, I. A., & Hopfer, C. J. (2016). Sources of prescription opioids for nonmedical use. *Journal of Addiction Medicine, 10*(2), 134. doi:10 .1097/ADM.0000000000000192.

Bava, S., & Tapert, S. F. (2010). Adolescent brain development and the risk for alcohol and other drug problems. *Neuropsychological Review, 20*(4), 398–413. doi:10.1007/s11065-010-9146-6.

Boyd, C. J., Young, A., Grey, M., & McCabe, S. E. (2009). Adolescents' nonmedical use of prescription medications and other problem behaviors. *Journal of Adolescent Health, 45*(6), 543–550. doi:10.1016/j.jadohealth.2009.03.023.

Boyd, C. J., Young, A., & McCabe, S. E. (2014). Psychological and drug abuse symptoms associated with nonmedical use of opioid analgesics among adolescents. *Substance Abuse, 35*(3), 284–289.

Brady, J. E., Wunsch, H., DiMaggio, C., Lang, B. H., Giglio, J., & Li, G. (2014). Prescription drug monitoring and dispensing of prescription opioids. *Public Health Rep, 129*(2), 139–147. doi:10.1177/003335491412900207.

Carlson, R. G., Nahhas, R. W., Martins, S. S., & Daniulaityte, R. (2016). Predictors of transition to heroin use among initially non-opioid dependent illicit pharmaceutical opioid users: A natural history study. *Drug and Alcohol Dependence, 160*, 127–134. doi:10.1016/j.drugalcdep.2015.12.026.

Carroll, B. C., McLaughlin, T. J., & Blake, D. R. (2006). Patterns and knowledge of nonmedical use of stimulants among college students. *Archives of Pediatric and Adolescent Medicine, 160*(5), 481–485. doi:10.1001/archpedi.160.5.481.

Center for Behavioral Health Statistics and Quality. (2015a). *2014 National Survey on Drug Use and Health: Detailed Tables*. Rockville, MD: Substance Abuse and Mental Health Services Administration.

Center for Behavioral Health Statistics and Quality. (2015b). *Behavioral Health Trends in the United States: Results from the 2014 National Survey on Drug Use and Health* (HHS Publication No. SMA 15-4927, NSDUH Series H-50). http://www.samhsa.gov/data.

Center for Behavioral Health Statistics and Quality. (2016a). *2015 National Survey on Drug Use and Health: Detailed Tables*. Rockville, MD: Substance Abuse and Mental Health Services Administration.

Center for Behavioral Health Statistics and Quality. (2016b). *Key Substance Use and Mental Health Indicators in the United States: Results from the 2015 National Survey on Drug Use and Health* (HHS Publication No. SMA 16-4984, NSDUH Series H-51). http://www.samhsa.gov/data.

Centers for Disease Control and Prevention. (2016). Prescription opioid overdose data. *Opioid Overdose*. https://www.cdc.gov/drugoverdose/data/overdose.html.

Centers for Disease Control and Prevention. (2017). Overdose death rates. *Trends and Statistics*. https://www.drugabuse.gov/related-topics/trends-statistics/overdose-death-rates.

Cerda, M., Santaella, J., Marshall, B. D., Kim, J. H., & Martins, S. S. (2015). Nonmedical prescription opioid use in childhood and early adolescence predicts transitions to heroin use in young adulthood: A national study. *Journal of Pediatrics, 167*(3), 605–612.e601–602. doi:10.1016/j.jpeds.2015.04.071.

Chen, L. Y., Crum, R. M., Strain, E. C., Alexander, G. C., Kaufmann, C., & Mojtabai, R. (2016). Prescriptions, nonmedical use, and emergency department visits involving prescription stimulants. *Journal of Clinical Psychiatry, 77*(3), e297–304. doi:10.4088/JCP.14m09291.

Chen, L. Y., Crum, R. M., Strain, E. C., Martins, S. S., & Mojtabai, R. (2015). Patterns of concurrent substance use among adolescent nonmedical ADHD stimulant users. *Addictive Behaviors, 49*, 1–6. doi:10.1016/j.addbeh.2015.05.007.

Chen, L. Y., Strain, E. C., Alexandre, P. K., Alexander, G. C., Mojtabai, R., & Martins, S. S. (2014). Correlates of nonmedical use of stimulants and methamphetamine use in a national sample. *Addictive Behaviors, 39*(5), 829–836. doi:10.1016/j.addbeh.2014.01.018.

Chen, L. Y., Strain, E. C., Crum, R. M., Storr, C. L., & Mojtabai, R. (2014). Sources of nonmedically used prescription stimulants: differences in onset, recency and severity of misuse in a population-based study. *Drug and Alcohol Dependence, 145*, 106–112. doi:10.1016/j.drugalcdep.2014.09.781.

Cole, J., & Logan, T. K. (2010). Nonmedical use of sedative-hypnotics and opiates among rural and urban women with protective orders. *Journal of Addictive Diseases, 29*(3), 395–409. doi:10.1080/10550887.2010.489453.

Cooper, R. J. (2013). Over-the-counter medicine abuse—A review of the literature. *Journal of Substance Use, 18*(2), 82–107. doi:10.3109/14659891.2011.615002.

Currie, C. L., & Wild, T. C. (2012). Adolescent use of prescription drugs to get high in Canada. *Canadian Journal of Psychiatry, 57*(12), 745–751. doi:10.1177/070674371205701206.

DeSantis, A. D., Webb, E. M., & Noar, S. M. (2008). Illicit use of prescription ADHD medications on a college campus: a multimethodological approach. *Journal of American College Health, 57*(3), 315–324. doi:10.3200/jach.57.3.315-324.

Dowell, D., Haegerich, T. M., & Chou, R. (2016). CDC guideline for prescribing opioids for chronic pain—United States, 2016. *JAMA, 315*(15), 1624–1645.

European School Survey on Alcohol and Other Drugs. (2015). Trends in substance use. http://www.espad.org/report/trends-1995-2015/trends-across-25-countries.

Fischer, B., Rehm, J., & Gittins, J. (2009). *An Overview of Non-medical Use of Prescription Drugs and Criminal Justice Issues in Canada.* Ottawa, Canada: Research and Statistics Division, Department of Justice Canada.

Ford, J. A. (2009). Nonmedical prescription drug use among adolescents: The influence of bonds to family and school. *Youth & Society, 40*(3), 336–352. doi:10.1177/0044118x08316345.

Ford, J. A., & Arrastia, M. C. (2008). Pill-poppers and dopers: A comparison of non-medical prescription drug use and illicit/street drug use among college students. *Addictive Behaviors, 33*(7), 934–941. doi:10.1016/j.addbeh.2008.02.016.

Garnier, L. M., Arria, A. M., Caldeira, K. M., Vincent, K. B., O'Grady, K. E., & Wish, E. D. (2009). Nonmedical prescription analgesic use and concurrent alcohol consumption among college students. *American Journal of Drug and Alcohol Abuse, 35*(5), 334–338. doi:10.1080/00952990903075059.

Ghandour, L. A., El Sayed, D. S., & Martins, S. S. (2012). Prevalence and patterns of commonly abused psychoactive prescription drugs in a sample of university students from Lebanon: An opportunity for cross-cultural comparisons. *Drug and Alcohol Dependence, 121*(1-2), 110–117. doi:10.1016 /j.drugalcdep.2011.08.021.

Ghandour, L. A., El Sayed, D. S., & Martins, S. S. (2013). Alcohol and illegal drug use behaviors and prescription opioids use: How do nonmedical and medical users compare, and does motive to use really matter? *European Addiction Research, 19*(4), 202–210. doi:10.1159/000345445.

Goldstein, S. (2008). Report from the National Survey on Drug Use and Health: Nonmedical stimulant use, other drug use, delinquent behaviors, and depression among adolescents. *Journal of Attention Disorders, 12*(1), 3. doi:10.1177/1087054708319106.

Gomes, A. A., Tavares, J., & de Azevedo, M. H. P. (2011). Sleep and academic performance in undergraduates: A multi-measure, multi-predictor approach. *Chronobiology International, 28*(9), 786–801.

Guo, L., Xu, Y., Deng, J., Huang, J., Huang, G., Gao, X., . . . Lu, C. (2016). Association between nonmedical use of prescription drugs and suicidal behavior among adolescents. *JAMA Pediatrics, 170*(10), 971–978. doi:10.1001 /jamapediatrics.2016.1802.

Hartung, C. M., Canu, W. H., Cleveland, C. S., Lefler, E. K., Mignogna, M. J., Fedele, D. A., . . . Clapp, J. D. (2013). Stimulant medication use in college students: comparison of appropriate users, misusers, and nonusers. *Psychology of Addictive Behaviors, 27*(3), 832–840. doi:10.1037/a0033822.

Herman-Stahl, M. A., Krebs, C. P., Kroutil, L. A., & Heller, D. C. (2007). Risk and protective factors for methamphetamine use and nonmedical use of prescription stimulants among young adults aged 18 to 25. *Addictive Behaviors, 32*(5), 1003–1015. doi:10.1016/j.addbeh.2006.07.010.

Huang, B., Dawson, D. A., Stinson, F. S., Hasin, D. S., Ruan, W. J., Saha, T. D., . . . Grant, B. F. (2006). Prevalence, correlates, and comorbidity of nonmedical prescription drug use and drug use disorders in the United States: Results of the National Epidemiologic Survey on Alcohol and Related Conditions. *Journal of Clinical Psychiatry, 67*(7), 1062–1073.

Hughes, A., Williams, M. R., Lipari, R. N., Bose, J., Copello, E. A. P., & Kroutil, L. A. (2016). *Prescription Drug Use and Misuse in the United States: Results from the 2015 National Survey on Drug Use and Health. NSDUH Data Review.* http://www.samhsa.gov/data.

Jeffers, A. J., & Benotsch, E. G. (2014). Non-medical use of prescription stimulants for weight loss, disordered eating, and body image. *Eating Behaviors, 15*(3), 414–418. doi:10.1016/j.eatbeh.2014.04.019.

Johnston, L. D., O'Malley, P. M., Bachman, J. G., Schulenberg, J. E., & Miech, R. A. (2016). *Monitoring the Future National Survey Results on Drug Use, 1975–2015.* Vol. 2, *College Students and Adults Ages 19–55.* Ann Arbor, MI: Institute for Social Research, University of Michigan.

Johnston, L. D., O'Malley, P. M., Miech, R. A., Bachman, J. G., & Schulenberg, J. E. (2016). *Monitoring the Future National Survey Results on Drug Use,*

1975–2015: 2015 Overview—Key Findings on Adolescent Drug Use. Ann Arbor, MI: Institute for Social Research, University of Michigan.

Johnston, L. D., O'Malley, P. M., Miech, R. A., Bachman, J. G., & Schulenberg, J. E. (2017). *Demographic Subgroup Trends among Adolescents in the Use of Various Licit and Illicit Drugs, 1975–2016.* Ann Arbor, MI: Institute for Social Research, University of Michigan.

Jones, C. M., Paulozzi, L. J., & Mack, K. A. (2014). Alcohol involvement in opioid pain reliever and benzodiazepine drug abuse-related emergency department visits and drug-related deaths—United States, 2010. *MMWR: Morbidity and Mortality Weekly Report, 63*(40), 881–885.

Kelly, B. C., & Parsons, J. T. (2007). Prescription drug misuse among club drug-using young adults. *American Journal of Drug and Alcohol Abuse, 33*(6), 875–884. doi:10.1080/00952990701667347.

Kokkevi, A., Fotiou, A., Arapaki, A., & Richardson, C. (2008). Prevalence, patterns, and correlates of tranquilizer and sedative use among European adolescents. *Journal of Adolescent Health, 43*(6), 584–592. doi:10.1016/j.jadohealth.2008.05.001.

Kraft, A. (2016). Adderall misuse rising among young adults. http://www.cbsnews.com/news/adderall-misuse-rising-among-young-adults.

Kuramoto, S. J., Chilcoat, H. D., Ko, J., & Martins, S. S. (2012). Suicidal ideation and suicide attempt across stages of nonmedical prescription opioid use and presence of prescription opioid disorders among U.S. adults. *Journal of Studies on Alcohol and Drugs, 73*(2), 178–184.

Lasopa, S. O., Striley, C. W., & Cottler, L. B. (2015). Diversion of prescription stimulant drugs among 10–18-year-olds. *Current Opinion in Psychiatry, 28*(4), 292–298. doi:10.1097/yco.0000000000000172.

Lieb, R., Pfister, H., & Wittchen, H. U. (1998). Use, abuse and dependence of prescription drugs in adolescents and young adults. *European Addiction Research, 4*(1-2), 67–74.

Lipari, R. N., Williams, M. R., Copello, E. A. P., & Pemberton, M. R. (2016). Risk and protective factors and estimates of substance use initiation: Results from the 2015 National Survey on Drug Use and Health. *NSDUH Data Review.* https://www.samhsa.gov/data/sites/default/files/NSDUH-PreventionandInit-2015/NSDUH-PreventionandInit-2015.htm.

Manchikanti, L., & Singh, A. (2008). Therapeutic opioids: A ten-year perspective on the complexities and complications of the escalating use, abuse, and nonmedical use of opioids. *Pain Physician, 11*(2 Suppl), S63–88.

Martins, S. S., & Ghandour, L. A. (2017). Nonmedical use of prescription drugs in adolescents and young adults: Not just a Western phenomenon. *World Psychiatry, 16*(1), 102–104. doi:10.1002/wps.20350.

Martins, S. S., Kim, J. H., Chen, L. Y., Levin, D., Keyes, K. M., Cerda, M., & Storr, C. L. (2015). Nonmedical prescription drug use among US young adults by educational attainment. *Social Psychiatry and Psychiatric Epidemiology, 50*(5), 713–724. doi:10.1007/s00127-014-0980-3.

Martins, S. S., Santaella-Tenorio, J., Marshall, B. D., Maldonado, A., & Cerda, M. (2015). Racial/ethnic differences in trends in heroin use and heroin-related risk behaviors among nonmedical prescription opioid users. *Drug and Alcohol Dependence, 151*, 278–283. doi:10.1016/j.drugalcdep.2015.03.020.

Martins, S. S., Segura, L. E., Santaella-Tenorio, J., Perlmutter, A., Fenton, M. C., Cerda, M., . . . Hasin, D. S. (2017). Prescription opioid use disorder and heroin use among 12–34-year-olds in the United States from 2002 to 2014. *Addictive Behaviors, 65*, 236–241. doi:10.1016/j.addbeh.2016.08.033.

Mateu-Gelabert, P., Guarino, H., Jessell, L., & Teper, A. (2015). Injection and sexual HIV/HCV risk behaviors associated with nonmedical use of prescription opioids among young adults in New York City. *Journal of Substance Abuse Treatment, 48*(1), 13–20. doi:10.1016/j.jsat.2014.07.002.

McCabe, S. E. (2005). Correlates of nonmedical use of prescription benzodiazepine anxiolytics: results from a national survey of U.S. college students. *Drug and Alcohol Dependence, 79*(1), 53–62. doi:10.1016/j.drugalcdep.2004.12.006.

McCabe, S. E., Boyd, C. J., & Teter, C. J. (2006). Medical use, illicit use, and diversion of abusable prescription drugs. *Journal of American College Health, 54*(5), 269–278.

McCabe, S. E., Boyd, C. J., & Teter, C. J. (2009). Subtypes of nonmedical prescription drug misuse. *Drug and Alcohol Dependence, 102*(1-3), 63–70. doi:10.1016/j.drugalcdep.2009.01.007.

McCabe, S. E., Cranford, J. A., & Boyd, C. J. (2006). The relationship between past-year drinking behaviors and nonmedical use of prescription drugs: Prevalence of co-occurrence in a national sample. *Drug and Alcohol Dependence, 84*(3), 281–288. doi:10.1016/j.drugalcdep.2006.03.006.

McCabe, S. E., Schulenberg, J. E., O'Malley, P. M., Patrick, M. E., & Kloska, D. D. (2014). Non-medical use of prescription opioids during the transition to adulthood: A multi-cohort national longitudinal study. *Addiction, 109*(1), 102–110. doi:10.1111/add.12347.

McCabe, S. E., & Teter, C. J. (2007). Drug use related problems among nonmedical users of prescription stimulants: A web-based survey of college students from a Midwestern university. *Drug and Alcohol Dependence, 91*(1), 69–76. doi:10.1016/j.drugalcdep.2007.05.010.

McCabe, S. E., Teter, C. J., & Boyd, C. J. (2004). The use, misuse and diversion of prescription stimulants among middle and high school students. *Substance Use & Misuse, 39*(7), 1095–1116.

McCabe, S. E., Teter, C. J., & Boyd, C. J. (2006a). Medical use, illicit use and diversion of prescription stimulant medication. *Journal of Psychoactive Drugs, 38*(1), 43–56.

McCabe, S. E., Teter, C. J., & Boyd, C. J. (2006b). Medical use, illicit use, and diversion of abusable prescription drugs. *Journal of American College Health, 54*(5), 269–278. doi:10.3200/jach.54.5.269-278.

McCabe, S. E., Teter, C. J., Boyd, C. J., Knight, J. R., & Wechsler, H. (2005). Nonmedical use of prescription opioids among U.S. college students: Prevalence and correlates from a national survey. *Addictive Behaviors, 30*(4), 789–805. doi:10.1016/j.addbeh.2004.08.024.

McCabe, S. E., & West, B. T. (2013). Medical and nonmedical use of prescription stimulants: Results from a national multicohort study. *Journal of American Academy of Child and Adolescent Psychiatry, 52*(12), 1272–1280. doi: 10.1016/j.jaac.2013.09.005.

McCabe, S. E., West, B. T., & Wechsler, H. (2007). Trends and college-level characteristics associated with the non-medical use of prescription drugs among US college students from 1993 to 2001. *Addiction, 102*(3), 455–465. doi:10.1111/j.1360-0443.2006.01733.x.

Mudur, G. (1999). Abuse of OTC drugs rising in South Asia. *BMJ: British Medical Journal, 318*(7183), 556.

Nargiso, J. E., Ballard, E. L., & Skeer, M. R. (2015). A systematic review of risk and protective factors associated with nonmedical use of prescription drugs among youth in the United States: A social ecological perspective. *Journal of Studies on Alcohol and Drugs, 76*(1), 5–20.

National Institute on Drug Abuse. (2014). Stimulant ADHD medications: Methylphenidate and amphetamines. https://www.drugabuse.gov/publications /drugfacts/stimulant-adhd-medications-methylphenidate-amphetamines.

Nattala, P., Murthy, P., Thennarasu, K., & Cottler, L. B. (2014). Nonmedical use of sedatives in urban Bengaluru. *Indian Journal of Psychiatry, 56*(3), 246.

Novak, S. P., Hakansson, A., Martinez-Raga, J., Reimer, J., Krotki, K., & Varughese, S. (2016). Nonmedical use of prescription drugs in the European Union. *BMC Psychiatry, 16*, 274. doi:10.1186/s12888-016-0909-3.

Opaleye, E. S., Noto, A. R., Sanchez, Z. M., Amato, T. C., Locatelli, D. P., Gossop, M., & Ferri, C. P. (2013). Nonprescribed use of tranquilizers or sedatives by adolescents: A Brazilian national survey. *BMC Public Health, 13*, 499. doi:10.1186/1471-2458-13-499.

Pulver, A., Davison, C., & Pickett, W. (2015). Time-use patterns and the recreational use of prescription medications among rural and small town youth. *Journal of Rural Health, 31*(2), 217–228. doi:10.1111/jrh.12103.

Roy, E., Nolin, M. A., Traore, I., Leclerc, P., & Vasiliadis, H. M. (2015). Nonmedical use of prescription medication among adolescents using drugs in Quebec. *Canadian Journal of Psychiatry, 60*(12), 556–563.

Rudd, R. A. (2016). Increases in drug and opioid-involved overdose deaths— United States, 2010–2015. *MMWR: Morbidity and Mortality Weekly Report, 65*, 1445–1452.

Schepis, T. S., & Krishnan-Sarin, S. (2008). Characterizing adolescent prescription misusers: A population-based study. *Journal of American Academy of Child and Adolescent Psychiatry, 47*(7), 745–754. doi:10.1097/CHI.0b013e 318172ef0ld.

Schepis, T. S., & Krishnan-Sarin, S. (2009). Sources of prescriptions for misuse by adolescents: Differences in sex, ethnicity, and severity of misuse in a population-based study. *Journal of American Academy of Child and Adolescent Psychiatry, 48*(8), 828–836. doi:10.1097/CHI.0b013e3181a8130d.

Simoni-Wastila, L., Yang, H. W., & Lawler, J. (2008). Correlates of prescription drug nonmedical use and problem use by adolescents. *Journal of Addiction Medicine, 2*(1), 31–39. doi:10.1097/ADM.0b013e31815b5590.

Stabler, M. E., Gurka, K. K., & Lander, L. R. (2015). Association between childhood residential mobility and non-medical use of prescription drugs among American youth. *Maternal and Child Health Journal, 19*(12), 2646–2653. doi:10.1007/s10995-015-1785-z.

Stewart, T. D., & Reed, M. B. (2015). Lifetime nonmedical use of prescription medications and socioeconomic status among young adults in the United States. *American Journal of Drug and Alcohol Abuse, 41*(5), 458–464. doi: 10.3109/00952990.2015.1060242.

Stock, M. L., Litt, D. M., Arlt, V., Peterson, L. M., & Sommerville, J. (2013). The prototype/willingness model, academic versus health-risk information, and risk cognitions associated with nonmedical prescription stimulant use among college students. *British Journal of Health Psychology, 18*(3), 490–507. doi:10.1111/j.2044-8287.2012.02087.x.

Striley, C. W., Kelso-Chichetto, N. E., & Cottler, L. B. (2016). Nonmedical prescription stimulant use among girls 10–18 years of age: Associations with other risky behavior. *Journal of Adolescent Health, 60*(3), 328–332. doi: 10.1016/j.jadohealth.2016.10.013.

Substance Abuse and Mental Health Services Administration. (2009). *The NSDUH Report: Nonmedical Use of Adderall® among Full-time College Students.* Rockville, MD: Substance Abuse and Mental Health Services Administration.

Substance Abuse and Mental Health Services Administration. (2010). *Results from the 2009 National Survey on Drug Use and Health: National Findings* (NSDUH Series H-38A, HHS Publication No. SMA 10–4586 Findings). Rockville, MD: Substance Abuse and Mental Health Services Administration.

Substance Abuse and Mental Health Services Administration. (2013). *The DAWN Report: Emergency Department Visits Involving Attention Deficit/Hyperactivity Disorder Stimulant Medications.* Rockville, MD: Substance Abuse and Mental Health Services Administration.

Sun, E. C., Dixit, A., Humphreys, K., Darnall, B. D., Baker, L. C., & Mackey, S. (2017). Association between concurrent use of prescription opioids and benzodiazepines and overdose: Retrospective analysis. *BMJ: British Medical Journal, 356*, j760. doi:10.1136/bmj.j760.

Tapscott, B. E., & Schepis, T. S. (2013). Nonmedical use of prescription medications in young adults. *Adolescent Medicine: State of the Art Reviews, 24*(3), 597–610.

Teter, C. J., Falone, A. E., Cranford, J. A., Boyd, C. J., & McCabe, S. E. (2010). Nonmedical use of prescription stimulants and depressed mood among college students: Frequency and routes of administration. *Journal of Substance Abuse Treatment, 38*(3), 292–298. doi:10.1016/j.jsat.2010.01.005.

Teter, C. J., McCabe, S. E., Cranford, J. A., Boyd, C. J., & Guthrie, S. K. (2005). Prevalence and motives for illicit use of prescription stimulants in an undergraduate student sample. *Journal of American College Health, 53*(6), 253–262. doi:10.3200/jach.53.6.253-262.

Teter, C. J., McCabe, S. E., LaGrange, K., Cranford, J. A., & Boyd, C. J. (2006). Illicit use of specific prescription stimulants among college students: Prevalence, motives, and routes of administration. *Pharmacotherapy, 26*(10), 1501–1510. doi:10.1592/phco.26.10.1501.

Treatment Episode Data Set. (2011). *Substance Abuse Treatment Admissions for Abuse of Benzodiazepines.* Rockville, MD: Substance Abuse and Mental Health Services Administration.

United Nations Office on Drugs and Crime. (2011a). *Misuse of Prescription Drugs: A South Asia Perspective.* Geneva, Switzerland: UNDOC. https://www.unodc .org/documents/southasia/reports/Misuse_of_Prescription_Drugs_-_A _South_Asia_Perspective_UNODC_2011.pdf.

United Nations Office on Drugs and Crime. (2011b). *The Non-medical Use of Prescription Drugs: Policy Direction Issues: Discussion Paper.* Geneva, Switzerland: UNDOC.

Van Zee, A. (2009). The promotion and marketing of OxyContin: Commercial triumph, public health tragedy. *American Journal of Public Health, 99*(2), 221–227. doi:10.2105/AJPH.2007.131714.

Vaughn, M. G., Nelson, E. J., Salas-Wright, C. P., Qian, Z., & Schootman, M. (2016). Racial and ethnic trends and correlates of non-medical use of prescription opioids among adolescents in the United States 2004–2013. *Journal of Psychiatric Research, 73*, 17–24.

Veliz, P. T., Boyd, C., & McCabe, S. E. (2013). Playing through pain: Sports participation and nonmedical use of opioid medications among adolescents. *American Journal of Public Health, 103*(5), e28–e30.

Warner, M., Trinidad, J. P., Bastian, B. A., Minino, A. M., & Hedegaard, H. (2016). Drugs most frequently involved in drug overdose deaths: United States, 2010–2014. *National Vital Statistics Reports, 65*(10), 1–15.

Weyandt, L. L., Janusis, G., Wilson, K. G., Verdi, G., Paquin, G., Lopes, J., . . . Dussault, C. (2009). Nonmedical prescription stimulant use among a sample of college students: Relationship with psychological variables. *Journal of Attention Disorders, 13*(3), 284–296. doi:10.1177/1087054709342212.

White, A. M., Hingson, R. W., Pan, I.-j., & Yi, H.-y. (2011). Hospitalizations for alcohol and drug overdoses in young adults ages 18–24 in the United States, 1999–2008: Results from the nationwide inpatient sample. *Journal of Studies on Alcohol and Drugs, 72*(5), 774–786.

White House. (2011). *Epidemic: Responding to America's Prescription Drug Abuse Crisis.* https://www.whitehouse.gov/sites/default/files/ondcp/policy-and -research/rx_abuse_plan.pdf.

Whiteside, L. K., Walton, M. A., Bohnert, A. S., Blow, F. C., Bonar, E. E., Ehrlich, P., & Cunningham, R. M. (2013). Nonmedical prescription opioid and sedative use among adolescents in the emergency department. *Pediatrics, 132*(5), 825–832. doi:10.1542/peds.2013-0721.

Wu, L. T., Pilowsky, D. J., Schlenger, W. E., & Galvin, D. M. (2007). Misuse of methamphetamine and prescription stimulants among youths and young adults in the community. *Drug and Alcohol Dependence, 89*(2-3), 195–205. doi:10.1016/j.drugalcdep.2006.12.020.

Wu, L. T., Ringwalt, C. L., Mannelli, P., & Patkar, A. A. (2008). Prescription pain reliever abuse and dependence among adolescents: A nationally representative study. *Journal of the American Academy of Child and Adolescent Psychiatry, 47*(9), 1020–1029. doi:10.1097/CHI.0b013e31817eed4d.

Wu, L. T., Swartz, M. S., Brady, K. T., Blazer, D. G., & Hoyle, R. H. (2014). Nonmedical stimulant use among young Asian-Americans, Native Hawaiians/Pacific Islanders, and mixed-race individuals aged 12–34 years in the United States. *Journal of Psychiatric Research, 59*, 189–199. doi:10.1016/j.jpsychires.2014.09.004.

Young, A., Grey, M., Boyd, C. J., & McCabe, S. E. (2011). Adolescent sexual assault and the medical and nonmedical use of prescription medication. *Journal of Addiction Nursing, 11*(1-2), 25–31. doi:10.3109/10884601003628138.

Young, A. M., Glover, N., & Havens, J. R. (2012). Nonmedical use of prescription medications among adolescents in the United States: a systematic review. *Journal of Adolescent Health, 51*(1), 6–17. doi:10.1016/j.jadohealth.2012.01.011.

Zosel, A., Bartelson, B. B., Bailey, E., Lowenstein, S., & Dart, R. (2013). Characterization of adolescent prescription drug abuse and misuse using the researched abuse diversion and addiction-related surveillance (RADARS®) system. *Journal of the American Academy of Child and Adolescent Psychiatry, 52*(2), 196–204.e192. doi:10.1016/j.jaac.2012.11.014.

Zullig, K. J., Divin, A. L., Weiler, R. M., Haddox, J. D., & Pealer, L. N. (2015). Adolescent nonmedical use of prescription pain relievers, stimulants, and depressants, and suicide risk. *Substance Use & Misuse, 50*(13), 1678–1689. doi:10.3109/10826084.2015.1027931.

Misuse of Prescription Drugs among Young Adults

Mark Pawson and Brian C. Kelly

Epidemiology and Trends of Prescription Drug Misuse among Young Adults

Although the prescription drug misuse (PDM) trend extends across a wide segment of the population, it has been particularly prevalent among young adults (Kelly et al., 2013b; McCabe, Teter, & Boyd, 2006). Recent statistics indicate that almost 19 million Americans reported the misuse of prescription drugs during the previous year, and young adults constituted the group with the highest prevalence of misuse (Substance Abuse and Mental Health Services Administration, 2016). As depicted in Figure 7.1, the prevalence of past-year misuse for young people between 18 and 29 well exceeds that for older age groups as well as adolescents. Over 15 percent of Americans between the ages of 18 and 25 reported the misuse of prescription drugs during the previous year (Substance Abuse and Mental Health Services Administration, 2016). This is a period of the life course when the misuse of these substances escalates considerably, as only 5.9 percent of adolescents reported such misuse. Furthermore, the prevalence of PDM among young Americans is greater than that for most illegal drugs; only marijuana has been more widely used than prescription drugs among young adults (Substance Abuse and Mental Health Services Administration, 2015). While the overall prescription drug trend has plateaued among U.S. young adults in recent years, misuse remains a significant public health problem in the United States and

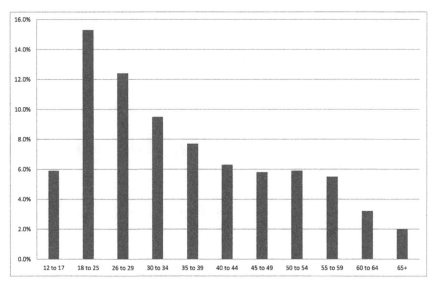

Figure 7.1   Prevalence of Past Year Misuse of Any Prescription Drug by Age

has increasingly become a global drug trend (United Nations Office on Drugs & Crime, 2011).

The first decade of the 21st century was the primary period for the diffusion of the PDM trend. Although the upward trend of misuse began during the 1990s, by the first few years of the 2000s, approximately 5.3 million Americans between the ages of 18 and 25 reported misusing prescription drugs within the previous year (Substance Abuse and Mental Health Services Administration, 2016). The growth in misuse among young adults was a notable driver of the general trend of growth in PDM among all age groups during this period of diffusion. In this regard, as has been the case for many other drug trends, young adults played an important role in the emergence and continued growth of PDM during the 21st century.

Rather than being focused on a particular type of prescription drug, young adults demonstrate elevated prevalence of misuse across several prescription drug classes. As highlighted in earlier chapters of this book, there are three prescription drug classes primarily associated with misuse: opioid painkillers (chapter 2), stimulants (chapter 3), and benzodiazepine and other sedative drugs (chapter 4). Young adults have the highest rates of misuse across all three of these classes of drugs in comparison with other age groups. As depicted in Figures 7.2 through 7.4, the prevalence of misuse peaks between the ages of 18 and 25 for any of these individual classes. While the figures for opioid painkillers and benzodiazepine/sedatives show that the trends in misuse are higher among young adults, the trend in the misuse of prescription stimulants in particular has been driven by young adults. The prevalence of stimulant misuse among young adults far exceeds that of Americans over the age of 30. This is perhaps unsurprising given their legitimate access to prescription stimulants, which are more commonly prescribed to individuals who are 18–25 years old (14.1%) in comparison with older adults (5.0%). Overall, the figures highlight the interesting age gradient of the PDM trend—rising sharply from adolescence to young adulthood before declining consistently after the age of 30. The motivations of young

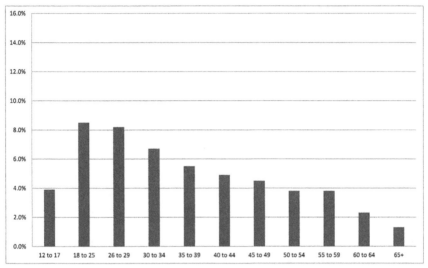

Figure 7.2   Prevalence of Past Year Misuse of a Prescription Pain Killer by Age

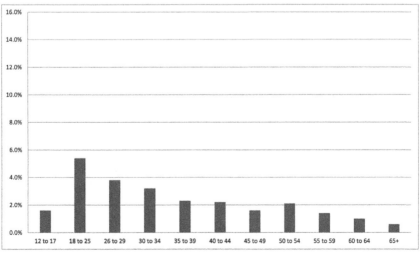

Figure 7.3   Prevalence of Past Year Misuse of a Tranquilizer by Age

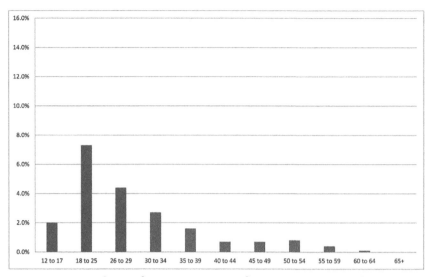

Figure 7.4   Prevalence of Past Year Misuse of a Prescription Stimulant by Age

adults who misuse prescription drugs are shaped by the particular stage of the life course they occupy, which provides the social and cultural context for how they think about the misuse of prescription drugs as well as the particular ways they misuse them.

Although many young adults misuse prescription drugs without major adverse consequences, some young adults experience a range of problems associated with PDM. Among these problems are social and interpersonal problems, risk of overdose, and dependence on prescription drugs. Notably, recent national data indicate that almost 1.5 percent of American young adults report indications of dependence on prescription medications (Substance Abuse and Mental Health Services Administration, 2016). Much like the elevated rates of misuse in general, young adults aged 18–25 report considerably higher prevalence of dependence symptoms than either adolescents (0.4%) or older adults (0.8%). While this represents only a small minority of young adults who misuse prescription drugs, this prevalence remains sizable and highlights the importance of intervening on problem patterns of misuse among the most at-risk young people, particularly given that substance dependence in early adulthood may produce long-term problems. This prevalence of dependence on prescription medications is higher than for all other substances, except for alcohol (4.7%) and marijuana use (3.7%), which are consumed by a far greater number of young people.

Transitions from Adolescence to Adulthood

While young adults are twice as likely to engage in PDM compared to other age cohorts, many initiated misuse as adolescents (Substance Abuse and Mental Health Services Administration, 2015). Yet, the misuse of prescription drugs accelerates dramatically from adolescence to young adulthood. As described in the previous section, adolescents (ages 12–17) have a considerably lower prevalence of past-year misuse in comparison with young adults (Manchikanti, 2007; Substance Abuse and Mental Health Services Administration, 2016). Although adolescence is an important period of experimentation for substance use, many young people begin misusing prescription drugs with regularity only after they reach young adulthood. Moreover, in recent years, many young people have been more likely to experiment first with misusing prescription drugs than with marijuana. This highlights a pattern that some describe as prescription drugs becoming the new "gateway drug" for 21st century U.S. youth (Manchikanti, 2007). Similarly, the dramatic increase in the number of youth legitimately prescribed psychotherapeutics throughout the 1990s and early 2000s has brought about a generational cohort some studies have referred to as "generation Rx," (Quintero, Peterson, & Young, 2006), although those most at risk for misusing prescription drugs also tend to have a history of using other substances (Sung, Richter, Vaughan, Johnson, & Thom, 2005).

Experimentation with psychoactive substances is common during adolescence and young adulthood (Schwartz, Côté, & Arnett, 2005). Although not all young people experiment with substances per se, experimentation more generally has been conceptualized as a key component of the experience of the developmental category of emerging adulthood (Arnett, 2015), which characterizes the shifting experience of young people reaching adulthood in the 21st century. Changes in the educational and occupational trajectories for young people navigating the transition to adulthood, along with larger economic shifts, have extended the life stage of "young adulthood." Many young people, particularly those in Western nations, now delay major life events that were traditionally viewed as hallmarks of adulthood, such as marriage, having children, and purchasing a home, until their late twenties or thirties (Arnett, 2015). The result is that many young people during the 21st century experience a period in which they achieve many of the rights and opportunities of adulthood while deferring many of its responsibilities.

In this manner, they experience a period of the life course in which they have a great degree of freedom to explore their identities, experiment with various roles and behaviors, and pursue their desires unencumbered by either adult responsibilities or parental oversight. The developmental and contextual changes (e.g., leaving for college, entering the workforce) that mark these transitions from adolescence to young adulthood can also shape the use of drugs and alcohol (Schulenberg & Maggs, 2002). The considerable instability of this life stage, often with rapid changes in living arrangements, parental supervision, academic expectations, and labor market involvement, along with changes in physical and cognitive development, has been linked with increases in alcohol consumption, substance use, and other risky health behaviors (Schulenberg & Maggs, 2002). Put simply, the great instability of this period not only creates a time of great opportunity but also great stress, which is alleviated by substance use in some young people.

The pursuit of adult goals also influences how emerging adults navigate substance use associated with this period of the life course. The life-course stage that young adults occupy is one in which they initiate the roles and responsibilities of adulthood, often feeling them out, as well as pursuing life goals in work, romance, and wider aspects of their social lives. Yet, in addition to the tremendous instability that produces stress, social pressures experienced by young adults in the workplace, the academic realm, and within friendship circles also lead them to misuse prescription drugs in particular ways (LeClair, Kelly, Pawson, Wells, & Parsons, 2015). A "work hard, play hard" narrative is engrained within the experiences of many contemporary young adults who perceive a need to pursue both a heightened state of productivity in the workplace and academic arena, while also fully devoting themselves to their social relationships and leisure pursuits. Navigating these simultaneously may be difficult for some young people. Many of the challenges of emerging adulthood, such as increases in feelings of instability and uncertainty, high stress, pressure to succeed, and fear of failure, also produce high rates of depression, anxiety, and insomnia (Arnett, 2015), which are legitimate targets of the prescription drugs misused by young adults.

The experience of negative affect generated by the experiences of emerging adulthood lend themselves to the misuse of various prescription drugs, including stimulants to manage and increase their abilities to take on workloads or benzodiazepines/sedatives to self-medicate the anxiety and stress experienced with increasing responsibilities and the simultaneous desire to manage social and romantic pursuits. In some instances, this spills over into what has been described as a "relax hard" attitude: the oxymoronic experience of heightening the intensity of relaxation through the misuse of medications (LeClair et al., 2015). As such, the particular features of the social contexts and life stages they inhabit—heightened pursuit of both life goals and social relationships—can motivate PDM among young people during this period of the life course (DeSantis & Hane, 2010; Racine & Forlini, 2010). Indeed, aspects of the life course are important backdrops that provide contexts for the misuse of prescription drugs.

Acquisition of Prescription Drugs

The acquisition of prescription drugs for misuse by young adults appears to be fairly easy. As a result of the wide availability of legally prescribed psychotherapeutic medications, the acquisition of these drugs among those who misuse them functions somewhat differently than for illicit markets. As noted earlier, the high level of legitimate prescriptions for stimulants received by young adults has shaped the high prevalence of their misuse relative to older cohorts. Some of this can be traced to misuse of one's own legitimate prescription, but also via the sharing, or diversion, of prescription pills within networks, which commonly occurs for many classes of prescription drugs. While research has identified that sources of prescription drugs are extremely varied, from doctors and pharmacists to dealers, theft, and the Internet, the majority of individuals who misuse prescription drugs acquire them through their social networks of friends and relatives (Boyd, McCabe, Cranford, & Young, 2006; Garnier-Dykstra, Caldeira, Vincent, O'Grady, & Arria, 2012; Inciardi, Surratt, Kurtz, & Cicero, 2007; McCabe & Boyd, 2005; Substance Abuse and Mental Health Services Administration, 2015; Twombly & Holtz, 2008). In this regard, the spillover from legitimate prescriptions and social networks are a key driver of the PDM problem among young adults, rather than a major illegitimate drug market. This aspect makes the prescription drug problem distinct from illicit drugs and particularly difficult with respect to policing the misuse of prescription drugs among young adults.

Sharing among peers is a key manner by which young adults obtain prescription drugs (Kelly, Vuolo, & Marin, 2017). Beyond providing a stable source of access, peer acquisition networks may also enable a process of social learning whereby the sharing of prescription medications becomes embedded, routinely integrated, and normalized within specific situational contexts (Parker, 2005). This may especially occur in situations where the suppliers are providing prescription drugs for misuse as a personal favor and not as a means to obtain profit (Parker, Aldridge, & Egginton, 2001). One of the manifestations of this normalizing drug trend is the ease with which these prescription drugs are obtained for free from friends (DuPont, Coleman, Bucher, & Wilford, 2008; Garnier-Dykstra et al., 2012). As young adults share these substances with friends and family, it is not surprising data suggests that almost half of those misusing in the past month obtained their prescription drugs through peer network sharing and not by purchasing them (Hurwitz, 2005). By sharing and promoting the misuse of prescription painkillers, stimulants, and sedatives, family members and peers invariably signal that misusing prescription drugs is both normative and safe. Misperceptions regarding the safety of prescription drugs continues to pose significant challenges as both young adults and adolescents have indicated they are more prone to misuse these medications because they believe them to be safer than illegal drugs (Manchikanti, 2007; Quintero, et al., 2006).

Although widely accessible and available within their social networks, a fairly low proportion (10.5%) of young adults who misuse prescription drugs report selling these substances to others (Vuolo, Kelly, Wells, & Parsons, 2014). This is fairly low given that approximately one-third (34.4%) of such young adults had been approached by others to sell prescription drugs. Yet, the patterns of selling were not consistent across groups of young adults.

Differing demographics were influential when considering actual and perceived selling. In particular, males were identified as important to reach to disrupt prescription drug sales among young adults (Vuolo et al., 2014). Personal access to prescriptions and their own frequency of misuse was also associated with involvement in prescription drug markets among young adults. In this manner, data on prescription drug selling suggests that most young adults who misuse prescription drugs are generally uninvolved in markets of prescription drug sales, a small proportion sell medications to others, and diversion often occurs as a favor to friends.

The Role of Peers in PDM

As is the case for many drug trends, peer networks play a key role in promoting PDM among young adults beyond simply providing a point of access. Peer influences on the misuse of prescription drugs have been less well studied than the role of peers in the use of other substances. Yet, a burgeoning literature indicates that peers similarly affect the misuse of prescription drugs among young people. Studies have identified that young people who have peers who misuse prescription drugs are more likely to misuse prescription drugs themselves (Ford, 2008). Other research has identified the importance of peers in shaping PDM through social learning processes, but it also indicated that social learning may be less influential than for illicit drug use (Schroeder & Ford, 2012). Peers may be more weakly associated because favorable definitions of prescription drugs circulate widely due to their legitimate medical uses, and thus peers' use may not be as important for the internalization of positive definitions of PDM. Nonetheless, it remains important to consider how peers may influence continuing patterns of PDM, particularly with respect to escalating drug practices and symptoms of dependence.

In a study considering the simultaneous influence of multiple peer factors, scholars identified several dimensions of peer effects on PDM among those endorsing regular misuse. Specifically, the research identified that network accessibility, the perceived peer normative context, and the motivation to misuse drugs to have a pleasant time with peers each played some role in shaping patterns of PDM while peer pressure did not (Kelly, Vuolo, & Marin, 2017). Importantly, this study identified that while many peer factors appear related to misuse when considered independently, only certain factors matter when they are considered as part of a wider constellation of peer influence. In this manner, peer pressure appears to matter for PDM among young adults only when considered outside of the wider peer context, but it does not maintain its effect once other dimensions of peer influence are considered alongside it. As such, peers influence patterns of PDM among young adults in a multifaceted manner, and peers shape prescription drug outcomes in several ways, particularly with respect to increasing frequency of misuse, escalation to nonoral modes of consumption, and heightened symptoms of dependence.

Prescription Drugs and Nightlife Involvement among Young Adults

While studies of college students have provided important information on the patterns of PDM among young adults, many young people, especially those beyond the age of 22, are not enrolled in higher education. As such, assessments of PDM among young adults active in various nightlife scenes, where the use of other drugs has been well established, have proven useful to identify patterns of misuse among young adults more broadly. Networks of young people come together for socializing, music, and other activities associated with nightlife participation, including substance use, and these have readily become environments tied to the PDM trend. Nightlife scenes have been characterized by some as environments where the social ecology and network ties facilitate substance use (Hunt, Moloney, & Evans, 2010). While prescription drugs have not been traditional substances within many of these nightlife scenes, they have been readily incorporated into the wider patterns of substance use among young adults.

Results from a venue-based study of young adults active in nightlife scenes found evidence that these young adults are at increased risk for misusing prescription drugs relative to other young people; they reported rates of lifetime misuse over 44 percent, which are considerably higher than national averages for young adults more generally (Kelly et al., 2013b). These data indicate that not only are nightlife scenes important sites for misuse among young adults but perhaps useful sites for intervention and harm reduction efforts as well. They are also particularly important sites for the consideration of the PDM trend, in part, because the nightlife arena is one from which other drug trends have often diffused among young adults (e.g., ecstasy).

Furthermore, nightlife scenes are highly varied in their form and function, and drug use trends do not necessarily occur in similar fashion across each of them; the PDM trend is no different from other drug trends in this regard. A varying prevalence of PDM occurs across distinct youth cultures tied to nightlife scenes, suggesting that the trend has not diffused equally among young people. Research has indicated that the prevalence of PDM is highest among young adults within the indie rock scene and electronic dance music scene (Kelly et al., 2013a, 2013b). Young adults who participate in hip-hop subcultures, on the other hand, consistently reported the lowest levels of PDM among all the nightlife scenes surveyed. Given that subcultures function with different social norms, we would expect to find such different patterns of PDM between youth cultural scenes. These differing prevalence rates also suggest that targeted approaches that account for the subculturally rooted differences in attitudes, social norms, and motivations for use among young people may be most efficacious.

With the growth in PDM among young adults, nightlife scenes provide particular contexts for this emerging drug trend and differentially shape patterns of misuse in accordance with the cultural milieus they provide. The phenomenon of PDM further highlights how youth cultures—as clusters of young people organized around specific activities, mind-sets, tastes, and styles—influence patterns of drug use beyond specific drug rituals through the routine practices engaged in by young people in their respective scenes. Research has also identified that the cultural dimensions of many youth cultures both enable and inhibit PDM and the particular ways that young people misuse these substances (Kelly, Trimarco et al., 2015). In this regard, although youth cultures are often portrayed as promoting drug use, they provide nuanced and varied influences on drug use and may inhibit PDM in some ways. For example, within the electronic dance music scene, the misuse of prescription drugs to moderate the effects of traditional drugs within that scene (e.g., ecstasy) may facilitate misuse, but the fact that prescription drugs are not traditional to this youth cultural scene may also inhibit their misuse.

As subcultural domains, the symbolic boundaries and subcultural capital within each nightlife scene set broader parameters for how young people conceive of drug use and enact drug use routines (Kelly, Trimarco et al., 2015). In this manner, young people involved in nightlife scenes generate particular ways of thinking about substance use on the basis of their strategies to create symbolic boundaries—between themselves and those on the "outside"—and to achieve status within their scenes by generating subcultural capital. Even when such boundaries and capital generation do not directly pertain to drugs, their broader cultural influences set the parameters for how young people think about drugs and how drugs fit into the dynamics of these scenes (Kelly, Trimarco et al., 2015). In this manner, their conceptions about prescription drugs may create conditions that in some ways facilitate the misuse of prescription drugs and in other ways inhibit the misuse of prescription drugs. These do not merely shape whether young people misuse prescription drugs but also the manner in which they misuse them.

As noted above in the example of the electronic dance music scene and described more fully below, of particular concern with regard to PDM among young adults active in nightlife scenes is their combined use with other drugs. Certain scenes make such combinations more sensible to those within that nightlife scene than other scenes. Many studies indicate that young adults reporting the misuse of a prescription drug are likely to do so in combination with another substance, the majority of which was done in combination with more than one substance (Firestone & Fischer, 2008; McCabe, Boyd, & Teter, 2009; Quintero, 2009). For instance, studies focusing on youth in electronic dance music scenes show that those engaged in polydrug use utilize particular prescription drugs to enhance or moderate the effects of other drugs in a desirable manner (Copeland, Dillon, & Gascoigne, 2006; Hunt, Evans, Moloney, & Bailey, 2009; Kelly & Parsons, 2007). The most common combination was the use of benzodiazepines to come down from the effects of such stimulant drugs as cocaine and MDMA (Bardhi, Sifaneck, Johnson, & Dunlap, 2007; Levy, O'Grady, Wish, & Arria, 2005; Topp, Hando, Dillon, Roche, & Solowij, 1999). As described within the next section, polydrug misuse places individuals at higher risk of adverse health outcomes. It is for these reasons that PDM remains an important issue within nightlife scenes, which are known for substance use more generally.

Incorporation of Prescription Pills into the Polydrug Routines of Young Adults

A key aspect of PDM is that young people have incorporated these medications into wider patterns of substance use. As noted above, young adulthood is often a period when individuals experiment with a wide range of substances. This extends to the misuse of prescription drugs as part of a wider substance use repertoire among young adults. Yet, the combination of prescription drugs with other psychoactive drugs has numerous health implications. Polydrug use has been linked to increased levels of intoxication and a greater likelihood of overdose (Collins, Ellickson, & Bell, 1998; Midanik, Tam, & Weisner, 2007). Additionally, studies have documented negative physical and psychological effects from polydrug use, including drug dependence (Leri, Bruneau, & Stewart, 2003); decreased cognitive functioning (Dillon, Copeland, & Jansen, 2003); and psychiatric comorbidity (Lynskey et al., 2006). Moreover, research has shown that polydrug use exacerbates problems associated with impaired driving (Thombs et al., 2009). Polydrug use with prescription drugs is of particular concern given that a majority of prescription drug-related emergency room visits and prescription drug overdoses involve coingestion with other substances (Cone et al., 2004).

A recent study among young adults involved in nightlife highlights the prevalent combination of illicit drugs with prescription drugs. An overwhelming majority—over 9 out of 10—of young adults who misuse prescription drugs also use illicit drugs (Kelly, Wells, Pawson, LeClair, & Parsons, 2014). Of concern is that approximately two-thirds of those engaged in PDM (65.9%) indicated that they had combined prescription drugs with an illegal drug. Recent combinations of PDM with alcohol were also quite prevalent among this group (71.2%). Among the wider general sample of young adults involved in nightlife, rather than specifically those who misuse prescription drugs, about 1 in 6 (16.4%) had combined an illegal drug with a prescription drug, indicating that this is a common practice among young people (Kelly et al., 2014).

Recent work (Pawson & Kelly, 2017) has identified that young adults' incorporation of prescription drugs into polydrug use repertoires is an embedded feature of how they are socialized into the world of pharmaceuticals, as youth go about "treating" physical and psychological discomforts from using uppers, psychedelics, and alcohol. The current visibility and ubiquity of pharmaceutical use spills over into young people's attempts to either extend and enhance the pleasure of other substances or counteract the discomfort and debilitation brought on by the use of alcohol and illegal drugs. Processes of normalization and pharmaceuticalization have contributed to young adults integrating prescription medications into their wider substance use routines. Both lax attitudes regarding misuse and the ease of accessing medications inform and influence young adults' perceptions of prescription drugs as suitable and reliable substances to navigate challenging aspects of nightlife participation and negotiate problematic elements of public intoxication. In this regard, prescription drugs have become part of the wider substance use patterns of young adults, in part, because they find them useful for managing other substance use.

Escalation

Beyond concerns about polydrug use among young adults is the issue of escalating to nonoral forms of consumption. Most PDM is accomplished by oral ingestion, as this is a normative means of ingestion for both medical and nonmedical use of pharmaceuticals. However, young adults also tamper with these substances to achieve a quicker and more intense effect (Budman, Serrano, & Butler, 2009; Raffa & Pergolizzi, 2010; Vosburg et al., 2012). By crushing the substance to a powder (Raffa & Pergolizzi, 2010), sniffing prescription drugs has become a common alternative route of administration among young adults. Sniffing is common enough, in fact, that companies have created formulas that are crush-resistant to prevent nonoral administration (Budman et al., 2009; Vosburg et al., 2012). Smoking prescription pills is also a common means of consumption, with the injection of prescription drugs quite uncommon among young adults. Along with health risks of alternative forms of consuming prescription drugs, having a quicker and more intense high from a substance has been shown to confer higher reinforcement and addictive potential than a drug that has been orally administered; such nonoral use may be more likely to produce dependence (Compton & Volkow, 2006; Kelly, Vuolo, Pawson, Wells, & Parsons, 2015). As such, the alternative consumption of prescription drugs is an indication of escalating misuse and heightened risk for related problems.

The sniffing of prescription drugs by young adults is associated with drug problems such as addiction and injection drug use. Epidemiological work by McCabe and colleagues suggests that young adults who transition to sniffing prescription drugs are more likely to experience substance-related problems (McCabe, Cranford, Boyd, & Teter, 2007). A qualitative study of high-risk youth and opioid misuse found that sniffing was marked as a transitional practice between prescription misuse and riskier practices, such as injection (Lankenau et al., 2012). Thus, the transition to sniffing prescription drugs is not insignificant, as such escalation has been shown to lead to drug problems and potentially riskier means of consumption.

Research has identified that social influences shape the transition to alternative forms of consumption (Kelly, Harris, & Vuolo, 2016). Experimentation with new routes of administering prescription drugs among young adults typically occurs in group settings among peers (Pawson, Kelly, Wells, & Parsons, 2016). More specifically, the peer normative context, desire to use drugs to have a pleasant time with friends, and stigma are significant factors in shaping the escalation to sniffing prescription drugs among young adults (Kelly et al., 2016; Pawson et al., 2016). In contrast, the psychological factors of sensation seeking and perceived coping are not influences on such escalation, once the effects of social influences are taken into account. Escalations to alternative routes of administration also have implications for polydrug use, as young adults may rely more on the faster rates of onset provided by sniffing or smoking prescription drugs when looking to counteract negative side effects from other drugs (Pawson et al., 2016). Opportunities for experimentation among young adults also shapes the practice of nonoral modes of consumption. Abundant access to psychotherapeutic pharmaceuticals coupled with high rates of substance use experimentation create a social context for young adults to be considered a high-risk group for misusing prescription drugs through such nonnormative routes of administration. In this regard, wider social influences play an important role not merely in the initiation of PDM but in escalating patterns among young adults who continue to misuse prescription drugs over time as well.

Conclusions

Within this chapter, we have highlighted the critical importance of the period of young adulthood for the PDM trend. Although a great deal of emphasis has historically been placed on the prevention of substance use among adolescents, the PDM phenomenon escalates considerably during young adulthood and merits a greater deal of attention. As illustrated in Figures 7.1 through 7.4, the prevalence of PDM remains highest among young adults in comparison with other age groups, and for certain substances, such as stimulants, misuse far outpaces those in other age categories. As such, it is individuals during the period of young adulthood who are driving the trend for stimulant misuse. Overall, young adults have been an important group shaping the PDM trend since its inception. The misuse of these substances coheres with a wider pattern of peaking substance use during this period of the life course.

While young adults' high rates of PDM also coincide with their high rates of substances in general, there are many specific facets of this age cohort that help to make meaning of their position as a high-risk population for misusing psychoactive medications. As emerging adulthood is framed as a transitional life stage where youth acclimate themselves to adulthood and learn to take on adult roles and responsibilities, exploring the potential benefits of prescription drugs may be becoming an embedded feature of young adults' social practices in the United States. PDM is context-specific, and studies focusing on young adults' utilization of these medications within their academic lives, leisure pursuits, coping strategies, and relaxation routines demonstrate the varied ways youth are socialized into the world of misusing pharmaceuticals. Moreover, the integration of PDM into the mundane practices of daily life may be a normalizing trend whose persistence may be increasing above and beyond the high-risk years of young adulthood.

As described above, it is not PDM alone that raises concern, but both the combination of prescription medications with other substances and the escalating patterns of misuse among young adults. Young people, particularly those involved in nightlife scenes, have demonstrated patterns of misuse in polydrug use and nonoral administration that may increase the possibility of harms, such as overdose and dependence. The combination of prescription drugs with substances widely utilized in these nightlife scenes may enhance risk. Yet, as noted above, there are also elements of these subcultures that temper PDM in certain ways. Overall, however, the pattern of polydrug use with prescription drugs as well as the escalation to nonoral modes of consumption remain key points for intervention and harm reduction.

Given their high prevalence of misuse and how they misuse prescription drugs, young adults remain a key population for prevention and intervention efforts focused on PDM. This is particularly important given that this is the age group reporting the highest prevalence of indicators of dependence (Substance Abuse and Mental Health Services Administration, 2016). A key area of focus may be the generation of *intraventions* within communities of young adults, subcultural or otherwise. As Friedman and colleagues describe, in contrast to traditional interventions, intraventions are "prevention activities that are conducted and sustained through processes within communities themselves" (Friedman et al., 2004, p. 251). Rather than being interventions imposed by professionals, intraventions have organic qualities and are nurtured within the community of participating individuals. They are public health promotion efforts that are fundamentally grounded within the community in an attempt to ameliorate harms in culturally sanctioned ways. Young people, particularly those involved in nightlife subcultures, may be especially receptive to such intraventions rather than those imposed from outside. By working within the social contexts of these groups, public health professionals may be able to promote intraventions that reduce the harms associated with PDM, particularly with respect to the ways they are integrated with other patterns of substance use among this age group.

References

Arnett, J. (2015). Emerging adulthood: The winding road through the late teens and twenties. New York: Oxford University Press.

Bardhi, F., Sifaneck, S. J., Johnson, B. D., & Dunlap, E. (2007). Pills, thrills and bellyaches: Case studies of prescription pill use and misuse among marijuana/blunt smoking middle class young women. *Contemporary Drug Problems, 34*(1), 53.

Boyd, C. J., McCabe, S. E., Cranford, J. A., & Young, A. (2006). Adolescents' motivations to abuse prescription medications. *Pediatrics, 118*(6), 2472–2480.

Budman, S. H., Serrano, J. M. G., & Butler, S. F. (2009). Can abuse deterrent formulations make a difference? Expectation and speculation. *Harm Reduction Journal, 6*(1), 8.

Collins, R. L., Ellickson, P. L., & Bell, R. M. (1998). Simultaneous polydrug use among teens: Prevalence and predictors. *Journal of Substance Abuse, 10*(3), 233–253.

Compton, W. M., & Volkow, N. D. (2006). Abuse of prescription drugs and the risk of addiction. *Drug and Alcohol Dependence, 83*, S4–S7.

Cone, E. J., Fant, R. V., Rohay, J. M., Caplan, Y. H., Ballina, M., Reder, R. F., & Haddox, J. D. (2004). Oxycodone involvement in drug abuse deaths. II. Evidence for toxic multiple drug-drug interactions. *Journal of Analytical Toxicology, 28*(4), 217–225.

Copeland, J., Dillon, P., & Gascoigne, M. (2006). Ecstasy and the concomitant use of pharmaceuticals. *Addictive Behaviors, 31*(2), 367–370.

DeSantis, A. D., & Hane, A. C. (2010). "Adderall is definitely not a drug": Justifications for the illegal use of ADHD stimulants. *Substance Use & Misuse, 45*(1-2), 31–46.

Dillon, P., Copeland, J., & Jansen, K. (2003). Patterns of use and harms associated with non-medical ketamine use. *Drug and Alcohol Dependence, 69*(1), 23–28.

DuPont, R. L., Coleman, J. J., Bucher, R. H., & Wilford, B. B. (2008). Characteristics and motives of college students who engage in nonmedical use of methylphenidate. *American Journal on Addictions, 17*(3), 167–171.

Firestone, M., & Fischer, B. (2008). A qualitative exploration of prescription opioid injection among street-based drug users in Toronto: Behaviours, preferences and drug availability. *Harm Reduction Journal, 5*(1), 30.

Ford, J. A. (2008). Social learning theory and nonmedical prescription drug use among adolescents. *Sociological Spectrum, 28*(3), 299–316.

Friedman, S. R., Maslow, C., Bolyard, M., Sandoval, M., Mateu-Gelabert, P., & Neaigus, A. (2004). Urging others to be healthy: "Intravention" by injection drug users as a community prevention goal. *AIDS Education and Prevention,* 16(3), 250–263.

Garnier-Dykstra, L. M., Caldeira, K. M., Vincent, K. B., O'Grady, K. E., & Arria, A. M. (2012). Nonmedical use of prescription stimulants during college: Four-year trends in exposure opportunity, use, motives, and sources. *Journal of American College Health,* 60(3), 226–234.

Harwood, H. J., & Bouchery, E. (2004). *The Economic Costs of Drug Abuse in the United States, 1992–2002.* Washington, D.C.: Executive Office of the President, Office of National Drug Control Policy.

Hunt, G., Evans, K., Moloney, M., & Bailey, N. (2009). Combining different substances in the dance scene: Enhancing pleasure, managing risk and timing effects. *Journal of Drug Issues,* 39(3), 495–522.

Hunt, G., Moloney, M., & Evans, K. (2010). *Youth, Drugs, and Nightlife.* London, England: Routledge.

Hurwitz, W. (2005). The challenge of prescription drug misuse: A review and commentary. *Pain Medicine,* 6(2), 152–161.

Inciardi, J. A., Surratt, H. L., Kurtz, S. P., & Cicero, T. J. (2007). Mechanisms of prescription drug diversion among drug-involved club- and street-based populations. *Pain Medicine,* 8(2), 171–183.

Kelly, B. C., Harris, E., & Vuolo, M. (2016). Psychosocial influences of the escalation of deviance: The case of prescription drug sniffing. *Deviant Behavior,* 1–16.

Kelly, B. C., & Parsons, J. T. (2007). Prescription drug misuse among club drug-using young adults. *American Journal of Drug and Alcohol Abuse,* 33(6), 875–884.

Kelly, B. C., Trimarco, J., LeClair, A., Pawson, M., Parsons, J. T., & Golub, S. A. (2015). Symbolic boundaries, subcultural capital and prescription drug misuse across youth cultures. *Sociology of Health & Illness,* 37(3), 325–339.

Kelly, B. C., Vuolo, M., & Marin, A. C. (2017). Multiple dimensions of peer effects and deviance: The case of prescription drug misuse among young adults. *Socius,* 3, 2378023117706819.

Kelly, B. C., Vuolo, M., Pawson, M., Wells, B. E., & Parsons, J. T. (2015). Chasing the bean: Prescription drug smoking among socially active youth. *Journal of Adolescent Health,* 56(6), 632–638.

Kelly, B. C., Wells, B. E., LeClair, A., Tracy, D., Parsons, J. T., & Golub, S. A. (2013a). Prescription drug misuse among young adults: Looking across youth cultures. *Drug and Alcohol Review,* 32(3), 288–294.

Kelly, B. C., Wells, B. E., LeClair, A., Tracy, D., Parsons, J. T., & Golub, S. A. (2013b). Prevalence and correlates of prescription drug misuse among socially active young adults. *International Journal of Drug Policy,* 24(4), 297–303.

Kelly, B. C., Wells, B. E., Pawson, M., LeClair, A., & Parsons, J. T. (2014). Combinations of prescription drug misuse and illicit drugs among young adults. *Addictive Behaviors,* 39(5), 941–944.

Lankenau, S. E., Teti, M., Silva, K., Bloom, J. J., Harocopos, A., & Treese, M. (2012). Patterns of prescription drug misuse among young injection drug users. *Journal of Urban Health,* 89(6), 1004–1016.

LeClair, A., Kelly, B. C., Pawson, M., Wells, B. E., & Parsons, J. T. (2015). Motivations for prescription drug misuse among young adults: Considering social and developmental contexts. *Drugs: Education, Prevention and Policy, 22*(3), 208–216.

Leri, F., Bruneau, J., & Stewart, J. (2003). Understanding polydrug use: Review of heroin and cocaine co-use. *Addiction, 98*(1), 7–22.

Levy, K. B., O'Grady, K. E., Wish, E. D., & Arria, A. M. (2005). An in-depth qualitative examination of the ecstasy experience: Results of a focus group with ecstasy-using college students. *Substance Use & Misuse, 40*(9-10), 1427–1441.

Manchikanti, L. (2007). National drug control policy and prescription drug abuse: Facts and fallacies. *Pain Physician, 10*(3), 399.

McCabe, S. E., & Boyd, C. J. (2005). Sources of prescription drugs for illicit use. *Addictive Behaviors, 30*(7), 1342–1350.

McCabe, S. E., Boyd, C. J., & Teter, C. J. (2009). Subtypes of nonmedical prescription drug misuse. *Drug and Alcohol Dependence, 102*(1), 63–70.

McCabe, S. E., Cranford, J. A., Boyd, C. J., & Teter, C. J. (2007). Motives, diversion and routes of administration associated with nonmedical use of prescription opioids. *Addictive Behaviors, 32*(3), 562–575.

McCabe, S. E., Teter, C. J., & Boyd, C. J. (2006). Medical use, illicit use, and diversion of abusable prescription drugs. *Journal of American College Health, 54*(5), 269–278.

Midanik, L. T., Tam, T. W., & Weisner, C. (2007). Concurrent and simultaneous drug and alcohol use: Results of the 2000 National Alcohol Survey. *Drug and Alcohol Dependence, 90*(1), 72–80.

Parker, H. (2005). Normalization as a barometer: Recreational drug use and the consumption of leisure by younger Britons. *Addiction Research & Theory, 13*(3), 205–215.

Parker, H., Aldridge, J., & Egginton, R. (2001). *UK Drugs Unlimited: New Research and Policy Lessons on Illicit Drug Use*. London, England: Palgrave Macmillan.

Pawson, M., & Kelly, B. C. (2017). *Presentations of Self in Nightlife and the Strategic Misuse of Prescription Drugs*. Paper presented at the Society for the Study of Symbolic Interaction, Montreal.

Pawson, M., Kelly, B. C., Wells, B. E., & Parsons, J. T. (2016). Becoming a prescription pill smoker: Revisiting Becker. *Criminology and Criminal Justice*, 1748895816677570.

Quintero, G. (2009). Rx for a party: A qualitative analysis of recreational pharmaceutical use in a collegiate setting. *Journal of American College Health, 58*(1), 64–72.

Quintero, G., Peterson, J., & Young, B. (2006). An exploratory study of sociocultural factors contributing to prescription drug misuse among college students. *Journal of Drug Issues, 36*(4), 903–931.

Racine, E., & Forlini, C. (2010). Cognitive enhancement, lifestyle choice or misuse of prescription drugs? *Neuroethics, 3*(1), 1–4.

Raffa, R. B., & Pergolizzi, J. V. (2010). Opioid formulations designed to resist/deter abuse. *Drugs, 70*(13), 1657–1675.

Schroeder, R. D., & Ford, J. A. (2012). Prescription drug misuse: A test of three competing criminological theories. *Journal of Drug Issues, 42*(1), 4–27.

Schulenberg, J. E., & Maggs, J. L. (2002). A developmental perspective on alcohol use and heavy drinking during adolescence and the transition to young adulthood. *Journal of Studies on Alcohol and Drugs, Supplement*(S14), 54–70.

Schwartz, S. J., Côté, J. E., & Arnett, J. J. (2005). Identity and agency in emerging adulthood two developmental routes in the individualization process. *Youth & Society, 37*(2), 201–229.

Substance Abuse and Mental Health Services Administration. (2010). *Results from the 2009 National Survey on Drug Use and Health.* Vol. I, *Summary of National Findings* (HHS Publication No. SMA 10-4856). Rockville, MD: Substance Abuse and Mental Health Services Administration Office of Applied Studies.

Substance Abuse and Mental Health Services Administration. (2015). *Behavioral Health Trends in the United States: Results from the 2014 National Survey on Drug Use and Health.* Rockville, MD: Substance Abuse and Mental Health Services Administration.

Substance Abuse and Mental Health Services Administration. (2016). *Results from the 2015 National Survey on Drug Use and Health: Summary of National Findings.* Rockville, MD: Substance Abuse and Mental Health Services Administration.

Sung, H.-E., Richter, L., Vaughan, R., Johnson, P. B., & Thom, B. (2005). Nonmedical use of prescription opioids among teenagers in the United States: Trends and correlates. *Journal of Adolescent Health, 37*(1), 44–51.

Thombs, D. L., O'Mara, R., Dodd, V. J., Merves, M. L., Weiler, R. M., Goldberger, B. A., . . . Gullet, S. E. (2009). Event-specific analyses of poly-drug abuse and concomitant risk behavior in a college bar district in Florida. *Journal of American College Health, 57*(6), 575–586.

Topp, L., Hando, J., Dillon, P., Roche, A., & Solowij, N. (1999). Ecstasy use in Australia: Patterns of use and associated harm. *Drug and Alcohol Dependence, 55*(1), 105–115.

Twombly, E. C., & Holtz, K. D. (2008). Teens and the misuse of prescription drugs: Evidence-based recommendations to curb a growing societal problem. *Journal of Primary Prevention, 29*(6), 503.

United Nations Office on Drugs and Crime. (2011). *The Nonmedical Use of Prescription Drugs: Policy Direction Issues.* Vienna, Austria: UNODC.

Vosburg, S. K., Jones, J. D., Manubay, J. M., Ashworth, J. B., Benedek, I. H., & Comer, S. D. (2012). Assessment of a formulation designed to be crush-resistant in prescription opioid abusers. *Drug and Alcohol Dependence, 126*(1), 206–215.

Vuolo, M., Kelly, B. C., Wells, B. E., & Parsons, J. T. (2014). Correlates of prescription drug market involvement among young adults. *Drug and Alcohol Dependence, 143,* 257–262.

CHAPTER EIGHT

Prescription Drug Misuse in Older Adults

Yu-Ping Chang

Prescription psychotherapeutic drug nonadherence (not taking a drug as prescribed) is a significant public health concern. In particular, the United States is in the midst of a growing and dangerous epidemic of prescription opioid misuse. Older adults are frequently prescribed psychotherapeutic drugs, including opioids (pain relievers) and central nervous system (CNS) depressants (sedatives and benzodiazepine and non-benzodiazepine tranquilizers). These medications can alter brain activity and are highly addictive. Compared with younger adults, adults over the age of 50 represent the largest consumers of prescription medications, and individuals in this age group are three times more likely to be prescribed opioids and benzodiazepines. Older adults are particularly susceptible to adverse medical outcomes from prescription drug misuse as well as drug interactions due to age-related physiologic changes in body composition and drug metabolism.

These negative consequences are even more adverse when older adults misuse more than one type of psychotherapeutic drug or simultaneously use psychotherapeutic drugs and alcohol (polysubstance use), which can lead to dangerous combination effects. Chronic pain is the second most common reason for primary care visits in patients age 65 and older and is associated with severe disability and comorbidities (e.g., depression, anxiety, insomnia), resulting in substantial health care costs (Makris, Abrams, Gurland, & Reid, 2014; Reid, Eccleston, & Pillemer, 2015). This chapter will review the scope of problems regarding prescription opioid misuse and abuse, prescription opioid misuse in older adults with chronic pain, issues related to use of benzodiazepines (BZD) in older adults, risk factors, consequences of prescription misuse and abuse, and behavioral interventions for prescription opioid misuse in older adults.

Opioid Epidemic in the United States

Opioid misuse continues to be an epidemic crisis in the United States. In the 2015 National Survey on Drug Use and Health (NSDUH; Lipari, Williams, & Van Horn, 2017), respondents provided information on their use and misuse of prescription analgesics, including hydrocodone (e.g., Vicodin); oxycodone (e.g., OxyContin, Percocet); and morphine. Approximately 91.8 million adults aged 18 or older reported using a prescription opioid in the past year in 2015, representing more than one-third (37.8%) of the adult population. Approximately 12.5 percent of these (11.5 million) adults reported misusing a prescription opioid at least once in the past year, meaning that 4.7 percent of all U.S. adults used an opioid in an unprescribed manner. Respondents also reported reasons for misuse, with the most common being to relieve physical pain (63.4%), although such pain relief was achieved without a prescription of one's own or by use at a higher dosage or more often than prescribed. Other commonly reported reasons were to feel good or get high (11.7%), to relax or relieve tension (10.9%), to help with sleep (4.5%), to help with feelings or emotions (3.2%), because they were "hooked" or had to have the drug (2.5%), to experiment or see what the drug was like (2.0%), and to increase or decrease the effects of other drugs (0.9%; Lipari et al., 2017).

Clearly, the misuse of prescribed opioids is common in those who do not have chronic pain, and the health consequences of opioid misuse were evident in increasing numbers of emergency department visits (Frank, Binswanger, Calcaterra, Brenner, & Levy, 2015), treatment admissions (Ling, Mooney, & Hillhouse, 2011), and overdose deaths (Center for Disease Control and Prevention; National Center for Health Statistics; National Vital Statistics System; Mortality File, 2015; Rudd, Seth, David, & Scholl, 2016). While many people benefit from using prescription opioids for pain management, improper use of prescription opioids is common. About 50.5 percent of people who misused prescription opioids obtained them from a friend or relative for free, and 22.1 percent obtained them from a doctor (Center for Behavioral Health Statistics and Quality, 2015).

Costs associated with prescription opioid misuse represent a substantial and growing economic burden for society. Total U.S. societal costs of prescription opioid misuse were estimated at $55.7 billion in 2007, with 45 percent accounted for by health care costs of $25 billion (Birnbaum et al.,

2011). The increasing prevalence of prescription opioid misuse suggests that there will be an even greater societal burden in the future (Birnbaum et al., 2011).

Overdose Death

In 2015, 52,404 persons in the United States died from a drug overdose, and 63.1 percent (33,091) of these deaths involved an opioid (Rudd et al., 2016). In 2016, the Centers for Disease Control and Prevention (CDC) reported that 78 people in the United States die from an opioid overdose daily, a number that has nearly quadrupled since 1999 (Centers for Disease Control and Prevention, 2016). These numbers continue to increase. According to CDC data from August 2017, 91 people die every day from an opioid overdose (Rudd et al., 2016). In attempting to understand the trend of opioid-related deaths over time, the CDC examined overall drug overdose death rates during 2010 to 2015 as well as opioid overdose death rates during 2014 to 2015 by subcategories: natural/semisynthetic opioids, methadone, heroin, and synthetic opioids other than methadone (Rudd et al., 2016). From 2014 to 2015, the death rate from synthetic opioids other than methadone, which included fentanyl, increased by 72.2 percent (Gladden, Martinez, & Seth, 2016; Peterson et al., 2016), and heroin death rates increased by 20.6 percent. Natural/semisynthetic opioid death rates increased by 2.6 percent, whereas methadone death rates decreased by 9.1 percent. It is important to note, although methadone death rates decreased overall, the rate increased among people aged 65 years or older (Rudd et al., 2016).

Opioid Misuse in Older Adults

According to the 2014 NSDUH, adults aged 50 or older were least likely to misuse opioids in the past year (2.0%), while young adults aged 18 and 25 were most likely (8.1%). Opioid misuse among adults aged 50 or older in 2014 was higher than most years between 2002 and 2011, with evidence of significantly increased rates from 2002 to 2013 (Schepis & McCabe, 2016). In contrast, opioid misuse among young adults decreased from 11.5 percent in 2002 to 8.1 percent in 2014. Although the rate of older adults who misuse opioids is relatively small compared to young adults, the NSDUH data suggest that opioid misuse is a growing problem among older adults. In particular, such misuse places them at risk for complications such as fractures and myocardial infarction, leads to poorer clinical outcomes, and can cause accidental injuries and mood or cognitive alterations (Ballantyne, 2012; Culberson & Ziska, 2008; Mailis-Gagnon et al., 2012). Of particular concern is when older adults mix opioids with alcohol or benzodiazepines (prescribed for anxiety and insomnia), which can lead to respiratory depression and death (Borges et al., 2005). During the past two decades, the greatest increase in hospital stays involving opioid overdose has been among people age 45 and older (Owens, Barrett, Weiss, Washington, & Kronick, 2014).

As the baby boomer generation (born between 1946 and 1964; aged 52–70 years) ages and more patients are prescribed opioids, the number of older individuals evidencing prescription opioid misuse is likely to become even greater. According to the 2014 U.S. Census, the number of Americans aged 65 and over is expected to grow to approximately 98 million individuals, and the number of Americans aged 85 and older is expected to grow to approximately 20 million by 2060. The projected increase in life expectancy provides more opportunities to use and potentially misuse prescription drugs and other substances, such as marijuana.

Prescription Opioid Misuse in Older Adults with Chronic Nonmalignant Pain

Although many studies of prescription opioid misuse have focused on adolescents and younger adults, researchers have begun to investigate misuse in older adults with chronic nonmalignant pain. Chronic nonmalignant pain that is unrelated to cancer and that persists beyond the usual course of disease or injury is one of the most common conditions encountered by health care professionals, particularly among patients 65 years and older (Johannes, Le, Zhou, Johnston, & Dworkin, 2010; van Hecke, Torrance, & Smith, 2013). Opioids are commonly prescribed to treat individuals with chronic pain (Chou, 2010; Kaye et al., 2017; White, Arnold, Norvell, Ecker, & Fehlings, 2011), but some patients misuse (e.g., take more than prescribed) or abuse (resulting in significant social, occupational, or health problems) their medication (Larance, Degenhardt, Lintzeris, Winstock, & Mattick, 2011). A review of 10 studies investigating opioid abuse, dependence, and related outcomes in chronic pain patients indicated that the prevalence of opioid abuse varies substantially, even after stratification by setting (Chou et al., 2015). Using DSM-IV criteria, in primary care settings, the prevalence of opioid abuse ranged from 0.6 percent to 8 percent and prevalence of dependence ranged from 3 percent to 26 percent (Chou et al., 2015).

A study in South Florida found that up to 80 percent of participants (aged 60 or older) had misused prescription opioids in the prior 90 days, and 34 percent reported substantial prescription opioid misuse (Levi-Minzi, Surratt, Kurtz, & Buttram, 2013). Participants also abused or misused other drugs, including alcohol (63.6%), benzodiazepines (48.9%), cocaine/crack (35.2%), marijuana (30.7%), heroin (14.8%), and other addictive medications (23.8%; Levi-Minzi et al., 2013). Similarly, a study conducted in western New York found that 35 percent of adults aged 50 and older with chronic pain misused their prescription opioids, and 28 percent reported alcohol consumption (Levi-Minzi et al., 2013). One study found that nearly 44 percent of ED patients aged 50 years and older who used prescription opioids within the past month also misused their prescription opioids, with taking prescription opioids in greater quantities or more often than prescribed being the most common types of misuse (Beaudoin, Merchant, & Clark, 2016).

Use of Benzodiazepines in Older Adults

The long-term use of benzodiazepines has been linked to adverse outcomes in older adults, including increased risks of cognitive impairment, falls, fractures, traffic accidents, delirium, and dependence (Buffett-Jerrott & Stewart, 2002; Clegg & Young, 2011; Cumming & Conteur, 2003; Hill & Wee, 2012; Meuleners et al., 2011; Voyer et al., 2011). The American Geriatrics Society 2012 Beers Criteria Update Expert Panel has recommended avoidance of benzodiazepine use for insomnia, agitation, or delirium in older adults because of their slower metabolism of and increased sensitivity to benzodiazepines (American Geriatrics Society Beers Criteria Update Expert Panel, 2012). Despite this, the use of benzodiazepines in older adults remains high, ranging from 12 percent to 32 percent (Dionne, Vasiliadis, Latimer, Berbiche, & Preville, 2013; Johnell & Fastbom, 2009), with a higher rate of use in those with psychiatric disorders (Martinsson, Fagerberg, Wiklund-Gustin, & Lindholm, 2012; Préville et al., 2011). It was estimated that 57–59 percent of older adults with psychiatric disorders used benzodiazepines (Martinsson et al., 2012), with higher rates in those with depression or anxiety disorder (Préville et al., 2011). However, very few studies were conducted to understand the scope of benzodiazepine misuse in older adults (Maree, Marcum, Saghafi, Weiner, & Karp, 2016). One study conducted in France found that 35.2 percent of their study subjects were addicted to benzodiazepines or equivalents (Landreat et al., 2010). Using face-to-face interviews with 2,785 community-dwelling older adults aged 65 years or older who were randomly selected from across the province of Quebec, Canada, researchers found that use of benzodiazepines was reported by 25.4 percent of their study respondents (Voyer, Preville, Cohen, Berbiche, & Beland, 2010). Approximately 9.5 percent of those met DSM-IV criteria for substance dependence, but 43 percent of individuals who used benzodiazepines reported being dependent and one-third agreed that it would be a good thing to stop taking benzodiazepines (Voyer et al., 2010).

Use of benzodiazepines continues to be high in older adults. This might be due to a lack of specialist knowledge about benzodiazepine prescribing in geriatric care; difficulties in translating prescribing guidelines into clinical practice (e.g., a perceived lack of alternative evidence-based treatments and unwillingness of older people to discontinue benzodiazepines); a perceived lack of priority for physicians (e.g., due to greater physical health needs); and physical and psychological dependence issues (Gould, Coulson, Patel,

Highton-Williamson, & Howard, 2014). Therefore, interventions targeting reduced benzodiazepine use, by withdrawing from them or changing prescribing, might help to reduce their use in older people (Gould et al., 2014).

Impact of Prescription Opioid Misuse in Older Adults

The aging process and its effects on body composition make older adults more sensitive to medications (Kaiser, 2009). For instance, older age (55 and older) has been identified as a risk factor for opioid-induced respiratory depression (Jarzyna et al., 2011). Also, misuse of opioids can lead to addiction and may cause accidents, mood changes, and cognitive decline (Ballantyne, 2012; Culberson & Ziska, 2008; Mailis-Gagnon et al., 2012). Nonmedical use of prescription opioids (use without a prescription of one's own or use only for the experience or feeling high) among older adults was found to be associated with falls, hip fracture, and traffic accidents (Buckeridge et al., 2010; Miller, Stürmer, Azrael, Levin, & Solomon, 2011). With respect to overdose and death, among adults aged 50 or older who visited the emergency department for prescription drug toxicity, pain relievers were most commonly involved (43.5%), with opioids being the most frequent type (Center for Behavioral Health Statistics and Quality, 2010), suggesting high rates of prescription opioid toxicity in this population. National data on hospital inpatient stays related to opioid overuse show that, from 1993 to 2012, the hospitalization rate increased more than five-fold for the three oldest age groups (45–64, 65–84, and 85 years and older), with the highest increase found in individuals 85 and older (Owens et al., 2014). A significant proportion of older adults receiving prescription opioids for chronic pain also consume other substances, with CNS depressants (alcohol and benzodiazepines) being the most common type. The combined use of alcohol and opioid drugs can have very detrimental effects on older adults' health and can quickly lead to respiratory depression and death (Borges et al., 2005).

Correlates of Prescription Opioid Misuse

Risk factors for prescription opioid misuse in general chronic pain patients receiving opioids are well documented, with a prior history of alcohol and illicit drug abuse being the most consistent predictor of misuse in patients with chronic pain, regardless of age (Jamison & Edwards, 2013; Sehgal, Manchikanti, & Smith, 2012; Turk, Swanson, & Gatchel, 2008). Other risk factors include pain-related functional limitations, cigarette smoking, family history of substance abuse, history of a mood disorder, history of childhood sexual abuse or neglect, legal system involvement, and significant psychosocial stressors (Boscarino et al., 2010; Broekmans, Dobbels, Milisen, Morlion, & Vanderschueren, 2010; Ives et al., 2006; Liebschutz et al., 2010; Wasan et al., 2007). Among female patients, those with more emotional distress were at increased risk of opioid misuse, whereas among males, those with legal problems tended to have a heightened risk of misuse (Jamison, Butler, Budman, Edwards, & Wasan, 2010). Other studies have suggested that opioid craving and catastrophic thinking are significantly associated with opioid misuse in chronic pain patients (Martel, Wasan, Jamison, & Edwards, 2013).

Several studies were conducted to examine risk factors of prescription opioid misuse in older adults with chronic pain. Lavin and Park (2011) found that higher levels of pain intensity, higher levels of depression, and lower levels of physical disability were associated with increased opioid misuse. Similar risk factors were found in a study conducted in western New York State, which found that older adults with illicit drug use, a moderate level of depression, and more functional pain interference had a greater risk of opioid misuse, defined as taking more than the prescribed dose (Chang, in press). Levi-Minzi and colleagues found that approximately 34 percent of their older adult participants reported substantial prescription opioid misuse (Levi-Minzi et al., 2013), supporting the finding of Chang (in press) that 35 percent of patients with chronic pain aged 50 or above reported misusing their prescription opioids in the past 30 days. Reflecting the national data, persistent pain patients aged 50–64 were more likely to misuse their prescription opioids than their older counterparts. In fact, more than 40 percent of participants in this age group reported prescription opioid misuse, which is slightly higher than the rate in general chronic pain patients (Boscarino et al., 2010; Vowles et al., 2015). Patients with chronic pain, aged 50–64, reflect the boomer generation; as this cohort ages, the prevalence of chronic pain will rise, with concern that increased opioid prescription use and misuse is likely to follow.

Those engaged in opioid misuse, particularly those that are middle-aged adults and older, often suffer from co-occurring mental health, chronic pain, and other substance use problems and likely to be high utilizers of hospital and community-based care services (Chang & Compton, 2013, 2016). Data from 2014 and 2015 Medicaid claims in eight western New York State counties suggested that those endorsing opioid misuse had significantly higher health care utilization across three types of services (emergency department (ED), outpatient, and inpatient) than those without opioid misuse, but older adults engaged in opioid misuse had significantly higher utilization across different types of health care services (Chang, Casucci, Xue, & Hewner, 2016). Higher ED use was correlated with sex, mental health comorbidities, smoking, other substance use disorders, and chronic pain (Chang et al., 2016). Furthermore, among adults with opioid misuse who were 50 or over, almost one-half (48.5%) had at least one type of mental health comorbidity, about 20 percent had chronic pain, 44.4 percent reported tobacco use, and about 3 percent reported other types substance use disorder. These results suggest that older adults with opioid misuse have higher health care needs due to the complexity of their comorbid chronic conditions.

A few studies have investigated reasons that older adults with chronic pain give for taking higher doses of prescription opioids than prescribed. Such reasons include accidental misuse, perhaps due to forgetfulness or confusion caused by multiple medication regimens; seeking immediate relief for poorly controlled pain; experiencing increased pain intensity due to poor activity pacing; wanting to be pain-free when spending time with family members and grandchildren; and experiencing negative emotions that intensify perceptions of pain (Chang, Compton, Almeter, & Fox, 2015). Older adults reported running out of prescription opioids due to overuse and then buying opioids from other sources or using over-the-counter analgesics to combat pain until their next appointment (Chang et al., 2015; Levi-Minzi et al., 2013). These findings highlight that self-management of chronic pain and multiple-medication regimens, social networks, and emotional status are important issues to be considered when delivering an intervention for prescription opioid misuse in older adults.

Behavioral Intervention to Reduce Prescription Opioid Misuse in Older Adults

Several factors make the primary care setting an important and unique one to address prescription opioid misuse in older adults with chronic pain. First, chronic pain is one of the most common reasons for primary care visits, and it has been estimated that more than 50 percent of chronic nonmalignant pain patients are managed in primary care settings (Breuer, Cruciani, & Portenoy, 2010). Second, chronic nonmalignant pain is highly prevalent in the geriatric population, and older adults often receive prescription opioids for their chronic pain. Third, compared to younger adults, older adults are more likely to misuse prescription opioids obtained from their regular doctors rather than from a drug dealer (Cicero, Surratt, Kurtz, Ellis, & Inciardi, 2012; Levi-Minzi et al., 2013). Finally, older adults presenting with mental health issues are more likely to seek and accept services in primary care versus specialty mental health care settings (Institute of Medicine, 2012). Thus, clinicians working in primary care settings are in a unique position to identify and intervene with older adult patients whose prescription opioid use may be hazardous to their health.

Brief interventions have been widely used in primary care to address a variety of behavioral health issues, including substance abuse and medication adherence in individuals with chronic conditions such as hypertension, diabetes, psychiatric disorders, and HIV (Barkhof, Meijer, de Sonneville, Linszen, & de Haan, 2012, 2013; Dray & Wade, 2012; Noordman, van der Weijden, & van Dulmen, 2012). Brief interventions for substance abuse in primary care typically range from 5 minutes of brief advice to 15–30 minutes of brief counseling (Substance Abuse and Mental Health Services Administration, 2014). Brief interventions in primary care are not designed to treat individuals with serious substance use disorders, but rather to manage problematic or risky substance use, like misuse (Substance Abuse and Mental Health Services Administration, 2014). The most commonly used types of brief behavioral interventions include brief cognitive behavioral therapy, motivational interviewing (MI), or their combination (Substance Abuse and Mental Health Services Administration, 2014).

Very little evidence has been found regarding the effects of behavioral interventions for older adults with prescription opioid misuse, with only one pilot study of MI in this population (Chang et al., 2015). The intervention included a diary to record medication taking and pain experience as well as education regarding pain management strategies, the risk of opioid misuse, and possible opioid-alcohol interactions. The intervention was delivered via an initial face-to-face session and three subsequent phone-delivered sessions.

This pilot study found that all participants completed the four intervention sessions and a one-month follow-up assessment; 5 of 30 did not complete the three-month follow-up. Participants reported high levels of satisfaction and found the MI intervention useful and the phone-delivered sessions convenient. Participants had a reduced risk of prescription opioid misuse immediately postintervention and at the one-month follow-up. From baseline to the one-month follow-up, participants reported improvement in self-efficacy for appropriate medication use as well as readiness to change medication use adherence. Pain intensity (rated for prior 24 hours for worst, least, average, and current levels) was reduced over time; statistically significant improvements were found for worst pain and least pain at one-month follow-up (Chang et al., 2015). The researchers also found that one-third of their study participants reported alcohol consumption. Those who used alcohol at baseline evidenced a reduction in alcohol use at immediately postintervention and the one-month follow-up.

There are significant gaps in the literature with regard to addressing the growing public health challenge of prescription opioid misuse in older adults: (1) interventions have targeted either opioid misuse or pain management, but evidence regarding the impact of interventions designed to simultaneously reduce prescription opioid misuse and promote pain self-management is lacking; (2) behavioral interventions for older adults with chronic pain have been examined only in a few feasibility studies, and brief interventions for reducing prescription opioid misuse in the primary care setting have not been developed in any age groups; (3) interventions developed for younger adults do not account for life-stage and aging process influences on older adults' reasons for misusing prescription opioids and motivations to change behavior (e.g., experiencing losses of a partner, occupation, family, and friends and desires to stay connected with remaining family while maintaining independence); and (4) mechanisms underlying the effects of behavioral interventions have not been well explored in the context of prescription opioid misuse or chronic pain management. Effective interventions for addressing prescription opioid misuse among older adults are urgently needed.

Strategies for Successful Management of Chronic Pain while Mitigating Opioid Misuse

In Chou's review (2015), substantial evidence was found to support the harms associated with opioid therapy across the population, including increased risk for overdose, opioid misuse and dependence, fractures, myocardial infarction, and sexual dysfunction. In addition, problematic side effects associated with opioid use, such as constipation, nausea, cognitive impairment, and potential opioid-induced hyperalgesia, limit the efficacy and utility of opioid therapy in the context of chronic pain. These findings suggest that opioid-sparing approaches be adopted, which concomitantly decrease the potential for the misuse of opioids in pain patients. Useful strategies for clinicians to balance the need to limit misuse with adequate pain management include a comprehensive patient assessment to identify patients at higher risk for substance use disorders and universal precautions to minimize opioid-related risks in all patients. These precautions incorporate the use of multimodal analgesia or abuse-deterrent opioid formulations (ADFs), random urine drug screening (UDS), participation in state-run prescription drug monitoring programs (PDMPs; see chapter 12 for more), and risk evaluation and mitigation strategy programs. Others include written opioid agreements and arranging frequent visits and use of specialty care for substance use treatment (McLellan & Turner, 2008).

Emerging signs of addiction can be identified and managed through regular monitoring, including UDS before every prescription is written, to assess for the presence of other opioids or drugs of abuse. Providers should be prepared to make a referral for specialty addiction treatment when indicated. Although addiction is a serious chronic condition, recovery is a predictable result of comprehensive, continuing care and monitoring (McLellan & Turner, 2008). In particular, the use of medication-assisted therapy significantly improves outcomes (e.g., methadone or buprenorphine) in those with both opioid addiction and co-occurring pain (Weiss, et al., 2015).

Conclusion

Currently, few studies have examined the efficacy of screening for risks or characteristics of older adults with prescription drug misuse in primary care settings, and few studies have assessed treatment or intervention strategies for opioid or benzodiazepine misuse in older adults. Older adults are at high risk for complications resulting from prescription opioid misuse. Inappropriate use of prescription opioids leads to poorer clinical outcomes and can cause injury, and neurocognitive alterations. Moreover, consuming other drugs, such as benzodiazepines or alcohol, with opioids increases the risk of drug-drug or drug-substance interactions and adverse reactions; this is especially true in older adults because of chronic illnesses and altered pharmacokinetics (Borges et al., 2005; Kaiser, 2009). The baby boomer generation representing 78 million Americans has shown the highest jump in prescription drug use. Prescription opioid misuse is likely to become an even greater problem as the baby boomer generation ages. Prevention and early behavioral intervention strategies are among the most promising and appropriate methods for maximizing health outcomes and minimizing health costs in this fast-growing population of older adults. Prescription opioid misuse and chronic pain both result in substantial health cost and often co-occur, therefore should be managed concurrently.

References

American Geriatrics Society Beers Criteria Update Expert Panel. (2012). American Geriatrics Society updated Beers Criteria for potentially inappropriate medication use in older adults. *Journal of the American Geriatrics Society, 60*(4), 616–631. doi:10.1111/j.1532-5415.2012.03923.x.

Ballantyne, J. C. (2012). "Safe and effective when used as directed": The case of chronic use of opioid analgesics. *Journal of Medical Toxicology, 8*(4), 417–423. doi:10.1007/s13181-012-0257-8.

Barkhof, E., Meijer, C. J., de Sonneville, L. M. J., Linszen, D. H., & de Haan, L. (2012). Interventions to improve adherence to antipsychotic medication in patients with schizophrenia—A review of the past decade. *European Psychiatry, 27*(1), 9–18. doi:https://doi.org/10.1016/j.eurpsy.2011.02.005.

Barkhof, E., Meijer, C. J., de Sonneville, L. M. J., Linszen, D. H., & de Haan, L. (2013). The effect of motivational interviewing on medication adherence and hospitalization rates in nonadherent patients with multi-episode schizophrenia. *Schizophrenia Bulletin, 39*(6), 1242–1251. doi:10.1093/schbul/sbt138.

Beaudoin, F. L., Merchant, R. C., & Clark, M. A. (2016). Prevalence and detection of prescription opioid misuse and prescription opioid use disorder among emergency department patients 50 years of age and older: Performance of the Prescription Drug Use Questionnaire, Patient Version. *American Journal of Geriatric Psychiatry, 24*(8), 627–636. doi:https://doi.org/10.1016/j.jagp.2016.03.010.

Birnbaum, H. G., White, A. G., Schiller, M., Waldman, T., Cleveland, J. M., & Roland, C. L. (2011). Societal costs of prescription opioid abuse, dependence, and misuse in the United States. *Pain Medicine, 12*(4), 657–667. doi:10.1111/j.1526-4637.2011.01075.x.

Borges, G., Mondragon, L., Medina-Mora, M. E., Orozco, R., Zambrano, J., & Cherpitel, C. (2005). A case-control study of alcohol and substance use disorders as risk factors for non-fatal injury. *Alcohol and Alcoholism, 40*(4), 257–262. doi:10.1093/alcalc/agh160.

Boscarino, J. A., Rukstalis, M., Hoffman, S. N., Han, J. J., Erlich, P. M., Gerhard, G. S., & Stewart W. F. (2010). Risk factors for drug dependence among out-patients on opioid therapy in a large US health-care system. *Addiction, 105*(10), 1776–1782. doi:10.1111/j.1360-0443.2010.03052.x.

Breuer, B., Cruciani, R., & Portenoy, R. K. (2010). Pain management by primary care physicians, pain physicians, chiropractors, and acupuncturists: A national survey. *Southern Medical Journal, 103*(8), 738–747. doi:10.1097 /SMJ.0b013e3181e74ede.

Broekmans, S., Dobbels, F., Milisen, K., Morlion, B., & Vanderschueren, S. (2010). Determinants of medication underuse and medication overuse in patients with chronic non-malignant pain: A multicenter study. *International Journal of Nursing Studies, 47*(11), 1408–1417. doi:https://doi .org/10.1016/j.ijnurstu.2010.03.014.

Buckeridge, D., Huang, A., Hanley, J., Kelome, A., Reidel, K., Verma, A., . . . Tamblyn, R. (2010). Risk of injury associated with opioid use in older adults. *Journal of the American Geriatrics Society, 58*(9), 1664–1670. doi:10 .1111/j.1532-5415.2010.03015.x.

Buffett-Jerrott, S. E., & Stewart, S. H. (2002). Cognitive and sedative effects of benzodiazepine use. *Current Pharmaceutical Design, 8*(1), 45–58.

Center for Behavioral Health Statistics and Quality. (2010). *The DAWN Report: Drug-related Emergency Department Visits Involving Pharmaceutical Misuse and Abuse by Older Adults.* Rockville, MD: Substance Abuse and Mental Health Services Administration.

Center for Behavioral Health Statistics and Quality. (2015). *Behavioral Health Trends in the United States: Results from the 2014 National Survey on Drug Use and Health* (HHS Publication No. SMA 15-4927, NSDUH Series H-50). http://www.samhsa.gov/data.

Centers for Disease Control and Prevention. (2016). *Wide-ranging Online Data for Epidemiologic Research (WONDER).* Atlanta, GA: CDC, National Center for Health Statistics http://wonder.cdc.gov.

Centers for Disease Control and Prevention, National Center for Health Statistics, National Vital Statistics System, Mortality File. (2015). *Number and Age-adjusted Rates of Drug-poisoning Deaths Involving Opioid Analgesics and Heroin: United States, 2000–2014.* Atlanta, GA: Centers for Disease Control and Prevention. http://www.cdc.gov/nchs/data/health_policy/AADR_drug _poisoning_involving_OA_Heroin_US_2000-2014.pdf.

Chang, Y. P. (in press). Factors associated with prescription opioid misuse in adults aged 50 or above. *Nursing Outlook*.doi:10.1016/j.outlook.2017.10.007.

Chang, Y. P., Casucci, S., Xue, Y., & Hewner, S. (2016). *Medicaid Utilization Patterns among Opioid Abusers in Western New York: Using Data Mining and Cluster Analysis to Customize Treatment Plans.* Paper presented at the 2016

National State of the Science Congress on Nursing Research, Washington, D.C., September 15–17.

Chang, Y. P., & Compton, P. (2013). Management of chronic pain with chronic opioid therapy in patients with substance use disorders. *Addiction Science & Clinical Practice, 8*(1), 21. doi:10.1186/1940-0640-8-21.

Chang, Y. P., & Compton, P. (2016). Opioid misuse/abuse and quality persistent pain management in older adults. *Journal of Gerontological Nursing, 42*(12), 21–30. doi:10.3928/00989134-20161110-06.

Chang, Y. P., Compton, P., Almeter, P., & Fox, C. H. (2015). The effect of motivational interviewing on prescription opioid adherence among older adults with chronic pain. *Perspectives in Psychiatric Care, 51*(3), 211–219. doi:10.1111/ppc.12082.

Chou, R. (2010). Pharmacological management of low back pain. *Drugs, 70*(4), 387–402. doi:10.2165/11318690-000000000-00000.

Chou, R., Turner, J. A., Devine, E. B., Hansen, R. D., Sullivan, S. D., Blazina, I., . . . Deyo, R. A. (2015). The effectiveness and risks of long-term opioid therapy for chronic pain: A systematic review for a national institutes of health pathways to prevention workshop. *Annals of Internal Medicine, 162*(4), 276–286. doi:10.7326/M14-2559.

Cicero, T. J., Surratt, H. L., Kurtz, S., Ellis, M. S., & Inciardi, J. A. (2012). Patterns of prescription opioid abuse and co-morbidity in an aging treatment population. *Journal of Substance Abuse Treatment, 42*(1), 87–94. doi:10.1016/j.jsat.2011.07.003.

Clegg, A., & Young, J. B. (2011). Which medications to avoid in people at risk of delirium: A systematic review. *Age and Ageing, 40*(1), 23–29. doi:10.1093/ageing/afq140.

Culberson, J. W., & Ziska, M. (2008). Prescription drug misuse/abuse in the elderly. *Geriatrics (Basel, Switzerland), 63*(9), 22–31.

Cumming, R. G., & Conteur, D. G. L. (2003). Benzodiazepines and risk of hip fractures in older people. *CNS Drugs, 17*(11), 825–837. doi:10.2165/00023210-200317110-00004.

Dionne, P. A., Vasiliadis, H. M., Latimer, E., Berbiche, D., & Preville, M. (2013). Economic impact of inappropriate benzodiazepine prescribing and related drug interactions among elderly persons. *Psychiatric Services, 64*(4), 331–338. doi:10.1176/appi.ps.201200089.

Dray, J., & Wade, T. D. (2012). Is the transtheoretical model and motivational interviewing approach applicable to the treatment of eating disorders? A review. *Clinical Psychology Review, 32*(6), 558–565. doi:https://doi.org/10.1016/j.cpr.2012.06.005.

Frank, J. W., Binswanger, I. A., Calcaterra, S. L., Brenner, L. A., & Levy, C. (2015). Non-medical use of prescription pain medications and increased emergency department utilization: Results of a national survey. *Drug and Alcohol Dependence, 157*, 150–157. doi:10.1016/j.drugalcdep.2015.10.027.

Gladden, R. M., Martinez, P., & Seth, P. (2016). Fentanyl law enforcement submissions and increases in synthetic opioid-involved overdose deaths—27 states, 2013–2014. *MMWR: Morbidity and Mortality Weekly Report, 65*(33), 837–843. doi:10.15585/mmwr.mm6533a2.

Gould, R. L., Coulson, M. C., Patel, N., Highton-Williamson, E., & Howard, R. J. (2014). Interventions for reducing benzodiazepine use in older people: Meta-analysis of randomised controlled trials. *British Journal of Psychiatry, 204*(2), 98–107. doi:10.1192/bjp.bp.113.126003.

Hill, K. D., & Wee, R. (2012). Psychotropic drug-induced falls in older people. *Drugs & Aging, 29*(1), 15–30. doi:10.2165/11598420-000000000-00000.

Institute of Medicine. (2012). The mental health and substance use workforce for older adults: In whose hands? http://www.iom.edu/Reports/2012/The-Mental-Health-and-Substance-Use-Workforce-for-Older-Adults.aspx.

Ives, T. J., Chelminski, P. R., Hammett-Stabler, C. A., Malone, R. M., Perhac, J. S., Potisek, N. M., . . . Pignone, M. P. (2006). Predictors of opioid misuse in patients with chronic pain: A prospective cohort study. *BMC Health Services Research, 6,* 46. doi:10.1186/1472-6963-6-46.

Jamison, R. N., Butler, S. F., Budman, S. H., Edwards, R. R., & Wasan, A. D. (2010). Gender differences in risk factors for aberrant prescription opioid use. *Journal of Pain, 11*(4), 312–320. doi:https://doi.org/10.1016/j.jpain.2009.07.016.

Jamison, R. N., & Edwards, R. R. (2013). Risk factor assessment for problematic use of opioids for chronic pain. *Clinical Neuropsychologist, 27*(1), 60–80. doi:10.1080/13854046.2012.715204.

Jarzyna, D., Jungquist, C. R., Pasero, C., Willens, J. S., Nisbet, A., Oakes, L., . . . Polomano, R. C. (2011). American Society for Pain Management Nursing guidelines on monitoring for opioid-induced sedation and respiratory depression. *Pain Management Nursing, 12*(3), 118–145.e110. doi:10.1016/j.pmn.2011.06.008.

Johannes, C. B., Le, T. K., Zhou, X., Johnston, J. A., & Dworkin, R. H. (2010). The prevalence of chronic pain in United States adults: Results of an Internet-based survey. *Journal of Pain, 11*(11), 1230–1239. doi:https://doi.org/10.1016/j.jpain.2010.07.002.

Johnell, K., & Fastbom, J. (2009). The use of benzodiazepines and related drugs amongst older people in Sweden: Associated factors and concomitant use of other psychotropics. *International Journal of Geriatric Psychiatry, 24*(7), 731–738. doi:10.1002/gps.2189.

Kaiser, R. M. (2009). Physiological and clinical considerations of geriatric patient care. In D. G. Blazer & D. C. Steffens (Eds.), *The American Psychiatric Publishing Textbook of Geriatric Psychiatry,* 45–62. Washington, D.C.: American Psychiatric Publishing.

Kaye, A. D., Jones, M. R., Kaye, A. M., Ripoll, J. G., Galan, V., Beakley, B. D., . . . Manchikanti L. (2017). Prescription opioid abuse in chronic pain: An updated review of opioid abuse predictors and strategies to curb opioid abuse: Part 1. *Pain Physician, 20*(2S), S93–S109.

Landreat, M. G., Vigneau, C. V., Hardouin, J. B., Bronnec, M. G., Marais, M., Venisse, J. L., & Jolliet, P. (2010). Can we say that seniors are addicted to benzodiazepines? *Substance Use & Misuse, 45*(12), 1988–1999. doi:10.3109 /10826081003777568.

Larance, B., Degenhardt, L., Lintzeris, N., Winstock, A., & Mattick, R. (2011). Definitions related to the use of pharmaceutical opioids: Extramedical use, diversion, non-adherence and aberrant medication-related behaviours. *Drug and Alcohol Review, 30*(3), 236–245. doi:10.1111/j.1465 -3362.2010.00283.x.

Lavin, R., & Park, J. (2011). Depressive symptoms in community-dwelling older adults receiving opioid therapy for chronic pain. *Journal of Opioid Management, 7*(4), 309–319.

Levi-Minzi, M. A., Surratt, H. L., Kurtz, S. P., & Buttram, M. E. (2013). Under treatment of pain: A prescription for opioid misuse among the elderly? *Pain Medicine (Malden, Mass.), 14*(11), 10.1111/pme.12189. doi:10.1111/pme.12189.

Liebschutz, J. M., Saitz, R., Weiss, R. D., Averbuch, T., Schwartz, S., Meltzer, E. C., . . . Samet, J. H. (2010). Clinical factors associated with prescription drug use disorder in urban primary care patients with chronic pain. *Journal of Pain, 11*(11), 1047–1055. doi:10.1016/j.jpain.2009.10.012.

Ling, W., Mooney, L., & Hillhouse, M. (2011). Prescription opioid abuse, pain and addiction: Clinical issues and implications. *Drug and Alcohol Review, 30*(3), 300–305. doi:10.1111/j.1465-3362.2010.00271.x.

Lipari, R. N., Williams, M., & Van Horn, S. L. (2017). *Why Do Adults Misuse Prescription Drugs? The CBHSQ Report*. Rockville, MD: Center for Behavioral Health Statistics and Quality, Substance Abuse and Mental Health Services Administration.

Mailis-Gagnon, A., Lakha, S. F., Furlan, A., Nicholson, K., Yegneswaran, B., & Sabatowski, R. (2012). Systematic review of the quality and generalizability of studies on the effects of opioids on driving and cognitive/psychomotor performance. *Clinical Journal of Pain, 28*(6), 542–555. doi:10.1097 /AJP.0b013e3182385332.

Makris, U. E., Abrams, R. C., Gurland, B., & Reid, M. C. (2014). Management of persistent pain in the older patient: A clinical review. *JAMA, 312*(8), 825–836. doi:10.1001/jama.2014.9405.

Maree, R. D., Marcum, Z. A., Saghafi, E., Weiner, D. K., & Karp, J. F. (2016). A systematic review of opioid and benzodiazepine misuse in older adults. *American Journal of Geriatric Psychiatry, 24*(11), 949–963. doi:https://doi .org/10.1016/j.jagp.2016.06.003.

Martel, M. O., Wasan, A. D., Jamison, R. N., & Edwards, R. R. (2013). Catastrophic thinking and increased risk for prescription opioid misuse in patients with chronic pain. *Drug and Alcohol Dependence, 132*(0), 335–341. doi:10.1016/j.drugalcdep.2013.02.034.

Martinsson, G., Fagerberg, I., Wiklund-Gustin, L., & Lindholm, C. (2012). Specialist prescribing of psychotropic drugs to older persons in Sweden—A register-based study of 188,024 older persons. *BMC Psychiatry, 12*(1), 197. doi:10.1186/1471-244x-12-197.

McLellan, A., & Turner, B. (2008). Prescription opioids, overdose deaths, and physician responsibility. *JAMA, 300*(22), 2672–2673. doi:10.1001/jama.2008.793.

Meuleners, L. B., Duke, J., Lee, A. H., Palamara, P., Hildebrand, J., & Ng, J. Q. (2011). Psychoactive medications and crash involvement requiring hospitalization for older drivers: A population-based study. *Journal of the American Geriatrics Society, 59*(9), 1575–1580. doi:10.1111/j.1532-5415.2011.03561.x.

Miller, M., Stürmer, T., Azrael, D., Levin, R., & Solomon, D. H. (2011). Opioid analgesics and the risk of fractures among older adults with arthritis. *Journal of the American Geriatrics Society, 59*(3), 430–438. doi:10.1111/j.1532-5415.2011.03318.x.

Noordman, J., van der Weijden, T., & van Dulmen, S. (2012). Communication-related behavior change techniques used in face-to-face lifestyle interventions in primary care: A systematic review of the literature. *Patient Education and Counseling, 89*(2), 227–244. doi:https://doi.org/10.1016/j.pec.2012.07.006.

Owens, P. L., Barrett, M. L., Weiss, A. J., Washington, R. E., & Kronick, R. (2014). Hospital inpatient utilization related to opioid overuse among adults, 1993–2012: Statistical Brief #177. *Healthcare Cost and Utilization Project (HCUP) Statistical Briefs.* Rockville, MD: Agency for Healthcare Research and Quality.

Peterson, A. B., Gladden, R. M., Delcher, C., Spies, E., Garcia-Williams, A., Wang, Y., et al. (2016). Increases in fentanyl-related overdose deaths— Florida and Ohio, 2013–2015. *MMWR: Morbidity and Mortality Weekly Report, 65*(33), 844–849. doi:10.15585/mmwr.mm6533a3.

Préville, M., Vasiliadis, H.-M., Bossé, C., Dionne, P.-A., Voyer, P., & Brassard, J. (2011). Pattern of psychotropic drug use among older adults having a depression or an anxiety disorder: Results from the Longitudinal ESA Study. *Canadian Journal of Psychiatry, 56*(6), 348–357. doi:10.1177/070674371105600606.

Reid, M. C., Eccleston, C., & Pillemer, K. (2015). Management of chronic pain in older adults. *BMJ: British Medical Journal, 350*, h532. doi:10.1136/bmj.h532.

Rudd, R. A., Seth, P., David, F., & Scholl, L. (2016). Increases in drug and opioid-involved overdose deaths—United States, 2010–2015. *MMWR: Morbidity and Mortality Weekly Report, 65*(5051), 1445–1452. doi:10.15585/mmwr.mm655051e1.

Schepis, T. S., & McCabe, S. E. (2016). Trends in older adult nonmedical prescription drug use prevalence: Results from the 2002–2003 and 2012–2013 National Survey on Drug Use and Health. *Addictive Behaviors, 60*, 219–222. doi:10.1016/j.addbeh.2016.04.020.

Sehgal, N., Manchikanti, L., & Smith, H. S. (2012). Prescription opioid abuse in chronic pain: A review of opioid abuse predictors and strategies to curb opioid abuse. *Pain Physician, 15*(3 Suppl), ES67–92.

Substance Abuse and Mental Health Services Administration. (2014). SBIRT: Brief intervention. http://www.integration.samhsa.gov/clinical-practice /sbirt/brief-interventions.

Turk, D. C., Swanson, K. S., & Gatchel, R. J. (2008). Predicting opioid misuse by chronic pain patients: A systematic review and literature synthesis. *Clinical Journal of Pain, 24*(6), 497–508. doi:10.1097/AJP.0b013e31816b1070.

van Hecke, O., Torrance, N., & Smith, B. H. (2013). Chronic pain epidemiology and its clinical relevance. *British Journal of Anaesthesia, 111*(1), 13–18. doi:10.1093/bja/aet123.

Vowles, K. E., McEntee, M. L., Julnes, P. S., Frohe, T., Ney, J. P., & van der Goes, D. N. (2015). Rates of opioid misuse, abuse, and addiction in chronic pain: A systematic review and data synthesis. *Pain, 156*(4), 569–576. doi: 10.1097/01.j.pain.0000460357.01998.f1.

Voyer, P., Preville, M., Cohen, D., Berbiche, D., & Beland, S. G. (2010). The prevalence of benzodiazepine dependence among community-dwelling older adult users in Quebec according to typical and atypical criteria. *Canadian Journal on Aging, 29*(2), 205–213. doi:10.1017/s0714980 810000115.

Voyer, P., Préville, M., Martin, L. S., Roussel, M. E., Béland, S. G., & Berbiche, D. (2011). Factors associated with self-rated benzodiazepine addiction among community-dwelling seniors. *Journal of Addictions Nursing, 22*(1-2), 46–56. doi:10.3109/10884602.2010.545087.

Wasan, A. D., Butler, S. F., Budman, S. H., Benoit, C., Fernandez, K., & Jamison, R. N. (2007). Psychiatric history and psychologic adjustment as risk factors for aberrant drug-related behavior among patients with chronic pain. *Clinical Journal of Pain, 23*(4), 307–315. doi:10.1097/AJP .0b013e3180330dc5.

Weiss, R. D., Potter, J. S., Griffin, M. L., Provost, S. E., Fitzmaurice, G. D., McDermott, K. A., et al. (2015). Long-term outcomes from the National Drug Abuse Treatment Clinical Trials Network Prescription Opioid Addiction Treatment Study. *Drug and Alcohol Dependence, 150*, 112–119. doi:10.1016/j.drugalcdep.2015.02.030.

White, A. P., Arnold, P. M., Norvell, D. C., Ecker, E., & Fehlings, M. G. (2011). Pharmacologic management of chronic low back pain: Synthesis of the evidence. *Spine, 36*(21 Suppl), S131–143. doi:10.1097/BRS.0b013e 31822f178f.

CHAPTER NINE

Opioids: Misuse and Guideline-Concordant Use in Pain Management

William C. Becker and Joanna L. Starrels

Introduction

For centuries, opioids have been effective in the treatment of acute pain and pain at the end of life. While these practices continued, the United States witnessed a marked surge in opioid prescribing for chronic pain from the 1990s into the 2010s, despite insufficient evidence of opioids' effectiveness for chronic pain and mounting evidence of harms.

Through a well-established neurohormonal cascade, opioids stimulate the reward center of the brain. Because this reward center evolved to encourage humans to perform such survival behaviors as eating and having sex, stimulating this pathway causes a dopamine surge that encourages continued behavior. In susceptible individuals, for example, those with a genetic predisposition due to allelic variation at the mu-opioid receptor, this response can lead to misuse and opioid use disorder. As opioid prescribing has increased and more susceptible individuals have been exposed, so too have prescription opioid misuse and its consequences. Furthermore, whether misused or taken as prescribed, opioid analgesics can have serious adverse effects, especially when taken at high doses or over long periods of time. It is important that clinicians treating patients with acute or chronic pain prescribe these medications cautiously to help mitigate the risks to patients and society.

This chapter reviews the epidemiology of prescription opioid use with a focus on individuals with chronic pain, our evolving understanding of opioids' role in chronic pain management, and strategies for clinicians to help prevent, identify, and manage prescription opioid misuse.

Terminology

The wide variety of terms related to opioid misuse can be confusing, impeding the ability of clinicians to communicate clearly with each other as well as with patients. Furthermore, imprecise terminology can compound challenges in diagnosis and treatment. Importantly, slang or non-person-centered terms can be stigmatizing (Kelly, Wakeman, & Saitz, 2015). For example, a *person with opioid misuse* or *a person with opioid use disorder* is preferred over the nouns *abuser* or *addict*. Stigmatizing language can discourage people from seeking treatment and alienate individuals in treatment, and it is inconsistent with ethical principles of beneficence and respect for persons. For all these reasons, we recommend consistent use of straightforward person-centered terms as described in this section.

Prescription opioid misuse is defined as any use of a prescribed opioid outside of the manner and intent for which it was prescribed. Among individuals prescribed opioids, this includes overuse (either in terms of frequency or dose), use to get high or achieve euphoria, diversion (sharing or selling to others), having multiple prescribers or nonprescribed sources of the medication, and concurrent use of alcohol, illicit substances, or nonprescribed controlled medications. The National Survey on Drug Use and Health (NSDUH), sponsored by the Substance Abuse and Mental Health Services Administration (SAMHSA), is the largest and longest-running U.S. household survey about drug use among individuals 12 years and older. In 2015, it eliminated its prior term "non-medical use of prescription opioids" in favor of the term *misuse*, which the survey defines as use in any way not directed by a doctor, including use without a prescription of one's own; use in greater amounts, more often, or longer than told to take a drug; or use in any other way not directed by a doctor.

Opioid use disorder is a criterion-based diagnosis from the DSM-5 that can be specified as mild, moderate, or severe and indicates compulsive use of opioids despite harm. In a person taking opioids as prescribed under medical supervision for chronic pain, two criteria—tolerance and withdrawal—should not be used in support of a diagnosis of opioid use disorder because they are expected among patients who take long-term opioids and do not necessarily suggest a use disorder. That said, instances where an individual overuses medication and runs out early, inducing withdrawal symptoms, could contribute to the diagnosis.

Epidemiology

Misuse

In the 2015 administration of the NSDUH, about 97.5 million people (36.4%) had used prescription opioids and approximately 12.5 million people (4.7%) had misused prescription opioids in the past year (Substance Abuse and Mental Health Services Administration, 2016). Among individuals reporting prescription opioid use in the past year, 16 percent reported misusing them. Among those with past-year prescription opioid misuse, the most commonly reported reason for their last misuse episode was to relieve physical pain (62.6%), and the most common source for the last pain reliever that was misused was either given by, bought from, or taken from a friend or relative (53.7%). Approximately one-third of individuals reporting past-year prescription opioid misuse misused a prescription from one doctor.

In a recent systematic review, the prevalence of opioid misuse among patients prescribed opioid analgesics for chronic pain was estimated to be 21–29 percent (Vowles et al., 2015), though published estimates vary widely due to differences in the populations and definitions of misuse among studies. Across studies, 16–78 percent of patients who were prescribed long-term opioid therapy (LTOT: generally, three months or greater) for chronic noncancer pain engaged in opioid misuse (Banta-Green, Merrill, Doyle, Boudreau, & Calsyn, 2009; Banta-Green et al., 2010; Fleming, Balousek, Klessig, Mundt, & Brown, 2007; Ives et al., 2006; Morasco & Dobscha, 2008; Reid et al., 2002). It is generally accepted that absolute numbers of individuals with prescription opioid misuse have increased due to the widespread surge in opioid prescribing for acute and chronic pain. Given efforts to educate prescribers on identification of misuse and their response to it, one might hypothesize a decrease in the proportion of individuals prescribed who exhibit misuse; this is not yet known. It is also not yet known whether recent data indicating declining opioid prescribing in some U.S. health systems have been accompanied by concomitant decreases in misuse (Mosher et al., 2015).

Of U.S. veterans treated in a primary care settings, 4.8 percent reported opioid analgesic misuse (Becker et al., 2009). Interestingly, the 2016 Monitoring the Future Survey, a survey funded by the National Institute on Drug Abuse (NIDA) of over 45,000 public and private high school students, found a marked decline in past-year misuse of prescription opioids among high school seniors over the previous five years: from 8.7 percent to 4.8 percent (National Institute on Drug Abuse, 2016).

Opioid Use Disorder

In the United States, the prevalence of opioid use disorder involving prescription opioids has dramatically increased. Among individuals seeking treatment for substance use disorder, 9.3 percent cited non-heroin opioids as their primary substance in 2013, compared to only 1.0 percent in 1995 (Substance Abuse and Mental Health Services Administration, 2015b; Wu, Zhu, & Swartz, 2016), most were white (88%; Substance Abuse and Mental Health Services Administration, 2015a, 2015b). Another shift is that, in 2010, individuals living in rural counties (10.6%) were more likely than those in urban counties (4.0%) to cite non-heroin opioids as their primary substance (Substance Abuse and Mental Health Services Administration, 2012).

In the 2015 NSDUH, approximately 0.7 percent of people 12 years old or older (2 million) reported criteria consistent with a prescription drug use disorder in the past year, with the majority of this driven by opioid misuse. In 2015, as part of their most recent substance use treatment, 822,000 people received treatment for the misuse of prescription opioids.

In a systematic review, the incidence of opioid use disorder among patients prescribed opioids for chronic pain was estimated to be 8–12 percent (Vowles et al., 2015). Cross-sectional studies have reported the prevalence of opioid abuse and dependence (terms from DSM-IV) among patients prescribed LTOT for chronic pain to range from 3 percent to 26 percent (Boscarino et al., 2010; Fleming et al., 2007; Liebschutz et al., 2010). In a 2007 study among veterans, the incidence of abuse and dependence diagnoses recorded in the medical record among patients prescribed long-term opioid therapy was 2 percent per year (Edlund, Steffick, Hudson, Harris, & Sullivan, 2007).

Morbidity and Mortality

Morbidity and mortality associated with opioid use have skyrocketed since the 1990s, leading many to use the term the *opioid epidemic*. In 2015, more than 52,000 deaths from drug overdose occurred in the United States, and more than 60 percent involved opioid analgesics (Kandel, Hu, Griesler, & Wall, 2017). Approximately 30 percent of overdose deaths involving prescription opioids also involved benzodiazepines (Kandel et al., 2017), which act synergistically with opioids to cause sedation and respiratory depression. Men have higher risk of overdose death than women, though between 1999 and 2014, overdose death involving opioid analgesics increased 516 percent among women and 300 percent among men (Centers for Disease Control and Prevention, 2013).

Importantly, overdose deaths involving prescription opioids reached a plateau between 2010 and 2015, but deaths involving illicit opioids such as heroin or illicit fentanyl continued to climb, driving the steady increase in overall opioid-related death (Rudd, Aleshire, Zibbell, & Gladden, 2016). Reasons for this are likely multifactorial. Individuals with opioid use disorder may transition to using illicit opioids due to lower cost or prescription opioids becoming unavailable, for example, if the prescriber stops prescribing (Compton, Jones, & Baldwin, 2016). In addition, the greater demand for opioids has led to an increasing supply of illicit opioids, making the latter easier to obtain in diverse geographic regions (Unick & Ciccarone, 2017). Further, the potency of illicit opioids is inconsistent; for example, heroin may be contaminated with potent opioids such as carfentanil, increasing the risk of accidental overdose death.

Although nonfatal and fatal overdose are the most catastrophic harms associated with opioid use and misuse, research suggests several other important harms are associated with opioids. A systematic review by Chou et al. (2015) identified good- and fair-quality observational studies suggesting that opioid therapy for chronic pain is associated with increased risk for fractures, motor vehicle accidents, myocardial infarction, and markers of sexual dysfunction.

Risk Factors for Opioid Misuse

Based on prior research, several factors increase a patient's risk of developing opioid misuse when prescribed opioids for chronic pain. The most significant risk factor is having a personal history of a substance use disorder, including a tobacco or alcohol use disorder (Edlund et al., 2007; Ives et al., 2006; Liebschutz et al., 2010; Morasco & Dobscha, 2008; Reid et al., 2002). Other important risk factors include a family history of a substance use disorder (Liebschutz et al., 2010); a mental health disorder, such as depression or posttraumatic stress disorder; a history of legal problems or incarceration; and age less than 40–45 years old. White race (compared with black race) is associated with prescription opioid misuse (Liebschutz et al., 2010); yet, studies have identified greater clinician concern and closer monitoring for black patients, suggesting evidence of clinician bias (Becker et al., 2011; Hausmann, Gao, Lee, & Kwoh, 2013; Vijayaraghavan, Penko, Guzman, Miaskowski, & Kushel, 2011). In addition, age over 65, multiple co-occurring conditions, high-dose prescription opioid use, and concurrent benzodiazepine use are associated with increased risk of overdose death.

Evolving Guidance on the Use of Opioids in the Treatment of Chronic Pain

In 2016, the Centers for Disease Control and Prevention (CDC) released the Guideline for Prescribing Opioids for Chronic Pain (Dowell, Haegerich, & Chou, 2016). Compared to the last major guideline, 2009's APS/AAPM Clinical Guidelines for the Use of Chronic Opioid Therapy in Chronic Noncancer Pain (Chou et al., 2009), the CDC guideline goes further to discourage use of opioids for chronic pain insofar as it promotes nonopioid and nonpharmacologic treatment options as preferred in the treatment of chronic pain; cautions against increasing opioid dose beyond specified limits; and advocates for regular monitoring of risks and benefits for indications to taper or discontinue opioids among patients already on LTOT. The CDC guideline also places much greater emphasis on the modest benefit LTOT has demonstrated and the clear evidence of harm, especially at higher doses.

The CDC guideline ushered in a growing appreciation that high-quality care for patients with chronic pain requires a blend of nonpharmacological and pharmacological options; that treatments where patients take an active role (e.g., yoga) are particularly valuable; that self-management skill building (i.e., teaching patients skills they can use on their own to combat pain flares, such as meditation, deep breathing, use of cold packs/hot packs, and guided imagery) is low-cost, effective, and promotes nonreliance on the health care system; and that it may be in patients' best interests in the near-, intermediate-, and especially long-term to avoid opioids. The recommendation to avoid LTOT for the treatment of chronic pain is not only to avoid risks of opioid use disorder or overdose but, importantly, in recognition of observational studies and emerging clinical trial data demonstrating that patients may experience accelerated decline in functional status and accrue s variety of bothersome and sometimes serious harms from LTOT.

That said, millions of Americans continue to use LTOT. Our goal below is to describe measures to prevent incident opioid misuse and opioid use disorder, techniques to monitor for misuse, and strategies for treatment should it arise.

Preventing Opioid Misuse in Chronic Pain

Assessing Risks and Benefits

Guidelines for opioid prescribing emphasize that opioids should only be prescribed when the benefits outweigh the risks for the individual patient (Dowell et al., 2016; Opioid Therapy for Chronic Pain Work Group, 2017). There is general agreement that current untreated substance use disorder, poorly controlled psychiatric illness, and inability or unwillingness to follow-up with the clinic for reassessment represent contraindications to prescribing opioids. In the absence of these contraindications, providers and patients must weigh the risks and benefits as best as they can, acknowledging some degree of uncertainty.

Though several tools have been developed to help predict a patient's risk of developing opioid misuse (Butler, Fernandez, Benoit, Budman, & Jamison, 2008; Compton, Wu, Schieffer, Pham, & Naliboff, 2008; Webster & Webster, 2005), few have been well validated, and none have been shown to improve outcomes. Whether a standardized tool is used or not, it is critical for a prescriber to collect data about opioid use and opioid-related risk from several sources. Interviewing the patient is the primary source, and the interview should include a complete pain, substance use, and mental health history as well as a family and social history. Physical examination can assess for signs of opioid use or withdrawal as well as signs of substance use, such as injection marks. Patient data can be supplemented by collateral information from other providers, family or friends, and objective data from urine drug tests (see "Drug Testing") and the state prescription drug monitoring program (PDMP).

A careful risk assessment helps the clinician decide whether to prescribe opioids, and if the decision is made to prescribe them, the risk assessment is important to guide care. For example, patients at elevated risk are likely to need higher intensity of monitoring, including more frequent visits; greater counseling and risk reduction, including prescription for naloxone; and additional support, such as behavioral health or pain management specialty care.

The risks must be considered alongside the benefits. Importantly, a patient's experience of pain is subjective, and each patient's experience of pain is unique. Further, the goal of managing chronic pain should be less to reduce pain intensity and more to improve a patient's function and quality of life. Therefore, it is recommended that clinicians use functional benchmarks to measure treatment outcomes. These may include specific patient-defined functional goals or standardized scales. The PEG scale is a validated three-item scale measuring pain intensity and pain-related interference with function and quality of life that can be used in diverse settings (Krebs et al., 2009).

Communicating with Patients

As with any pharmacotherapy, clinicians should discuss the potential risks, benefits, and treatment alternatives before prescribing opioids. Written treatment agreements help guide the conversation between prescribers and patients about risks of controlled substances and the strategies that will be used to monitor for and respond to any harms that become apparent during treatment. Though evidence is lacking for the effectiveness of using treatment agreements in reducing opioid misuse (Starrels et al., 2010), most experts recommend them as a platform for documenting a discussion about risks and benefits, setting patient goals, and outlining the monitoring plan and expectations if concerning behaviors arise (Chou et al., 2009).

Limiting Opioid Exposure

For acute pain, such as pain associated with an injury or procedure, it is recommended that prescribers prescribe the lowest effective dose and no more than a three- to seven-day supply (Dowell et al., 2016). Higher daily doses of prescribed opioids and greater numbers of prescriptions per month have been associated with increased risk of overdose death when compared to lower daily doses and fewer prescriptions (Bohnert, Ilgen, Galea, McCarthy, & Blow, 2011; Dunn et al., 2010; Paulozzi et al., 2012). This is likely due to greater respiratory depression at higher doses for patients with insufficient tolerance. Having an excess of pills is also likely to increase opportunities for diversion or misuse, and intermittent pill counts can be useful to identify or dissuade from diversion. The CDC recommends limiting a patient's daily dose to the lowest effective dose.

Monitoring for Prescription Opioid Misuse

Clinicians should monitor patients to whom they prescribe opioids for misuse and adverse events (Dowell et al., 2016; Federation of State Medical Boards, 2013; Opioid Therapy for Chronic Pain Work Group, 2017). This is important to determine whether the risks exceed the benefits. Experts recommend a standard prescribing and monitoring framework for all patients prescribed opioids (Gourlay, Heit, & Almahrezi, 2005). Monitoring should occur in an ongoing way throughout treatment and should include information from multiple sources. Patient interviews are essential to obtain information about how they are taking their medications and any use of alcohol or other substances. Physical examination is important to observe intoxication, oversedation, signs of opioid withdrawal, or evidence of drug injection or intranasal drug use. Objective data from drug testing and PDMPs can identify opioid misuse and are described in more detail below. Finally, collateral history from family, friends, and other providers can be helpful. The CDC recommends that regular visits occur at least every three months and within one to four weeks of a dose adjustment (Dowell, Haegerich, & Chou, 2016). U.S. practitioners should adhere to federal and state law and policies of state boards, which may include specific actions not discussed here.

Drug Testing

Drug testing is increasingly used and recommended to obtain objective data that can confirm use of prescribed medication and help to identify use of nonprescribed substances that can increase the risks associated with opioid use. Urine is the most commonly used because collection is noninvasive and tests are widely available, though drug testing of oral fluid, serum, and hair is also available. The CDC recommends drug testing at the time of initiating or continuing LTOT and suggests that clinicians consider testing at least annually; others recommend more frequent testing, particularly when risk factors are present. Drug testing that is ordered at random times rather than on a fixed schedule may be more likely to detect misuse. Urine drug testing is more sensitive than self-report or physician observation for identifying illicit and nonprescribed drug use, though studies of the impact of routine drug testing on opioid misuse are lacking (Starrels et al., 2010). In one study, 60 percent of patients who were considered by their clinicians not to have misused had a urine drug test result indicating either use of an illicit drug or absence of a prescribed medication (Bronstein, Passik, Munitz, & Leider, 2011).

Currently, urine drug testing can include point-of-care or lab-based immunoassay tests and confirmatory tests using gas or liquid chromatography and mass spectrometry. It is essential that clinicians are aware of the limitations of the tests that they use because the interpretation of results is complicated by false positive and false negative results. Misinterpreting results could lead to poorly informed conclusions about a patient's risks and could have negative outcomes for patient care or the physician-patient relationship (Reisfield, Webb, Bertholf, Sloan, & Wilson, 2007; Starrels, Fox, Kunins, & Cunningham, 2012).

Prescription Drug Monitoring Programs (PDMPs)

Clinicians should query PDMP records for a patient before prescribing opioids, in accordance with CDC recommendations and state policies. This allows a prescriber to check whether a patient has received undisclosed prescriptions for controlled substances, to confirm the doses of disclosed prescriptions (e.g., if a patient is changing practices), and to determine the dispensing date or pharmacy when needed. Undisclosed opioid use is a type of misuse and raises concerns about opioid use disorder, diversion, drug-drug interactions, and overdose. Evidence about the effectiveness of PDMPs in preventing misuse and overdose is mixed; while PDMP use appears to be associated with reduced opioid prescribing and some studies have found an association between state PDMP introduction and slowing of opioid-related overdose (Reifler et al., 2012), others have not found this association (Finley et al., 2017). For more on PDMPs, see chapter 12 of this book.

Addressing Opioid Misuse

Providers and practices should have a standardized approach to addressing opioid misuse. The standardized approach should be communicated to patients, for example, when initiating opioids or as part of a written treatment agreement. Having a standardized approach reduces room for provider biases to impact clinical decision making.

Opioid misuse behaviors range in severity, with more severe behaviors indicating a higher level or risk. For example, a less severe behavior would include one episode of running out of medication early, and a more severe behavior would include selling medication or injecting heroin. A clinician's response to misuse should be based on severity. For example, a response to a less severe behavior may be to review the treatment agreement and monitor more closely, and a response to a more severe behavior may be to taper or discontinue opioid therapy if the risks exceed the benefits of continuing. Opioid tapering should generally be slow enough to avoid clinically significant withdrawal symptoms. When opioid misuse occurs, it is important to assess the patient for a DSM-5–defined opioid use disorder and consider referring the patient for evaluation by an addiction specialist. Effective treatments for opioid use disorder are available, including treatment with methadone or buprenorphine.

Patient-Centered Tapering

As health systems, payers, and individual clinicians have considered responses to the opioid overdose crisis, one strategy that has emerged has been *unilateral tapering*, whereby even patients who may perceive a benefit from opioids and are not experiencing present harm are tapered off involuntarily (Kertesz, 2017). We oppose that approach as it runs contrary to the CDC guideline, the most authoritative and current guideline available. We recommend a biopsychosocially informed, interdisciplinary approach to chronic pain management where patient's functional goals are the guideposts of treatment. In this approach, patients for whom benefit is outweighing harm should be continued on the therapy at the lowest effective dose. Patients assessed to have benefit not outweighing harm should be counseled on treatment options that include an opioid taper; a taper in some situations may need to become unilateral, but even such a unilateral taper should be done at a speed commensurate with the risk at hand while offering viable treatment alternatives.

Conclusions

In the midst of a public health crisis of opioid use disorder and overdose, guidelines recommend that clinicians prescribe opioids for pain judiciously. This includes assessing the risks and benefits of opioids, communicating effectively with patients, limiting opioid exposure, monitoring for and addressing prescription opioid misuse, and identifying and treating opioid use disorder. It is important for clinicians to consider each individual's particular risks and benefits throughout treatment and in decisions about whether opioid tapering is indicated. Evidence comparing tapering strategies for patients on LTOT for chronic pain is lacking, though a patient-centered approach includes engaging the patient in a voluntary taper and reducing the dose slowly enough to avoid severe opioid withdrawal symptoms. Finally, it is important that clinicians keep current with the evolving evidence, guidelines, and regulations regarding prescription opioid use in pain management.

References

Banta-Green, C. J., Merrill, J. O., Doyle, S. R., Boudreau, D. M., & Calsyn, D. A. (2009). Measurement of opioid problems among chronic pain patients in a general medical population. *Drug and Alcohol Dependence, 104*(1), 43–49.

Banta-Green, C. J., Von Korff, M., Sullivan, M. D., Merrill, J. O., Doyle, S. R., & Saunders, K. W. (2010). The prescribed opioids difficulties scale: A patient-centered assessment of problems and concerns. *Clinical Journal of Pain, 26*(6), 489–497. doi:10.1097/AJP.0b013e3181e103d9.

Becker, W. C., Fiellin, D. A., Gallagher, R. M., Barth, K. S., Ross, J. T., & Oslin, D. W. (2009). The association between chronic pain and prescription drug abuse in veterans. *Pain Medicine, 10*(3), 531–536.

Becker, W. C., Starrels, J. L., Heo, M., Li, X., Weiner, M. G., & Turner, B. J. (2011). Racial differences in primary care opioid risk reduction strategies. *Annals of Family Medicine, 9*(3), 219–225.

Bohnert, A. S., Ilgen, M. A., Galea, S., McCarthy, J. F., & Blow, F. C. (2011). Accidental poisoning mortality among patients in the Department of Veterans Affairs Health System. *Medical Care, 49*(4), 393–396.

Boscarino, J. A., Rukstalis, M., Hoffman, S. N., Han, J. J., Erlich, P. M., Gerhard, G. S., & Stewart, W. F. (2010). Risk factors for drug dependence among out-patients on opioid therapy in a large US health-care system. *Addiction, 105*(10), 1776–1782. doi:10.1111/j.1360-0443.2010.03052.x.

Bronstein, K., Passik, S., Munitz, L., & Leider, H. (2011). Can clinicians accurately predict which patients are misusing their medications? *Journal of Pain, 12*(4), P3.

Butler, S. F., Fernandez, K., Benoit, C., Budman, S. H., & Jamison, R. N. (2008). Validation of the revised Screener and Opioid Assessment for Patients with Pain (SOAPP-R). *Journal of Pain, 9*(4), 360–372.

Centers for Disease Control and Prevention. (2013). Vital signs: Overdoses of prescription opioid pain relievers and other drugs among women—United States, 1999-2010. *MMWR: Morbidity and Mortality Weekly Report, 62*(26), 537.

Chou, R., Fanciullo, G. J., Fine, P. G., Adler, J. A., Ballantyne, J. C., Davies, P., . . . American Pain Society–American Academy of Pain Medicine Opioids Guidelines Panel. (2009). Clinical guidelines for the use of chronic opioid therapy in chronic noncancer pain. *Journal of Pain, 10*(2), 113–130.

Chou, R., Turner, J. A., Devine, E. B., Hansen, R. N., Sullivan, S. D., Blazina, I., . . . Deyo, R. A. (2015). The effectiveness and risks of long-term opioid therapy for chronic pain: A systematic review for a National Institutes of Health Pathways to Prevention Workshop. *Annals of Internal Medicine, 162*(4), 276–286.

Compton, P. A., Wu, S. M., Schieffer, B., Pham, Q., & Naliboff, B. D. (2008). Introduction of a self-report version of the prescription drug use questionnaire and relationship to medication agreement noncompliance. *Journal of Pain and Symptom Management, 36*(4), 383–395.

Compton, W. M., Jones, C. M., & Baldwin, G. T. (2016). Relationship between nonmedical prescription-opioid use and heroin use. *New England Journal of Medicine, 2016*(374), 154–163.

Dowell, D., Haegerich, T. M., & Chou, R. (2016). CDC guideline for prescribing opioids for chronic pain—United States, 2016. *JAMA, 315*(15), 1624–1645.

Dunn, K. M., Saunders, K. W., Rutter, C. M., Banta-Green, C. J., Merrill, J. O., Sullivan, M. D., . . . Von Korff, M. (2010). Opioid prescriptions for chronic pain and overdose. *Annals of Internal Medicine, 152,* 85–92.

Edlund, M. J., Steffick, D., Hudson, T., Harris, K. M., & Sullivan, M. (2007). Risk factors for clinically recognized opioid abuse and dependence among veterans using opioids for chronic non-cancer pain. *Pain, 129*(3), 355–362.

Federation of State Medical Boards. (2013). *Model Policy on the Use of Opioid Analgesics in the Treatment of Chronic Pain.* http://www.fsmb.org/pdf/pain _policy_july2013.pdf.

Finley, E. P., Garcia, A., Rosen, K., McGeary, D., Pugh, M. J., & Potter, J. S. (2017). Evaluating the impact of prescription drug monitoring program implementation: A scoping review. *BMC Health Services Research, 17*(1), 420.

Fleming, M. F., Balousek, S. L., Klessig, C. L., Mundt, M. P., & Brown, D. D. (2007). Substance use disorders in a primary care sample receiving daily opioid therapy. *Journal of Pain, 8*(7), 573–582.

Gourlay, D. L., Heit, H. A., & Almahrezi, A. (2005). Universal precautions in pain medicine: A rational approach to the treatment of chronic pain. *Pain Medicine, 6*(2), 107–112.

Hausmann, L. R., Gao, S., Lee, E. S., & Kwoh, C. K. (2013). Racial disparities in the monitoring of patients on chronic opioid therapy. *Pain, 154*(1), 46–52.

Ives, T. J., Chelminski, P. R., Hammett-Stabler, C. A., Malone, R. M., Perhac, J. S., Potisek, N. M., . . . Pignone, M. P. (2006). Predictors of opioid misuse in patients with chronic pain: a prospective cohort study. *BMC Health Services Research, 6,* 46.

Kandel, D. B., Hu, M.-C., Griesler, P., & Wall, M. (2017). Increases from 2002 to 2015 in prescription opioid overdose deaths in combination with other substances. *Drug and Alcohol Dependence, 178,* 501–511.

Kelly, J. F., Wakeman, S. E., & Saitz, R. (2015). Stop talking "dirty": Clinicians, language, and quality of care for the leading cause of preventable death in the United States. *American Journal of Medicine, 128*(1), 8–9.

Kertesz, S. G. (2017). Turning the tide or riptide? The changing opioid epidemic. *Substance Abuse, 38*(1), 3–8.

Krebs, E. E., Lorenz, K. A., Bair, M. J., Damush, T. M., Wu, J., Sutherland, J. M., . . . Kroenke, K. (2009). Development and initial validation of the PEG, a three-item scale assessing pain intensity and interference. *Journal of General Internal Medicine, 24*(6), 733–738.

Liebschutz, J. M., Saitz, R., Weiss, R. D., Averbuch, T., Schwartz, S., Meltzer, E. C., . . . Samet, J. H. (2010). Clinical factors associated with prescription drug use disorder in urban primary care patients with chronic pain. *Journal of Pain, 11*(11), 1047–1055.

Morasco, B. J., & Dobscha, S. K. (2008). Prescription medication misuse and substance use disorder in VA primary care patients with chronic pain. *General Hospital Psychiatry, 30*(2), 93–99.

Mosher, H., Krebs, E., Carrel, M., Kaboli, P., Vander Weg, M., & Lund, B. (2015). Trends in prevalent and incident opioid receipt: an observational study in Veterans Health Administration 2004–2012. *Journal of General Internal Medicine, 30*(5), 597–604.

National Institute on Drug Abuse. (2016). Teen substance use shows promising decline. https://www.drugabuse.gov/news-events/news-releases/2016 /12/teen-substance-use-shows-promising-decline.

Opioid Therapy for Chronic Pain Work Group. (2017). VA/DoD clinical practice guideline for opioid therapy for chronic pain. http://www.healthquality .va.gov/guidelines/Pain/cot.

Paulozzi, L. J., Kilbourne, E. M., Shah, N. G., Nolte, K. B., Desai, H. A., Landen, M. G., . . . Loring, L. D. (2012). A history of being prescribed controlled substances and risk of drug overdose death. *Pain Medicine, 13*(1), 87–95.

Reid, M. C., Engles-Horton, L. L., Weber, M. B., Kerns, R. D., Rogers, E. L., & O'Connor, P. G. (2002). Use of opioid medications for chronic noncancer pain syndromes in primary care. *Journal of General Internal Medicine, 17*(3), 173–179.

Reifler, L. M., Droz, D., Bailey, J. E., Schnoll, S. H., Fant, R., Dart, R. C., & Bucher Bartelson, B. (2012). Do prescription monitoring programs impact state trends in opioid abuse/misuse? *Pain Medicine, 13*(3), 434–442. doi:10.1111/j.1526-4637.2012.01327.x.

Reisfield, G. M., Webb, F. J., Bertholf, R. L., Sloan, P. A., & Wilson, G. R. (2007). Family physicians' proficiency in urine drug test interpretation. *Journal of Opioid Management, 3*(6), 333–337.

Rudd, R. A., Aleshire, N., Zibbell, J. E., & Matthew Gladden, R. (2016). Increases in drug and opioid overdose deaths—United States, 2000–2014. *American Journal of Transplantation, 16*(4), 1323–1327.

Starrels, J. L., Becker, W. C., Alford, D. P., Kapoor, A., Williams, A. R., & Turner, B. J. (2010). Systematic review: Treatment agreements and urine drug testing to reduce opioid misuse in patients with chronic pain. *Annals of Internal Medicine, 152*(11), 712–720.

Starrels, J. L., Fox, A. D., Kunins, H. V., & Cunningham, C. O. (2012). They don't know what they don't know: Internal medicine residents' knowledge and confidence in urine drug test interpretation for patients with chronic pain. *Journal of General Internal Medicine, 27*(11), 1521–1527.

Substance Abuse and Mental Health Services Administration. (2012). *A Comparison of Rural and Urban Substance Abuse Treatment Admissions.* https:// www.samhsa.gov/sites/default/files/teds-short-report043-urban-rural -admissions-2012.pdf.

Substance Abuse and Mental Health Services Administration. (2015a). *Treatment Episode Data Set (TEDS) 2001–2011. State Admissions to Substance Abuse*

Treatment Services. https://www.samhsa.gov/data/sites/default/files/TED S2011St_Web/TEDS2011St_Web/TEDS2011St_Web.pdf.

Substance Abuse and Mental Health Services Administration. (2015b). *Treatment Episode Data Set (TEDS): 2003–2013. State Admissions to Substance Abuse Treatment Services.* Rockville, MD: SAMHSA.

Substance Abuse and Mental Health Services Administration. (2016). *Prescription Drug Use and Misuse in the United States: Results from the 2015 National Survey on Drug Use and Health.* https://www.samhsa.gov/data/sites/default /files/NSDUH-FFR2-2015/NSDUH-FFR2-2015.htm.

Unick, G. J., & Ciccarone, D. (2017). US regional and demographic differences in prescription opioid and heroin-related overdose hospitalizations. *International Journal of Drug Policy, 46*, 112–119.

Vijayaraghavan, M., Penko, J., Guzman, D., Miaskowski, C., & Kushel, M. B. (2011). Primary care providers' judgments of opioid analgesic misuse in a community-based cohort of HIV-infected indigent adults. *Journal of General Internal Medicine, 26*(4), 412–418.

Vowles, K. E., McEntee, M. L., Julnes, P. S., Frohe, T., Ney, J. P., & van der Goes, D. N. (2015). Rates of opioid misuse, abuse, and addiction in chronic pain: A systematic review and data synthesis. *Pain, 156*(4), 569–576.

Webster, L. R., & Webster, R. M. (2005). Predicting aberrant behaviors in opioid-treated patients: Preliminary validation of the opioid risk tool. *Pain Medicine, 6*(6), 432–442.

Wu, L. T., Zhu, H., & Swartz, M. S. (2016). Treatment utilization among persons with opioid use disorder in the United States. *Drug and Alcohol Dependence, 169*, 117–127.

CHAPTER TEN

Opioids in the Emergency Setting

Travis L. Hase and Francesca L. Beaudoin

Pain is the most common reason to seek emergency care, and it is often treated with opioid medications, with just over 30 percent of patients discharged with a prescription (Cordell et al., 2002; Mazer-Amirshahi, Mullins, Rasooly, van den Anker, & Pines, 2014a). Pain is a highly subjective experience fraught with challenges in objective assessment, cultural and social differences of expression, and bias among providers. Practitioners have a responsibility to treat pain and ease suffering; however, it is important to balance this against the potential for negative sequelae, including the risk of misuse, abuse, dependence, and diversion of prescribed opioid medications. The axiom *primum non nocere* (Latin, translating to "first, do no harm" and alluding to the bioethical principal of nonmaleficence) is of little guidance to this complex, multifactorial issue that remains under heightened legal, social, and political scrutiny (Venkat, Fromm, Isaacs, Ibarra, & Committee, 2013). As such, it is critical that practitioners use their best judgment, utilize the best evidence in treatment decisions, and always keep the patient's best interests in mind. Indeed, there is a risk-benefit analysis that must be continually addressed in a patient-centered manner.

Since the 1980s, there has been a significant paradigm shift in the management of pain in the United States; at one time grossly underrecognized and undertreated, there has since been a dichotomous shift from an epidemic of untreated pain to an epidemic of opioid overdose (Centers for Disease Control and Prevention, 2012). Through the efforts of the pharmaceutical industry, marketing campaigns, and patient advocacy groups, pain assessment emerged as a "fifth vital sign" to address the issue of oligoanalgesia, resulting in increased use of opioids (Kirschner, Ginsburg, Sulmasy, Health, & Public Policy Committee of the American College of, 2014; Tompkins, Hobelmann, & Compton, 2017; Van Zee, 2009). And while there has been a dramatic increase in opioid prescribing from both the adult and pediatric acute care settings, there has only been a modest increase in pain-related presentations (Mazer-Amirshahi, et al., 2014a; Mazer-Amirshahi, Mullins, Rasooly, van den Anker, & Pines, 2014b).

This surge in opioid prescribing has been paralleled by an unprecedented increase in opioid-related deaths, which has increased nearly five-fold since 1999 (Hedegaard, Warner, & Minino, 2017; Rudd, Seth, David, & Scholl, 2016). Opioids now play a role in over 75 percent of all pharmaceutical-related mortality, and overdose is now the leading cause of accidental death in the United States (Jones, Mack, & Paulozzi, 2013; Warner, Chen, Makuc, Anderson, & Minino, 2011). It is unlikely that a significant change in the population's susceptibility to overdose has taken place during this time. Indeed, we are in the midst of a public health crisis, with prescription opioid misuse, abuse, and overdose placing an enormous burden on communities across the country.

Pain management, addiction, and overdose are complex issues with multifactorial etiologies. As potentially interrelated phenomena, it is imperative that practitioners prescribe appropriately, employ risk reduction strategies, and maximize nonopioid and nonpharmacologic adjuvants when possible. The iatrogenic (i.e., health care–related) contribution to this crisis is increasingly recognized, but prescribers need not unwittingly contribute. In this chapter, we will discuss the use of opioids for the management of acute pain and the risks associated with their use. We will summarize responsible prescribing practices useful in the emergency department (ED) setting. Further, we will explore the complex dilemma of managing pain in patients with opioid use disorders, undergoing medication-assisted treatment, or with high potential for abuse. We will highlight some nonopioid therapies available for optimizing pain control. Lastly, we will conclude by reviewing best practices for the management of patients presenting to the ED after an opioid overdose.

Opioids for Acute Pain

Nearly two-thirds of patients who present to the ED do so for acute pain or an exacerbation of a chronic pain condition (Cordell et al., 2002). The use of opioids is common, and emergency physicians are among the most frequent prescribers of these medicines, with nearly one-third of ED patients now discharged with a prescription opioid (Mazer-Amirshahi et al., 2014a). Opioids are an accepted treatment for the management of acute pain and have an excellent therapeutic effect when optimally dosed. As such, they are often used as a first-line treatment for moderate to severe pain.

Pain management is a key component in treating emergency patients. This begins with obtaining the best objective measurement of pain severity, usually with a 0 to 10 numerical rating scale (Mohan, Ryan, Whelan, & Wakai, 2010). The same tool can be used to assess opioid response and need for additional dosing. As with outpatient treatment, it is essential to utilize non-opioid and nonpharmacologic adjuvant therapies when possible in a multimodal approach. Furthermore, the management of patient expectations regarding pain is crucial to their overall treatment and to maintaining a therapeutic doctor-patient relationship. The goal of therapy is not complete alleviation of symptoms, but rather pain reduction to a level that facilitates functional status. Most acute pain improves in days; therefore, we suggest a short-term course of short-acting medication (three to five days) that can be used on an as needed basis (Cantrill et al., 2012; Dowell, Haegerich, & Chou, 2016; Weiner, Perrone, & Nelson, 2013). These medications should be used in conjunction with nonopioid adjuvants to maximize the synergistic effect from a multimodal approach, and it may be beneficial to do so on a standing basis (Raffa, 2001). Patients with continued severe pain or pain that persists beyond this short-term period warrant reevaluation.

Many patients will require continuing management of their pain symptoms once discharged. While there is limited research investigating the risk of opioid misuse and abuse associated with the use of opioids within the emergency department, there is a growing body of evidence to suggest potential risk in patients discharged with a prescription for opioid medications, which will be discussed. Given this evolving body of evidence, it is ever more prudent that acute care providers be diligent in their safe prescribing practices and that they utilize risk-reduction tools. Nevertheless, patients with obvious painful conditions or injuries where ongoing pain is expected warrant appropriate management of their symptoms, even when there are ongoing concerns for abuse liability. This is often achieved with opioid analgesics. While there should be extra care when prescribing to at-risk and high-risk populations, opioid medications should not be withheld in the acute setting when otherwise warranted.

Opioids and Chronic Pain

In contrast to acute pain, opioids have less clear benefit for the treatment of chronic pain, and most evidence supports their use as first-line or routine therapy only in active cancer, palliative care, or end-of-life care (Chou et al., 2015; Dowell et al., 2016). Apart from the adverse events associated with chronic use, there are two commonly observed phenomena that complicate long-term treatment. Opioid tolerance is a normal physiologic response resulting in reduced effectiveness at a given dose and thus requiring higher doses to achieve the same result. This is a predictable phenomenon that should be anticipated. Additionally, opioid-induced hyperalgesia, a response by which regular opioid use results in pain out of proportion to a given stimulus, is a well-observed effect (Yi & Pryzbylkowski, 2015). These compounding variables can be difficult to clinically distinguish, result in a cycle of poor pain control and escalating dosing, and may contribute to the transition to chronic opioid use and dependence. As this occurs, there is a dramatic shift in the balance of benefit to harm, especially with respect to high doses, long-acting formulations, and the use of methadone for pain (Dunn et al., 2010; Gomes, Mamdani, Dhalla, Paterson, & Juurlink, 2011; M. Miller et al., 2015; Webster et al., 2011). Indeed, there is strong evidence to suggest a dose-dependent risk (Bohnert et al., 2011). Although there are no high-quality studies addressing the risk of transitioning to misuse and addiction, there is a growing body of evidence that highlights these concerns in those chronically using opioids, and we will discuss this evidence in the following section.

Despite limited evidence to support the efficacy of such tools, recent guidelines for the use of opioids in managing chronic pain seem to agree on a number of risk-mitigation strategies. These include pain contracts, urine drug screening, upper dose limitations, and the use of various screening tools (Nuckols et al., 2014). Most of the guideline recommendations (especially related to maximum dosage) are based on epidemiologic and observational studies regarding risk association and do not specifically show a reduction in opioid-related harm. The generally accepted dose limitation is 100–200 morphine equivalents per day. There has also been an increased focus on safety with concomitant benzodiazepine use, which is a factor in half of fatal overdoses (Jones, Paulozzi, Mack, Centers for Disease Control and Prevention, 2014; Nuckols et al., 2014; Park, Saitz, Ganoczy, Ilgen, & Bohnert, 2015; Webster et al., 2011). Additionally, the use of methadone for pain has also been of particular concern given its significantly higher association with overdose death (Centers for Disease Control and Prevention, 2012b; Webster et al., 2011).

While more commonly used in the outpatient setting, many of the above tools are either beyond the scope of emergency medicine practice or not practical for use in that setting. When chronic pain patients present to the emergency setting, it is important to assess for their involvement in a pain clinic and the existence of a pain contract. These contracts vary by provider and clinic but often restrict a patient's access to opioids outside of those provided by their pain specialist through pharmacy agreements, dose and pill restrictions, and agreements that lost or stolen prescriptions will not be replaced (Arnold, Han, & Seltzer, 2006). Some contracts may detail previously agreed upon interventions to trial in a stepwise fashion or include the contact information of the clinic/provider so that management can be discussed or approved. For patients on chronic opioid therapy who are not involved with a pain specialist, a referral can be provided.

As we will discuss in a later section, it is important to reference a prescription drug monitoring program (PDMP) database (Cantrill et al., 2012). This may help providers in determining whether the patient demonstrates concerning signs that may signal misuse. For more on PDMPs, also see chapter 12.

Table 10.1 Signs of Potential Opioid Misuse or Diversion

Demonstrates Opioid Misuse	Potential for Opioid Misuse
Report of opioid addiction	Frequent visits or refills
Report of opioid diversion	Continuing dose escalations
Obtains drugs from dealer	Reports of lost or stolen medication
Obtains drugs through others	History of substance use
Obtains drugs by theft	Declines other treatments or testing
Prescription forging	Symptom inconsistency or distractibility
Use of false identification or name	Decline in social function

Signs of concerning use and historical features that should raise concern for the possibility of misuse or diversion are reviewed in Table 10.1 (Brady, McCauley, & Back, 2016; Cheatle, 2015).

Many chronic pain patients may request opioids to manage an acute exacerbation of their symptoms, but this may not always be in the patient's best interest from both a safety and efficacy standpoint. Chronic pain can worsen, not because of a lack of increased opioids but through tolerance and hyperalgesia. As always, nonopioid options should be maximized in these patients. As we will discuss, ketamine may be an excellent option for chronic pain patients, given its effectiveness at treating severe pain. Additionally, it is known to improve opioid-induced hyperalgesia.

An opioid medication may sometimes be used in the acute setting to improve symptoms and functional status to facilitate discharge, but it is generally not advisable to discharge a patient on chronic opioids with a prescription for more opioids (Cantrill et al., 2012). Changes to a patient's regimen are best made by the primary provider. Given the increased risk of overdose seen in this population, it is prudent to coprescribe naloxone for these patients, which can be a lifesaving intervention (Coffin et al., 2016). For more on naloxone use, see chapter 13.

Risk of Use

Addiction is a complex, multifactorial phenomenon that is thought to require repeated drug exposure in the context of abuse liability of a drug, environmental factors, and genetic risk. To date, the ways by which prescription opioid use leads to harm have yet to be well characterized by robust studies, and there are no randomized trials characterizing the rate of iatrogenic addiction. Nevertheless, the abuse liability of opioids is well established, and progression to opioid use disorders and use of illegitimate opioids has been documented as a consequence of what started as legitimate medical use.

Some individuals will intentionally misuse opioids, and their initial exposure may be entirely of their own volition; however, the transition from appropriate medical opioid use for pain relief to nonmedical use, misuse, and addiction is poorly understood. One study of treatment-seeking, opioid-dependent patients showed that 29 percent were introduced to opioids by a physician for the treatment of pain, suggesting mere treatment may be a pathway for some who become addicted (Tsui et al., 2010).

The risk of an incident opioid use disorder is likely small when these medications are used on an acute basis, and opioids should not be withheld when indicated for the short-term management of moderate to severe painful conditions. There is reasonable evidence, however, to suggest that iatrogenic addiction may result from the prescribed use of opioids, especially as it pertains to chronic pain (Edlund et al., 2014; Fishbain, Cole, Lewis, Rosomoff, & Rosomoff, 2008). This effect of both chronicity and total daily dose have important impacts on this risk (Deyo et al., 2017; Shah, Hayes, & Martin, 2017). Risk is further increased in patients with a history of substance use disorder and in those with mental health disorders (Becker, Sullivan, Tetrault, Desai, & Fiellin, 2008; Boscarino et al., 2010; Edlund et al., 2010; Sun, Darnall, Baker, & Mackey, 2016). It is important to consider the degree of aberrant prescription opioid use, as this is more common than the development of a diagnosable opioid use disorder (Fishbain et al., 2008; Martell et al., 2007; Sullivan et al., 2010). Furthermore, the nonmedical use of prescription opioids is particularly concerning because of its association with intravenous heroin use (Cicero, Ellis, Surratt, & Kurtz, 2014; Compton, Jones, & Baldwin, 2016; Lankenau et al., 2012).

Given the high proportion of painful conditions seen in the ED as well as the frequency at which opioids are prescribed, it is important to consider this unique environment when discussing the potential for iatrogenic addiction (Mazer-Amirshahi et al., 2014a). While it has been commonly assumed that brief exposures for acute pain play a negligible role in the development of iatrogenic addition, there is now a growing body of literature that has begun to challenge this assertion (Alam et al., 2012; Carroll et al., 2012). Despite the fact that emergency providers are likely to prescribe in accordance with guideline recommendations for short durations and for lower daily doses, recent data suggests that prescriptions specifically from the emergency setting play a role in initial exposure and recurrent use, which may precede addiction (Barnett, Olenski, & Jena, 2017; Butler et al., 2016; Hoppe, Kim, & Heard, 2015; Hoppe, Nelson et al., 2015; Jeffery et al., 2017).

In addition to the concern for iatrogenic addiction, it is clear that prescribers contribute significantly to the availability of prescription opioids for illicit use. A nationally representative 2015 U.S. survey estimated that 34 percent of people who used opioid medication nonmedically received the drug from just one doctor (Substance Abuse and Mental Health Services Administration, 2016). Less than 2 percent used more than one doctor to obtain medication, further highlighting the misconception of frequent "doctor shopping" (McDonald & Carlson, 2013). Additionally, 54 percent of individuals acquired the drugs from a friend or relative (either for free, by purchase, or theft). According to 2013 data, among those receiving medication from a friend, 83 percent said their source obtained the drug from a single doctor (Substance Abuse and Mental Health Services Administration, 2014). Only 5 percent of misused opioids are obtained from a dealer. As such, it is especially important prescribers be prudent, especially with respect to the quantity of medication prescribed, as leftover medication is a significant source for nonmedical use (Beaudoin, Straube, Lopez, Mello, & Baird, 2014; Bicket, Long, Pronovost, Alexander, & Wu, 2017; Lewis, Cucciare, & Trafton, 2014; Wang, Fiellin, & Becker, 2014).

Responsible Prescribing Practices

Even when used as prescribed, opioids are associated with potential harms, and it appears that the most significant risk factor for opioid dependence, addiction, and overdose is receiving a prescription. Consequently, it is critical that prescribers employ risk-reduction strategies when prescribing these medications. Practices such as considering PDMP reports, counseling patients about risks of addiction and overdose, educating patients about the importance of taking medication as prescribed, advising patients on proper medication storage and disposal, and monitoring patients for aberrant use behaviors are among the risk management options that prescribers should utilize.

While there are myriad guidelines from various organizations offering best practices for risk reduction and mitigation, many of these practices are not easily applied in the acute care setting (Haegerich, Paulozzi, Manns, & Jones, 2014). Indeed, a unique challenge facing emergency providers is a lack of continuity with their patients. Patients present in an undifferentiated fashion, and it is not uncommon to have little information about their medical and prescription histories. Further, it is especially laborious and burdensome to obtain outside records and imaging, which may lend insight and provide objective data. Complicating the picture more is the difficulty in quickly establishing good rapport and a therapeutic relationship with patients who are in pain, especially in a population often stigmatized and inappropriately mislabeled as "drug seeking." But perhaps the most challenging clinical scenario involves patients truly engaging in deceitful acts.

One of the easiest tools that emergency providers can rely on to assist with clinical decision making is a PDMP database (Cantrill et al., 2012). Briefly, these are often state-run databases that collect pharmacy data on controlled substances that are dispensed. Unfortunately, at present, PDMPs remain underutilized by emergency providers (Greenwood-Ericksen, Poon, Nelson, Weiner, & Schuur, 2016). While this is related, in part, to a lack of standardization and some well-characterized limitations, we argue that these databases are one of the best tools available in the emergency setting to assess for presence of risk factors for misuse and concerning use patterns (Greenwood-Ericksen et al., 2016). The literature supporting the efficacy of these programs is largely limited to observational studies, but there is reasonable data demonstrating that the use of PDMPs are a useful tool in reducing opioid addiction, diversion, and overdose (Albert et al., 2011; Delcher, Wagenaar, Goldberger, Cook, & Maldonado-Molina, 2015; Haegerich et al., 2014; Reifler et al., 2012).

Evidence shows that providers are poor at detecting patients at risk for opioid misuse or overdose (Greenwood-Ericksen et al., 2016). Furthermore, subjective impressions may lead to stigma and inappropriate withholding of necessary opioid analgesia. PDMPs offer objective data that clinicians can use in the context of history, examination, and overall clinical picture to make an informed decision about abuse liability (Weiner, Griggs et al., 2013). PDMP consultation may result in a treatment plan change for a patient at high risk, but it may also help to provide appropriate treatment to a patient inappropriately misjudged or mislabeled as drug seeking. Overall, there is state-level data to suggest that PDMP use reduces opioid prescribing and opioid use (Rutkow et al., 2015). While it remains unclear what patient-specific factors have led to this decline, presumably this is because PDMPs are enabling providers to better identify high-risk features and concerning use patterns. Specifically, there is data that demonstrates this effect in the emergency setting and shows that the use of PDMP alters prescribing behavior both positively and negatively (Baehren et al., 2010). For a more comprehensive review and assessment of PDMPs, see chapter 12.

There are a number of validated screening tools available for use to aid clinicians in early detection of problematic substance use, including Screener and Opioid Assessment for Patients with Pain, Revised (SOAPP-R); Current Opioid Misuse Measure (COMM); Opioid Risk Tool (ORT); and Prescription Drug Use Questionnaire (PDUQ) (Brady et al., 2016; Butler et al., 2007; Butler, Fernandez, Benoit, Budman, & Jamison, 2008; Compton, Darakjian, & Miotto, 1998; Webster & Webster, 2005). These tools are an important first step in screening, brief intervention, and referral to treatment (SBIRT; Babor et al., 2007). Although these specific screening tools can be difficult to implement in the emergency department setting, particularly because of their length, they highlight one option to aid the clinician in identifying patients at increased risk (Delgado et al., 2011). Recent data demonstrates improved implementation with electronic screening as part of the triage and check-in process (Johnson, Woychek, Vaughan, & Seale, 2013; Weiner, Horton, Green, & Butler, 2015). Additionally, data shows improved detection of concerning use patterns beyond that of screening with a PDMP alone (Weiner, Horton, Green, & Butler, 2016).

As a best practice, patients should be provided with educational materials regarding the safe use, storage, and disposal of controlled substances they are prescribed, and the provision of such information should be documented within the medical record (Haegerich et al., 2014). Although there is no data to support these interventions, these discussions are not only prudent, but, as with prescribing any medication, an important aspect of overall care. There is research that demonstrates education strategies to be useful as a component piece of broad overdose prevention strategies (Dwyer et al., 2015; Reifler et al., 2012).

Pain Management in Patients with Substance Use Disorders

Acute pain management in patients actively misusing opioids with a history of misuse or in those on opioid agonist replacement therapies (e.g., methadone, buprenorphine) is particularly challenging, in part due to some common misconceptions we will discuss. Patients with clearly painful conditions or traumatic injury warrant effective and expeditious pain management, and opioid medications should not be withheld if otherwise indicated. While providers should always be prudent and aggressively utilize nonopioid and nonpharmacologic modalities, many acute episodes of moderate to severe pain will require treatment with opioid medications. Indeed, adequate treatment of acute painful conditions is an essential component of quality care.

It is worth addressing the emotion-laden topic of drug-seeking behavior, as this leads to stigmatization and often the gross undertreatment of acute pain in this population. Drug-seeking behaviors are broadly defined as concerted efforts to obtain opioid medications. An important distinction is that these efforts may not always be ill-intended and may represent pain relief–seeking behavior by efforts to ensure an adequate supply of medication to treat poorly controlled pain (pseudoaddiction) or related to anxiety and fear of medication discontinuation, changes to their current regimen, or the emergence of withdrawal symptoms (Weissman & Haddox, 1989). Pain is a subjective experience that is difficult to assess, even with the use of standardized and validated tools. The patient's anxiety about being stigmatized or not having their pain relieved further complicates this process. Complaints of acute pain with objective findings are less likely to be manipulative, especially in patients on maintenance therapies. As previously discussed, the use of a PDMP may be particularly useful in these situations (Weiner et al., 2016). It is of the upmost importance that clinicians approach these patients with an open mind, carefully search for objective findings and etiologies of pain, validate the patient's concerns and fears, openly and nonjudgmentally discuss concerns about abuse liability and a plan for pain management, and reassure the patient that their misuse history will not prevent their pain from being treated.

Discussing the use of opioids in patients recovering or in remission from opioid use disorders is particularly important, as these individuals may wish to decline treatment with opioid medications to prevent relapse or loss of progress toward recovery, even in the presence of acutely painful conditions. This special circumstance requires reassurance and an aggressive use of nonopioid adjuncts. Furthermore, it is useful to note that no data supports the concern that the use of opioids to treat an episode of acute pain results in relapse (Kantor, Cantor, & Tom, 1980; Manfredi, Gonzales, Cheville, Kornick, & Payne, 2001). In fact, untreated pain is thought to be a more likely trigger (Karasz et al., 2004).

It is especially important to understand that maintenance opioid agonists do not provide adequate analgesia, as the pharmacokinetics of their analgesic and addiction treatment (i.e., withdrawal prevention) properties differ. Maintenance therapies such as methadone and buprenorphine are dosed every 24 to 48 hours, but the duration of analgesic action is only 4–8 hours, a substantially shorter time frame. As such, maintenance therapy cannot be relied upon to provide adequate analgesia for acute pain. Additionally, it is especially important to remember that tolerance and cross-tolerance significantly diminish the analgesic and euphoric effects of these medicines. Hyperalgesia from long-term opioid exposure further complicates the picture. For these reasons, when opioids are used, there is often a requirement for higher and more frequent dosing. The effect of treatment and need for redosing or dose escalation, as well as any signs of oversedation or respiratory depression, should be frequently reassessed in a standardized fashion. The risk of respiratory depression is of less concern in patients on maintenance therapies, especially buprenorphine, secondary to the rapid development of tolerance to central and respiratory system depression (Inturrisi, 2002; McNicol et al., 2003). The additive effect may be less predictable in patients using heroin, given the variability in its composition and difficulty with calculating equivalent dosing.

Various management strategies have been described for patients on methadone and buprenorphine. In general, it is best to first confirm the timing and dosing with the distributing clinic or pharmacy, to inform the program or prescriber of any administration of opioids or other substances that may be the subject of drug testing, and to notify them of admission and discharge. Second, ensure that the daily opioid treatment requirement has been met before attempting to achieve analgesia, as attempts otherwise will be ineffective secondary to tolerance. Plan to aggressively treat pain using a multimodal approach, which includes short-acting opioids, and consider using scheduled dosing rather than as-needed orders. Avoid combination products to avoid hepatotoxicity and nephrotoxicity so that adjuvant medication such as acetaminophen can be maximally dosed on a scheduled basis. The recommended maximum daily doses of acetaminophen and ibuprofen in adults are 4,000 mg and 3,200 mg, respectively.

In general, it is best to continue methadone maintenance dosing (Alford, Compton, & Samet, 2006; Mitra & Sinatra, 2004). In patients not tolerating or with contraindications to oral intake, methadone can be given parenterally and is most safely done by administering half to two-thirds of the maintenance dose divided into two to four equal doses (Fishman, Wilsey, Mahajan, & Molina, 2002). There is less data and clinical experience regarding buprenorphine; however, the two easiest methods described are to either continue buprenorphine and titrate short-acting opioids to analgesic effect or to discontinue buprenorphine, replace it with a standing equivalent dose (potentially with a sustained release formulation), and then titrate to analgesic effect using short-acting opioids (Huxtable, Roberts, Somogyi, & MacIntyre, 2011; Mitra & Sinatra, 2004). Previously, there was some low-quality data that suggested routine buprenorphine discontinuation given concern for an analgesic ceiling effect, but this has since been disproven (Macintyre, Russell, Usher, Gaughwin, & Huxtable, 2013; Pergolizzi et al., 2010). Alternatively, there is data to suggest that dividing the total daily maintenance dose and administering it every six to eight hours is useful, as the pharmacokinetics of this approach takes advantage of the analgesic properties (Johnson, Fudala, & Payne, 2005).

Pain management in patients taking naltrexone, especially depot formulations, is exceedingly difficult, as naltrexone is a complete opioid antagonist and blocks the effects of even substantial doses of opioids (Vickers & Jolly, 2006). It is important to note that this medication is used not only for MAT but also for the treatment of alcoholism. There are currently no options available for reversal of this medication, and pain management will depend on nonopioid options. Ketamine may be especially beneficial in this patient population. Patients who recently discontinued naltrexone are at increased risk of oversedation, respiratory depression, and overdose secondary to opioid receptor upregulation (Gibson & Degenhardt, 2007; Yoburn, 1988).

Alternatives and Nonopioid Adjuncts

Given the ubiquity of pain, the magnitude of pain-related patient presentations to emergent and urgent settings is unsurprising. As pain management is a fundamental component of care to these patients, it is important for clinicians to have a diverse armamentarium of analgesic options, as opioids may not be the best or only option for any given clinical scenario. Regarding severe pain and opioid tolerant patients, where repeat and escalating doses of opioids are likely to be used, it is notable that high doses of opioids are associated with potentially life-threatening adverse effects related to respiratory depression. As such, a multimodal approach to the management of both acute and chronic painful conditions is important, and this should include both pharmacologic and nonpharmacologic modalities. Not only may such an approach have an opioid-sparing effect and be a safer option than giving an additional dose of an opioid, but it may provide more analgesia to the patient than using opioids alone. Further, having a diversity of options is especially important for appropriately managing conditions for which opioids are not indicated, have been shown to have limited efficacy, or in those patients with allergies, intolerances, at high risk for complication, or with other contraindications. Here, we will review nonopioid alternatives that may be practically used in the acute care setting. Our purpose is to provide an overview of alternatives, and this overview is not exhaustive. Further, a complete discussion regarding dosing, pharmacokinetics, and side-effect profiles is beyond our scope. Providers should consult appropriate reference materials or pharmacists as needed.

Nonpharmacologic modalities are often underappreciated but are generally very beneficial as well as simple and cost-effective. In the emergency settings, these include simple interventions, such as ice, heat, elevation, positioning, splinting, and compression. These same tools can be used in the outpatient setting, and it is important to not underestimate the effect they can have on improving comfort and healing. Furthermore, patients can be recommended massage, stretching activities, specific exercises, and orthotic/brace devices for a number of painful conditions.

Popular transdermal alternatives, such as lidocaine and diclofenac patches, are excellent options for localized pain, especially of a musculoskeletal nature (Derry et al., 2017). These products are available both by prescription and over-the-counter. They come in a variety of transdermal formulations other than patches, such as creams and ointments. Counterirritant preparations are other popular commercial products.

There are a variety of nerve blocks that can be incorporated into a pain management strategy. If pain is localized to a specific area amenable to a nerve block and is expected to be short-lived or procedure-related, complete analgesia can be provided with an appropriate anesthetic agent without the use of opioids. When pain is expected to be ongoing, there is evidence demonstrating not only superior pain control but an opioid-sparing effect when nerve blocks are incorporated in the emergency setting (Beaudoin, Haran, & Liebmann, 2013). It is prudent to document a thorough neurologic examination prior to the use of a nerve block. Some relatively simple and commonly performed blocks include various dental/maxillofacial, median, ulnar, digital, femoral or fascia iliaca, posterior tibial, and intercostal nerves. There are numerous quality resources detailing the specifics of these procedures elsewhere. It may be beneficial to anesthetize with a combination of a shorter- and longer-acting medication, such as with lidocaine for immediate analgesia and bupivacaine for a sustained effect. If clinically appropriate, formulations with the addition of epinephrine will also have a longer duration of action.

Two of the most common nonopioid analgesics are acetaminophen and nonsteroidal anti-inflammatory drugs (NSAIDs), such as ibuprofen and naproxen. These medications are generally well tolerated and should be used as first-line therapies in mildly to moderately painful conditions or as an adjunct for the treatment of moderate to severe pain. These medications are especially useful for the management of inflammatory and musculoskeletal conditions. In fact, a recent randomized controlled trial has demonstrated no difference in the amount of pain reduction offered by either ibuprofen or acetaminophen alone versus hydrocodone-acetaminophen, oxycodone-acetaminophen, or codeine-acetaminophen for the treatment of extremity pain (Chang, Bijur, Esses, Barnaby, & Baer, 2017). There are both oral and intravenous formulations of acetaminophen and NSAIDs, and data supports the combination of these medicines to achieve a synergistic response (Derry, Derry, & Moore, 2013; Raffa, 2001).

When the addition of opioids is necessary, there is evidence to support the use of opioid combinations with either ibuprofen or acetaminophen rather than an opioid alone for the treatment of pain (Derry, Derry, & Moore, 2013; Gaskell, Derry, Moore, & McQuay, 2009). Combining opioids with either of these medicines may lead to better analgesia than if opioids are used alone; however, the available formulations can lead to underdosing of the non-opioid component, reducing the overall efficacy of their analgesic and anti-inflammatory properties. To optimize the dosing of nonopioid adjuvants, clinicians can consider using noncombination formulations. Alternatively, additional dosing of the combined medication can be administered to achieve therapeutic dosing. Discharging a patient with a prescription or specific instructions to take scheduled doses of nonopioid medications such as acetaminophen or ibuprofen not only emphasizes these medicines as an important component of pain control but may provide better overall pain relief.

Intravenous lidocaine and dexmedetomidine are additional options for the management of severe pain. While most of the literature supporting their use is from studies in the perioperative setting, there is good evidence to support their use for pain control in conscious patients (Peng, Liu, Wu, Cheng, & Ji, 2015; Yousefshahi, Predescu, & Francisco Asenjo, 2017). The use of these medications is often only available within the emergency department or intensive care setting, but this is institution-specific. Although these agents are not first-line, they are an important consideration for pain that is poorly controlled by opioids, chronic pain, or in those patients for whom an opioid alternative is desirable or necessary.

Ketamine is perhaps the most widely accepted nonopioid option for the intravenous treatment of severe pain. Its use has grown in popularity over the past several years, in part because of its ease of administration and favorable adverse-effect profile. There is strong data specifically from the emergency department setting that demonstrates its efficacy, utility, and safety (Beaudoin, Lin, Guan, & Merchant, 2014; Miller, Schauer, Ganem, & Bebarta, 2015; Motov et al., 2015). When used at subdissociative dosing (typically 0.15–0.3 mg/kg), the goal is analgesia without the effect of dissociation seen at higher doses. At these lower doses, ketamine is an excellent option for severe pain, pain refractory to opioids, or in those patients with high opioid tolerance. Because of its favorable hemodynamic profile, it may be a useful agent for injured patients with hypotension. Additionally, there is data to suggest a resensitization effect of opioid receptors, resulting in improved response to these medicines and decreased hyperalgesia (Gupta, Devi, & Gomes, 2011; Himmelseher & Durieux, 2005).

The use of benzodiazepines carries with it similar concerns to opioids regarding abuse liability, and their use in conjunction with opioids is controversial. It is well established that concomitant use potentiates the sedating effects of opioids and is associated with an increase in adverse events, including overdose (Webster et al., 2011). Nevertheless, there are indications for the use of these medicines, such as muscle strain and spasm or to facilitate muscular relaxation, in the acute setting. Furthermore, it is not uncommon that alcohol-intoxicated patients present with injuries requiring pain control who will then require benzodiazepines to control symptoms and prevent sequela of alcohol withdrawal. Patients with indications for the use of both benzodiazepines and opioids warrant additional monitoring above that of patients requiring either medication alone. The ongoing use of both agents upon discharge is more controversial.

A variety of spasmolytics, although generally less efficacious than benzodiazepines, acetaminophen, and NSAIDs, are widely used to treat muscle spasms, cramps, and myofascial pain (van Tulder, Touray, Furlan, Solway, & Bouter, 2003). Antidepressants are frequently used for the management of chronic pain, and their analgesic effect is thought to be independent of their antidepressant features. While duloxetine is the only antidepressant approved by the FDA for management of chronic pain, many patients are treated off-label by other dual serotonin and norepinephrine reuptake inhibitors (SNRIs). Anticonvulsants, specifically gabapentin and pregabalin, are approved for the treatment of neuropathic conditions. While these agents are not typically started in the acute care setting, it is important to understand the role they play given their widespread use. Clinicians should be aware of the growing concern regarding the abuse liability of gabapentin (Smith, Havens, & Walsh, 2016).

A variety of devices, such as implantable pumps and internal and external neuromodulators, are used in patients with chronic pain. Again, while these are not often utilized in the acute setting, it is prudent to be informed of their applications, especially as it pertains to the medical complications related thereto.

While incorporating physical therapy, behavioral therapy, psychiatric and psychologic services, and complementary and alternative medicine (CAM) options into the care of patients in the emergency setting is impractical, it is important to recognize that these are validated and effective approaches to the management for patients with chronic pain. There is good data that supports the efficacy of a multidisciplinary approach for the management of chronic pain (Flor, Fydrich, & Turk, 1992; Kamper et al., 2015). While access to these multidisciplinary clinics is now quite limited, the components of these individual modalities are available. Emergency providers play an important role in referring when appropriate, recommending various modalities as indicated, and discussing these options with primary providers. Further, there is growing availability of pain clinics, and providers should be familiar with their institutional and local referral options. Pain clinics may incorporate some of the modalities above, provide interventional options, or be opioid-focused. They play an especially important role for patients being managed on chronic opioid therapy for both the purposes of continuity and monitoring.

Best Practices in Opioid Overdose

As discussed previously, the rates of opioid overdose have reached epidemic proportions in the United States. Given the high number of nonfatal overdoses presenting to emergency departments each year, this represents a significant opportunity to intervene. Data demonstrates that emergency physicians are willing to engage with opiate harm reduction (OHR) interventions, an essential step to ensuring the success of these programs (Samuels, 2014). Many patients may decline resources offered to them after an overdose is reversed, but it is incumbent upon providers, as well as potentially lifesaving, to offer resources for counseling, medication-assisted treatment (MAT; i.e., treatment with methadone or buprenorphine), and overdose prevention. There is a significant amount of quality data that shows that MAT has a mortality benefit, reduces opioid use, reduces rates of human immunodeficiency and hepatitis C virus infection, and reduces incarceration (Gowing, Farrell, Bornemann, Sullivan, & Ali, 2011; Mattick, Breen, Kimber, & Davoli, 2009; Schwartz et al., 2013; Schwartz et al., 2015; Volkow, Frieden, Hyde, & Cha, 2014). More recently, there is emerging promising evidence that the initiation of buprenorphine treatment from the emergency department may improve outcomes (D'Onofrio et al., 2017; D'Onofrio et al., 2015).

Patients presenting to the ED with overdose should always be counseled using motivational interviewing techniques, as this is a unique opportunity to prevent repeat overdose and encourage treatment. Approaching this as a teachable moment is a critical intervention given that these patients are at high risk of repeat overdose and death, with recent, yet-to-be published data suggesting 10 percent of these patients will die within a year (American College of Emergency Physicians, 2017). In addition to the community models available, peer-based models of behavioral intervention have been described (Samuels, 2014).

There is a growing body of compelling data that shows that overdose education and community naloxone distribution (OEND) programs are effective in changing some of these same outcomes measures, especially pertaining to mortality (Albert et al., 2011; McAuley, Aucott, & Matheson, 2015; R. McDonald & Strang, 2016; Walley, Doe-Simkins et al., 2013; Walley, Xuan et al., 2013). These programs typically involve education about opioid risk awareness, education about the signs of overdose, and training on the use of rescue naloxone administration (Clark, Wilder, & Winstanley, 2014; Kerensky & Walley, 2017). OEND programs play an important role of overdose prevention education, and data supports their efficacy at reducing risky behaviors when implemented in the emergency setting (Bohnert et al., 2016). Furthermore, more recent data demonstrates a significant reduction in opioid-related emergency department visits (Coffin et al., 2016).

In addition to focusing especially on patients at high risk for overdose, these programs should be targeted toward individuals who may be likely to witness an overdose. In fact, the Centers for Disease Control and Prevention (CDC) recommends overdose prevention education and a consideration of naloxone prescription for both patients and household members for all people with a history of overdose, history of substance use disorder, those taking high doses (greater than 50 morphine equivalents daily), or those with concurrent use of benzodiazepines (Dowell et al., 2016). This is consistent with the guidelines of the World Health Organization (WHO), which recommend naloxone access for individuals likely to witness an overdose (WHO, 2014). A significant number of overdoses occur in patients using opioids as prescribed, and this is a particularly important population that need not be ignored, as data supports the coprescription of naloxone in those engaged in chronic opioid use and in those taking high doses (Coffin et al., 2016). As with similar public health campaigns, despite the concerns of some, there is absolutely no data to suggest an increase in risk-taking behavior with implementation of this risk-reduction strategy (Doe-Simkins et al., 2014).

Naloxone is an opioid antagonist that rapidly reverses the respiratory depression and decreased consciousness that occur during an opioid overdose. It is available by prescription, from pharmacies directly in some jurisdictions, directly from an emergency department, and through community programs (Green, Dauria, Bratberg, Davis, & Walley, 2015; Lim, Bratberg, Davis, Green, & Walley, 2016). While community-based programs have traditionally been the primary source for naloxone distribution, there has been a marked uptick in prescription use (Jones, Lurie, & Compton, 2016). The legal environment in which OEND programs exist has significant impact on their effectiveness. There has been a shift in the legal environment in most jurisdictions, which now allow not only the prescriptions for third parties likely to witness overdose but make naloxone available from pharmacies without a prescription (Jones et al., 2016). As always, it is important for providers to be familiar with the regulations affecting their individual practice.

In the United States, there are now four different ways a rescue dose of naloxone can be delivered: Luer-Jet needless syringe of naloxone for intramuscular or intravenous use (also commonly used with the attachment of a mucosal atomizer), a branded intranasal device (Narcan Nasal Spray), a multidose flip-top vial of naloxone and syringe with needle, or a branded autoinjector device (EVZIO) that uses an English voice-prompting system (Lim et al.,

2016). Providers should note that nasal naloxone delivered via syringe or nasal atomizer is not FDA approved. Intranasal naloxone is just as effective as intravenous formulations for reversing respiratory and central nervous system depression (Sabzghabaee, Eizadi-Mood, Yaraghi, & Zandifar, 2014). Most OEND programs favor either nasal atomized or intramuscular injections because they are cost-effective, and intranasal delivery has several benefits, namely, ease of use by laypersons and decreased risk of needle stick (Kerr, Dietze, & Kelly, 2008). As of 2015, the American Heart Association has incorporated naloxone into its algorithms, and this represents a ripe area for bystander training (Lavonas et al., 2015). There are a multitude of reasons to equip those using opioids with naloxone kits, and providers should embrace their position to help patients prevent and respond to opioid overdose. As a leading cause of accidental death, it is arguable that providers have a moral imperative to educate and improve access to this lifesaving public health intervention. See chapter 13 for more on community-based harm-reduction approaches, including naloxone distribution.

Conclusion

In our attempt to address oligoanalgesia, promote increased pain control, improve functional status in chronic pain patients, and increase patient satisfaction, providers have undoubtedly—and in most cases, unknowingly—contributed to the epidemic of opioid-related morbidity and mortality. Indeed, the pendulum has swung to an extreme of opioid prescribing and an unprecedented surge in opioid-related deaths and other harms. But the illumination of the medical community's contributions to this epidemic is not action enough. While opioids remain the first-line treatment for acute episodes of moderate to severe pain, providers need not unwittingly contribute to this public health crisis. Rampant misuse and diversion of opioids is, in part, an unintended consequence of inappropriate prescribing practices, and we are now just beginning to understand our contribution to addiction.

Undoubtedly, there is a requirement for a multifaceted and comprehensive response, but prescribers have a duty to act now. To that end, as a significant source of opioid prescriptions, emergency providers have both a professional and moral obligation to utilize responsible and evidenced-based prescribing practices, maximize nonopioid and nonpharmacologic adjuvants, and to employ risk-reduction strategies with respect to both abuse liability and overdose. Indeed, there must exist a balance between effective pain management and patient safety. This change in our practice is not intended to limit appropriate and necessary prescribing and restrict access to opioid analgesics; rather, its purpose is to improve the safety and benefits of these medications. The metric of our success should be a reduction in opioid-related morbidity and mortality. These commonsense practice changes are formidable steps in engaging emergency providers in addressing an epidemic fueled by inappropriate prescribing practices—a problem iatrogenic at its core.

References

Alam, A., Gomes, T., Zheng, H., Mamdani, M. M., Juurlink, D. N., & Bell, C. M. (2012). Long-term analgesic use after low-risk surgery: A retrospective cohort study. *Archives of Internal Medicine, 172*(5), 425–430. doi:10.1001/archinternmed.2011.1827.

Albert, S., Brason, F. W., II, Sanford, C. K., Dasgupta, N., Graham, J., & Lovette, B. (2011). Project Lazarus: Community-based overdose prevention in rural North Carolina. *Pain Medicine, 12 Suppl 2*, S77–S85. doi:10.1111/j.1526-4637.2011.01128.x.

Alford, D. P., Compton, P., & Samet, J. H. (2006). Acute pain management for patients receiving maintenance methadone or buprenorphine therapy. *Annals of Internal Medicine, 144*(2), 127–134.

American College of Emergency Physicians. (2017). *Research Offers New Insights into the Opioid Crisis.* Washington, D.C.: American College of Emergency Physicians.

Arnold, R. M., Han, P. K., & Seltzer, D. (2006). Opioid contracts in chronic non-malignant pain management: Objectives and uncertainties. *American Journal of Medicine, 119*(4), 292–296. doi:10.1016/j.amjmed.2005.09.019.

Babor, T. F., McRee, B. G., Kassebaum, P. A., Grimaldi, P. L., Ahmed, K., & Bray, J. (2007). Screening, brief intervention, and referral to treatment (SBIRT): Toward a public health approach to the management of substance abuse. *Substance Abuse, 28*(3), 7–30. doi:10.1300/J465v28n03_03.

Baehren, D. F., Marco, C. A., Droz, D. E., Sinha, S., Callan, E. M., & Akpunonu, P. (2010). A statewide prescription monitoring program affects emergency department prescribing behaviors. *Annals of Emergency Medicine, 56*(1), 19–23 e11–13. doi:10.1016/j.annemergmed.2009.12.011.

Barnett, M. L., Olenski, A. R., & Jena, A. B. (2017). Opioid-prescribing patterns of emergency physicians and risk of long-term use. *New England Journal of Medicine, 376*(7), 663–673. doi:10.1056/NEJMsa1610524.

Beaudoin, F. L., Haran, J. P., & Liebmann, O. (2013). A comparison of ultrasound-guided three-in-one femoral nerve block versus parenteral opioids alone for analgesia in emergency department patients with hip fractures: A randomized controlled trial. *Academic Emergency Medicine, 20*(6), 584–591. doi:10.1111/acem.12154.

Beaudoin, F. L., Lin, C., Guan, W., & Merchant, R. C. (2014). Low-dose ketamine improves pain relief in patients receiving intravenous opioids for acute pain in the emergency department: Results of a randomized, double-blind, clinical trial. *Academic Emergency Medicine, 21*(11), 1193–1202. doi:10.1111/acem.12510.

Beaudoin, F. L., Straube, S., Lopez, J., Mello, M. J., & Baird, J. (2014). Prescription opioid misuse among ED patients discharged with opioids. *American Journal of Emergency Medicine, 32*(6), 580–585. doi:10.1016/j.ajem.2014 .02.030.

Becker, W. C., Sullivan, L. E., Tetrault, J. M., Desai, R. A., & Fiellin, D. A. (2008). Non-medical use, abuse and dependence on prescription opioids among U.S. adults: Psychiatric, medical and substance use correlates. *Drug and Alcohol Dependence, 94*(1-3), 38–47. doi:10.1016/j.drugalcdep.2007.09.018.

Bicket, M. C., Long, J. J., Pronovost, P. J., Alexander, G. C., & Wu, C. L. (2017). Prescription opioid analgesics commonly unused after surgery: A systematic review. *JAMA Surgery, 152*(11), 1066–1071. doi:10.1001/ jamasurg.2017.0831.

Bohnert, A. S., Bonar, E. E., Cunningham, R., Greenwald, M. K., Thomas, L., Chermack, S., . . . Walton, M. (2016). A pilot randomized clinical trial of an intervention to reduce overdose risk behaviors among emergency department patients at risk for prescription opioid overdose. *Drug and Alcohol Dependence, 163*, 40–47. doi:10.1016/j.drugalcdep.2016.03.018.

Bohnert, A. S., Valenstein, M., Bair, M. J., Ganoczy, D., McCarthy, J. F., Ilgen, M. A., & Blow, F. C. (2011). Association between opioid prescribing patterns and opioid overdose-related deaths. *JAMA, 305*(13), 1315–1321. doi:10.1001/jama.2011.370.

Boscarino, J. A., Rukstalis, M., Hoffman, S. N., Han, J. J., Erlich, P. M., Gerhard, G. S., & Stewart, W. F. (2010). Risk factors for drug dependence among out-patients on opioid therapy in a large US health-care system. *Addiction, 105*(10), 1776–1782. doi:10.1111/j.1360-0443.2010.03052.x.

Brady, K. T., McCauley, J. L., & Back, S. E. (2016). Prescription opioid misuse, abuse, and treatment in the United States: An update. *American Journal of Psychiatry, 173*(1), 18–26. doi:10.1176/appi.ajp.2015.15020262.

Butler, M. M., Ancona, R. M., Beauchamp, G. A., Yamin, C. K., Winstanley, E. L., Hart, K. W., . . . Lyons, M. S. (2016). Emergency department prescription opioids as an initial exposure preceding addiction. *Academic Emergency Medicine, 68*(2), 202–208. doi:10.1016/j.annemergmed.2015.11.033.

Butler, S. F., Budman, S. H., Fernandez, K. C., Houle, B., Benoit, C., Katz, N., & Jamison, R. N. (2007). Development and validation of the current opioid misuse measure. *Pain, 130*(1-2), 144–156. doi:10.1016/j.pain.2007.01.014.

Butler, S. F., Fernandez, K., Benoit, C., Budman, S. H., & Jamison, R. N. (2008). Validation of the revised screener and opioid assessment for patients with pain (SOAPP-R). *Journal of Pain, 9*(4), 360–372. doi:10.1016/j.jpain .2007.11.014.

Cantrill, S. V., Brown, M. D., Carlisle, R. J., Delaney, K. A., Hays, D. P., Nelson, L. S., . . . Whitson, R. R. (2012). Clinical policy: Critical issues in the prescribing of opioids for adult patients in the emergency department. *Academic Emergency Medicine, 60*(4), 499–525. doi:10.1016/j .annemergmed.2012.06.013.

Carroll, I., Barelka, P., Wang, C. K., Wang, B. M., Gillespie, M. J., McCue, R., . . . Mackey, S. (2012). A pilot cohort study of the determinants of longitudinal opioid use after surgery. *Anesthesia & Analgesia, 115*(3), 694–702. doi:10.1213/ANE.0b013e31825c049f.

Centers for Disease Control and Prevention. (2012a). CDC grand rounds: Prescription drug overdoses—A U.S. epidemic. *MMWR: Morbidity and Mortality Weekly Report, 61*(1), 10–13.

Centers for Disease Control and Prevention. (2012b). Vital signs: Risk for overdose from methadone used for pain relief—United States, 1999–2010. *MMWR: Morbidity and Mortality Weekly Report, 61*(26), 493–497.

Chang, A. K., Bijur, P. E., Esses, D., Barnaby, D. P., & Baer, J. (2017). Effect of a single dose of oral opioid and nonopioid analgesics on acute extremity pain in the emergency department: A randomized clinical trial. *JAMA, 318*(17), 1661–1667. doi:10.1001/jama.2017.16190.

Cheatle, M. D. (2015). Prescription opioid misuse, abuse, morbidity, and mortality: Balancing effective pain management and safety. *Pain Medicine, 16 Suppl 1*, S3–S8. doi:10.1111/pme.12904.

Chou, R., Turner, J. A., Devine, E. B., Hansen, R. N., Sullivan, S. D., Blazina, I., . . . Deyo, R. A. (2015). The effectiveness and risks of long-term opioid therapy for chronic pain: a systematic review for a National Institutes of Health Pathways to Prevention Workshop. *Annals of Internal Medicine, 162*(4), 276–286. doi:10.7326/M14-2559.

Cicero, T. J., Ellis, M. S., Surratt, H. L., & Kurtz, S. P. (2014). The changing face of heroin use in the United States: A retrospective analysis of the past 50 years. *JAMA Psychiatry, 71*(7), 821–826. doi:10.1001/jamapsychiatry.2014.366.

Clark, A. K., Wilder, C. M., & Winstanley, E. L. (2014). A systematic review of community opioid overdose prevention and naloxone distribution programs. *Journal of Addiction Medicine, 8*(3), 153–163. doi:10.1097/ADM.0000000000000034.

Coffin, P. O., Behar, E., Rowe, C., Santos, G. M., Coffa, D., Bald, M., & Vittinghoff, E. (2016). Nonrandomized intervention study of naloxone coprescription for primary care patients receiving long-term opioid therapy for pain. *Annals of Internal Medicine, 165*(4), 245–252. doi:10.7326/M15-2771.

Compton, P., Darakjian, J., & Miotto, K. (1998). Screening for addiction in patients with chronic pain and "problematic" substance use: Evaluation of a pilot assessment tool. *Journal of Pain and Symptom Management, 16*(6), 355–363.

Compton, W. M., Jones, C. M., & Baldwin, G. T. (2016). Relationship between nonmedical prescription-opioid use and heroin use. *New England Journal of Medicine, 374*(2), 154–163. doi:10.1056/NEJMra1508490.

Cordell, W. H., Keene, K. K., Giles, B. K., Jones, J. B., Jones, J. H., & Brizendine, E. J. (2002). The high prevalence of pain in emergency medical care. *American Journal of Emergency Medicine, 20*(3), 165–169.

D'Onofrio, G., Chawarski, M. C., O'Connor, P. G., Pantalon, M. V., Busch, S. H., Owens, P. H., & Fiellin, D. A. (2017). Emergency department-initiated buprenorphine for opioid dependence with continuation in primary care: Outcomes during and after intervention. *Journal of General Internal Medicine, 32*(6), 660–666. doi:10.1007/s11606-017-3993-2.

D'Onofrio, G., O'Connor, P. G., Pantalon, M. V., Chawarski, M. C., Busch, S. H., Owens, P. H., . . . Fiellin, D. A. (2015). Emergency department-initiated buprenorphine/naloxone treatment for opioid dependence: A randomized clinical trial. *JAMA, 313*(16), 1636–1644. doi:10.1001/jama.2015.3474.

Delcher, C., Wagenaar, A. C., Goldberger, B. A., Cook, R. L., & Maldonado-Molina, M. M. (2015). Abrupt decline in oxycodone-caused mortality after implementation of Florida's prescription drug monitoring program. *Drug and Alcohol Dependence, 150*, 63–68. doi:10.1016/j.drugalcdep.2015.02.010.

Delgado, M. K., Acosta, C. D., Ginde, A. A., Wang, N. E., Strehlow, M. C., Khandwala, Y. S., & Camargo, C. (2011). National survey of preventive health services in US emergency departments. *Annals of Emergency Medicine, 57*(2), 104–108 e102. doi:10.1016/j.annemergmed.2010.07.015.

Derry, C. J., Derry, S., & Moore, R. A. (2013). Single dose oral ibuprofen plus paracetamol (acetaminophen) for acute postoperative pain. *Cochrane Database of Systematic Reviews, 6*, D010210. doi:10.1002/14651858.CD010210.pub2.

Derry, S., Derry, C. J., & Moore, R. A. (2013). Single dose oral ibuprofen plus oxycodone for acute postoperative pain in adults. *Cochrane Database of Systematic Reviews, 6*, CD010289. doi:10.1002/14651858.CD010289.pub2.

Derry, S., Wiffen, P. J., Kalso, E. A., Bell, R. F., Aldington, D., Phillips, T., . . . Moore, R. A. (2017). Topical analgesics for acute and chronic pain in adults—An overview of Cochrane Reviews. *Cochrane Database of Systematic Reviews, 5*, CD008609. doi:10.1002/14651858.CD008609.pub2.

Deyo, R. A., Hallvik, S. E., Hildebran, C., Marino, M., Dexter, E., Irvine, J. M., . . . Millet, L. M. (2017). Association between initial opioid prescribing patterns and subsequent long-term use among opioid-naïve patients: A statewide retrospective cohort study. *Journal of General Internal Medicine, 32*(1), 21–27. doi:10.1007/s11606-016-3810-3.

Doe-Simkins, M., Quinn, E., Xuan, Z., Sorensen-Alawad, A., Hackman, H., Ozonoff, A., & Walley, A. Y. (2014). Overdose rescues by trained and untrained participants and change in opioid use among substance-using participants in overdose education and naloxone distribution programs: A retrospective cohort study. *BMC Public Health, 14*, 297. doi:10.1186/1471-2458-14-297.

Dowell, D., Haegerich, T. M., & Chou, R. (2016). CDC guideline for prescribing opioids for chronic pain—United States, 2016. *JAMA, 315*(15), 1624–1645. doi:10.1001/jama.2016.1464.

Dunn, K. M., Saunders, K. W., Rutter, C. M., Banta-Green, C. J., Merrill, J. O., Sullivan, M. D., . . . Von Korff, M. (2010). Opioid prescriptions for chronic pain and overdose: A cohort study. *Annals of Internal Medicine, 152*(2), 85–92. doi:10.7326/0003-4819-152-2-201001190-00006.

Dwyer, K., Walley, A. Y., Langlois, B. K., Mitchell, P. M., Nelson, K. P., Cromwell, J., & Bernstein, E. (2015). Opioid education and nasal naloxone rescue kits in the emergency department. *Western Journal of Emergency Medicine, 16*(3), 381–384. doi:10.5811/westjem.2015.2.24909.

Edlund, M. J., Martin, B. C., Fan, M. Y., Devries, A., Braden, J. B., & Sullivan, M. D. (2010). Risks for opioid abuse and dependence among recipients of chronic opioid therapy: Results from the TROUP study. *Drug and Alcohol Dependence, 112*(1-2), 90–98. doi:10.1016/j.drugalcdep.2010.05.017.

Edlund, M. J., Martin, B. C., Russo, J. E., DeVries, A., Braden, J. B., & Sullivan, M. D. (2014). The role of opioid prescription in incident opioid abuse and dependence among individuals with chronic noncancer pain: The role of opioid prescription. *Clinical Journal of Pain, 30*(7), 557–564. doi:10.1097/AJP.0000000000000021.

Fishbain, D. A., Cole, B., Lewis, J., Rosomoff, H. L., & Rosomoff, R. S. (2008). What percentage of chronic nonmalignant pain patients exposed to chronic opioid analgesic therapy develop abuse/addiction and/or aberrant drug-related behaviors? A structured evidence-based review. *Pain Medicine, 9*(4), 444–459. doi:10.1111/j.1526-4637.2007.00370.x.

Fishman, S. M., Wilsey, B., Mahajan, G., & Molina, P. (2002). Methadone reincarnated: Novel clinical applications with related concerns. *Pain Medicine, 3*(4), 339–348. doi:10.1046/j.1526-4637.2002.02047.x.

Flor, H., Fydrich, T., & Turk, D. C. (1992). Efficacy of multidisciplinary pain treatment centers: A meta-analytic review. *Pain, 49*(2), 221–230.

Gaskell, H., Derry, S., Moore, R. A., & McQuay, H. J. (2009). Single dose oral oxycodone and oxycodone plus paracetamol (acetaminophen) for acute postoperative pain in adults. *Cochrane Database of Systematic Reviews, 3*, CD002763. doi:10.1002/14651858.CD002763.pub2.

Gibson, A. E., & Degenhardt, L. J. (2007). Mortality related to pharmacotherapies for opioid dependence: A comparative analysis of coronial records. *Drug and Alcohol Review, 26*(4), 405–410. doi:10.1080/09595230701373834.

Gomes, T., Mamdani, M. M., Dhalla, I. A., Paterson, J. M., & Juurlink, D. N. (2011). Opioid dose and drug-related mortality in patients with nonmalignant pain. *Archives of Internal Medicine, 171*(7), 686–691. doi:10.1001/archinternmed.2011.117.

Gowing, L., Farrell, M. F., Bornemann, R., Sullivan, L. E., & Ali, R. (2011). Oral substitution treatment of injecting opioid users for prevention of HIV infection. *Cochrane Database of Systematic Reviews, 8*, CD004145. doi:10.1002/14651858.CD004145.pub4.

Green, T. C., Dauria, E. F., Bratberg, J., Davis, C. S., & Walley, A. Y. (2015). Orienting patients to greater opioid safety: Models of community pharmacy-based naloxone. *Harm Reduction Journal, 12*, 25. doi:10.1186/s12954-015-0058-x.

Greenwood-Ericksen, M. B., Poon, S. J., Nelson, L. S., Weiner, S. G., & Schuur, J. D. (2016). Best practices for prescription drug monitoring programs in the emergency department setting: Results of an expert panel. *Annals of Emergency Medicine, 67*(6), 755–764 e754. doi:10.1016/j.annemergmed.2015.10.019.

Gupta, A., Devi, L. A., & Gomes, I. (2011). Potentiation of mu-opioid receptor-mediated signaling by ketamine. *Journal of Neurochemistry, 119*(2), 294–302. doi:10.1111/j.1471-4159.2011.07361.x.

Haegerich, T. M., Paulozzi, L. J., Manns, B. J., & Jones, C. M. (2014). What we know, and don't know, about the impact of state policy and systems-level interventions on prescription drug overdose. *Drug and Alcohol Dependence, 145*, 34–47. doi:10.1016/j.drugalcdep.2014.10.001.

Hedegaard, H., Warner, M., & Minino, A. M. (2017). Drug overdose deaths in the United States, 1999–2015. *NCHS Data Brief* (273), 1–8.

Himmelseher, S., & Durieux, M. E. (2005). Ketamine for perioperative pain management. *Anesthesiology, 102*(1), 211–220.

Hoppe, J. A., Kim, H., & Heard, K. (2015). Association of emergency department opioid initiation with recurrent opioid use. *Annals of Emergency Medicine, 65*(5), 493–499 e494. doi:10.1016/j.annemergmed.2014.11.015.

Hoppe, J. A., Nelson, L. S., Perrone, J., Weiner, S. G., & Prescribing Opioids Safely in the Emergency Department (POSED) Study Investigators. (2015). Opioid prescribing in a cross section of US emergency departments. *Annals of Emergency Medicine, 66*(3), 253–259 e251. doi:10.1016/j.annemergmed.2015.03.026.

Huxtable, C. A., Roberts, L. J., Somogyi, A. A., & MacIntyre, P. E. (2011). Acute pain management in opioid-tolerant patients: a growing challenge. *Anaesthesia and Intensive Care, 39*(5), 804–823.

Inturrisi, C. E. (2002). Clinical pharmacology of opioids for pain. *Clinical Journal of Pain, 18*(4 Suppl), S3–S13.

Jeffery, M. M., Hooten, W. M., Hess, E. P., Meara, E. R., Ross, J. S., Henk, H. J., . . . Bellolio M. F. (2017). Opioid prescribing for opioid-naive patients in emergency departments and other settings: Characteristics of prescriptions and association with long-term use. *Annals of Emergency Medicine.* doi:10.1016/j.annemergmed.2017.08.042.

Johnson, J. A., Woychek, A., Vaughan, D., & Seale, J. P. (2013). Screening for at-risk alcohol use and drug use in an emergency department: Integration of screening questions into electronic triage forms achieves high screening rates. *Annals of Emergency Medicine, 62*(3), 262–266. doi:10.1016/j.annemergmed.2013.04.011.

Johnson, R. E., Fudala, P. J., & Payne, R. (2005). Buprenorphine: Considerations for pain management. *Journal of Pain and Symptom Management, 29*(3), 297–326. doi:10.1016/j.jpainsymman.2004.07.005.

Jones, C. M., Lurie, P. G., & Compton, W. M. (2016). Increase in naloxone prescriptions dispensed in US retail pharmacies since 2013. *American Journal of Public Health, 106*(4), 689–690. doi:10.2105/AJPH.2016.303062.

Jones, C. M., Mack, K. A., & Paulozzi, L. J. (2013). Pharmaceutical overdose deaths, United States, 2010. *JAMA, 309*(7), 657–659. doi:10.1001/jama .2013.272.

Jones, C. M., Paulozzi, L. J., Mack, K. A., & Centers for Disease Control and Prevention. (2014). Alcohol involvement in opioid pain reliever and benzodiazepine drug abuse-related emergency department visits and drug-related deaths—United States, 2010. *MMWR: Morbidity and Mortality Weekly Report, 63*(40), 881–885.

Kamper, S. J., Apeldoorn, A. T., Chiarotto, A., Smeets, R. J., Ostelo, R. W., Guzman, J., & Van Tulder, M. W. (2015). Multidisciplinary biopsychosocial rehabilitation for chronic low back pain: Cochrane systematic review and meta-analysis. *BMJ: British Medical Journal, 350*, h444. doi:10.1136/bmj.h444.

Kantor, T. G., Cantor, R., & Tom, E. (1980). A study of hospitalized surgical patients on methadone maintenance. *Drug and Alcohol Dependence, 6*(3), 163–173.

Karasz, A., Zallman, L., Berg, K., Gourevitch, M., Selwyn, P., & Arnsten, J. H. (2004). The experience of chronic severe pain in patients undergoing methadone maintenance treatment. *Journal of Pain and Symptom Management, 28*(5), 517–525. doi:10.1016/j.jpainsymman.2004.02.025.

Kerensky, T., & Walley, A. Y. (2017). Opioid overdose prevention and naloxone rescue kits: What we know and what we don't know. *Addiction Science & Clinical Practice, 12*(1), 4. doi:10.1186/s13722-016-0068-3.

Kerr, D., Dietze, P., & Kelly, A. M. (2008). Intranasal naloxone for the treatment of suspected heroin overdose. *Addiction, 103*(3), 379–386. doi:10.1111/j .1360-0443.2007.02097.x.

Kirschner, N., Ginsburg, J., Sulmasy, L. S., Health, & Public Policy Committee of the American College of Physicians. (2014). Prescription drug abuse: Executive summary of a policy position paper from the American College of Physicians. *Annals of Internal Medicine, 160*(3), 198. doi:10.7326/M13-2209.

Lankenau, S. E., Teti, M., Silva, K., Jackson Bloom, J., Harocopos, A., & Treese, M. (2012). Initiation into prescription opioid misuse amongst young injection drug users. *International Journal of Drug Policy, 23*(1), 37–44. doi:10.1016/j.drugpo.2011.05.014.

Lavonas, E. J., Drennan, I. R., Gabrielli, A., Heffner, A. C., Hoyte, C. O., Orkin, A. M., . . . Donnino, M. W. (2015). Part 10: Special circumstances of resuscitation: 2015 American Heart Association guidelines update for cardiopulmonary resuscitation and emergency cardiovascular care. *Circulation, 132*(18 Suppl 2), S501–S518. doi:10.1161/CIR.0000000000000264.

Lewis, E. T., Cucciare, M. A., & Trafton, J. A. (2014). What do patients do with unused opioid medications? *Clinical Journal of Pain, 30*(8), 654–662. doi:10.1097/01.ajp.0000435447.96642.f4.

Lim, J. K., Bratberg, J. P., Davis, C. S., Green, T. C., & Walley, A. Y. (2016). Prescribe to prevent: Overdose prevention and naloxone rescue kits for prescribers and pharmacists. *Journal of Addiction Medicine, 10*(5), 300–308. doi:10.1097/ADM.0000000000000223.

Macintyre, P. E., Russell, R. A., Usher, K. A., Gaughwin, M., & Huxtable, C. A. (2013). Pain relief and opioid requirements in the first 24 hours after surgery in patients taking buprenorphine and methadone opioid substitution therapy. *Anaesthesia and Intensive Care, 41*(2), 222–230.

Manfredi, P. L., Gonzales, G. R., Cheville, A. L., Kornick, C., & Payne, R. (2001). Methadone analgesia in cancer pain patients on chronic methadone maintenance therapy. *Journal of Pain and Symptom Management, 21*(2), 169–174.

Martell, B. A., O'Connor, P. G., Kerns, R. D., Becker, W. C., Morales, K. H., Kosten, T. R., & Fiellin, D. A. (2007). Systematic review: Opioid treatment for chronic back pain: Prevalence, efficacy, and association with addiction. *Annals of Internal Medicine, 146*(2), 116–127.

Mattick, R. P., Breen, C., Kimber, J., & Davoli, M. (2009). Methadone maintenance therapy versus no opioid replacement therapy for opioid dependence. *Cochrane Database of Systematic Reviews, 3*, CD002209. doi:10.1002/14651858.CD002209.pub2.

Mazer-Amirshahi, M., Mullins, P. M., Rasooly, I., van den Anker, J., & Pines, J. M. (2014a). Rising opioid prescribing in adult U.S. emergency department visits: 2001–2010. *Academic Emergency Medicine, 21*(3), 236–243. doi:10.1111/acem.12328.

Mazer-Amirshahi, M., Mullins, P. M., Rasooly, I. R., van den Anker, J., & Pines, J. M. (2014b). Trends in prescription opioid use in pediatric emergency department patients. *Pediatric Emergency Care, 30*(4), 230–235. doi:10.1097/PEC.0000000000000102.

McAuley, A., Aucott, L., & Matheson, C. (2015). Exploring the life-saving potential of naloxone: A systematic review and descriptive meta-analysis of take home naloxone (THN) programmes for opioid users. *International Journal of Drug Policy, 26*(12), 1183–1188. doi:10.1016/j.drugpo.2015.09.011.

McDonald, D. C., & Carlson, K. E. (2013). Estimating the prevalence of opioid diversion by "doctor shoppers" in the United States. *PLoS One, 8*(7), e69241. doi:10.1371/journal.pone.0069241.

McDonald, R., & Strang, J. (2016). Are take-home naloxone programmes effective? Systematic review utilizing application of the Bradford Hill criteria. *Addiction, 111*(7), 1177–1187. doi:10.1111/add.13326.

McNicol, E., Horowicz-Mehler, N., Fisk, R. A., Bennett, K., Gialeli-Goudas, M., Chew, P. W., . . . Carr, D. (2003). Management of opioid side effects in cancer-related and chronic noncancer pain: A systematic review. *Journal of Pain, 4*(5), 231–256.

Miller, J. P., Schauer, S. G., Ganem, V. J., & Bebarta, V. S. (2015). Low-dose ketamine vs morphine for acute pain in the ED: A randomized controlled trial. *American Journal of Emergency Medicine, 33*(3), 402–408. doi:10.1016/j.ajem.2014.12.058.

Miller, M., Barber, C. W., Leatherman, S., Fonda, J., Hermos, J. A., Cho, K., & Gagnon, D. R. (2015). Prescription opioid duration of action and the risk of unintentional overdose among patients receiving opioid therapy. *JAMA Internal Medicine, 175*(4), 608–615. doi:10.1001/jamainternmed .2014.8071.

Mitra, S., & Sinatra, R. S. (2004). Perioperative management of acute pain in the opioid-dependent patient. *Anesthesiology, 101*(1), 212–227.

Mohan, H., Ryan, J., Whelan, B., & Wakai, A. (2010). The end of the line? The Visual Analogue Scale and Verbal Numerical Rating Scale as pain assessment tools in the emergency department. *Emergency Medical Journal, 27*(5), 372–375. doi:10.1136/emj.2007.048611.

Motov, S., Rockoff, B., Cohen, V., Pushkar, I., Likourezos, A., McKay, C., . . . Fromm, C. (2015). Intravenous subdissociative-dose ketamine versus morphine for analgesia in the emergency department: A randomized controlled trial. *Annals of Emergency Medicine, 66*(3), 222–229 e221. doi:10.1016/j.annemergmed.2015.03.004.

Nuckols, T. K., Anderson, L., Popescu, I., Diamant, A. L., Doyle, B., Di Capua, P., & Chou, R. (2014). Opioid prescribing: A systematic review and critical appraisal of guidelines for chronic pain. *Annals of Internal Medicine, 160*(1), 38–47. doi:10.7326/0003-4819-160-1-201401070-00732.

Park, T. W., Saitz, R., Ganoczy, D., Ilgen, M. A., & Bohnert, A. S. (2015). Benzodiazepine prescribing patterns and deaths from drug overdose among US veterans receiving opioid analgesics: Case-cohort study. *BMJ: British Medical Journal, 350*, h2698. doi:10.1136/bmj.h2698.

Peng, K., Liu, H. Y., Wu, S. R., Cheng, H., & Ji, F. H. (2015). Effects of combining dexmedetomidine and opioids for postoperative intravenous patient-controlled analgesia: A systematic review and meta-analysis. *Clinical Journal of Pain, 31*(12), 1097–1104. doi:10.1097/AJP.0000000000000219.

Pergolizzi, J., Aloisi, A. M., Dahan, A., Filitz, J., Langford, R., Likar, R., et al. (2010). Current knowledge of buprenorphine and its unique pharmacological profile. *Pain Practice, 10*(5), 428–450. doi:10.1111/j.1533-2500.2010.00378.x.

Raffa, R. B. (2001). Pharmacology of oral combination analgesics: rational therapy for pain. *Journal of Clinical Pharmacy and Therapeutics, 26*(4), 257–264.

Reifler, L. M., Droz, D., Bailey, J. E., Schnoll, S. H., Fant, R., Dart, R. C., & Bartelson, B. B. (2012). Do prescription monitoring programs impact state trends in opioid abuse/misuse? *Pain Medicine, 13*(3), 434–442. doi:10 .1111/j.1526-4637.2012.01327.x.

Rudd, R. A., Seth, P., David, F., & Scholl, L. (2016). Increases in drug and opioid-involved overdose deaths—United States, 2010–2015. *MMWR: Morbidity and Mortality Weekly Report, 65*(5051), 1445–1452. doi:10.15585/mmwr .mm655051e1.

Rutkow, L., Chang, H. Y., Daubresse, M., Webster, D. W., Stuart, E. A., & Alexander, G. C. (2015). Effect of Florida's prescription drug monitoring program and pill mill laws on opioid prescribing and use. *JAMA Internal Medicine, 175*(10), 1642–1649. doi:10.1001/jamainternmed.2015.3931.

Sabzghabaee, A. M., Eizadi-Mood, N., Yaraghi, A., & Zandifar, S. (2014). Naloxone therapy in opioid overdose patients: Intranasal or intravenous? A randomized clinical trial. *Archives of Medical Science, 10*(2), 309–314. doi:10.5114/aoms.2014.42584.

Samuels, E. (2014). Emergency department naloxone distribution: A Rhode Island department of health, recovery community, and emergency department partnership to reduce opioid overdose deaths. *Rhode Island Medical Journal, 97*(10), 38–39.

Schwartz, R. P., Gryczynski, J., O'Grady, K. E., Sharfstein, J. M., Warren, G., Olsen, Y., . . . Jaffe, J. H. (2013). Opioid agonist treatments and heroin overdose deaths in Baltimore, Maryland, 1995–2009. *American Journal of Public Health, 103*(5), 917–922. doi:10.2105/AJPH.2012.301049.

Schwartz, R. P., Kelly, S. M., Gryczynski, J., Mitchell, S. G., O'Grady, K. E., & Jaffe, J. H. (2015). Heroin use, HIV-risk, and criminal behavior in Baltimore: Findings from clinical research. *Journal of Addictive Diseases, 34*(2-3), 151–161. doi:10.1080/10550887.2015.1059222.

Shah, A., Hayes, C. J., & Martin, B. C. (2017). Characteristics of initial prescription episodes and likelihood of long-term opioid use—United States, 2006–2015. *MMWR: Morbidity and Mortality Weekly Report, 66*(10), 265–269. doi:10.15585/mmwr.mm6610a1.

Smith, R. V., Havens, J. R., & Walsh, S. L. (2016). Gabapentin misuse, abuse and diversion: A systematic review. *Addiction, 111*(7), 1160–1174. doi:10.1111/add.13324.

Substance Abuse and Mental Health Services Administration. (2014). *Results from the 2013 National Survey on Drug Use and Health: Summary of National Findings* (NSDUH Series H-48, HHS Publication No. (SMA) 14-4863). Rockville, MD: Center for Behavioral Health Statistics and Quality, Substance Abuse and Mental Health Services Administration.

Substance Abuse and Mental Health Services Administration. (2016). *Key Substance Use and Mental Health Indicators in the United States: Results from the 2015 National Survey on Drug Use and Health* (NSDUH Series H-51, HHS Publication No. (SMA) 16-4984). Rockville, MD: Center for Behavioral Health Statistics and Quality, Substance Abuse and Mental Health Services Administration, United States Department of Health and Human Services.

Sullivan, M. D., Edlund, M. J., Fan, M. Y., Devries, A., Brennan Braden, J., & Martin, B. C. (2010). Risks for possible and probable opioid misuse among recipients of chronic opioid therapy in commercial and medicaid insurance plans: The TROUP Study. *Pain, 150*(2), 332–339. doi:10.1016/j.pain.2010.05.020.

Sun, E. C., Darnall, B. D., Baker, L. C., & Mackey, S. (2016). Incidence of and risk factors for chronic opioid use among opioid-naive patients in the postoperative period. *JAMA Internal Medicine, 176*(9), 1286–1293. doi:10.1001/jamainternmed.2016.3298.

Tompkins, D. A., Hobelmann, J. G., & Compton, P. (2017). Providing chronic pain management in the "Fifth Vital Sign" Era: Historical and treatment perspectives on a modern-day medical dilemma. *Drug and Alcohol Dependence, 173*(Suppl 1), S11–S21. doi:10.1016/j.drugalcdep.2016.12.002.

Tsui, J. I., Herman, D. S., Kettavong, M., Alford, D., Anderson, B. J., & Stein, M. D. (2010). Physician introduction to opioids for pain among patients with opioid dependence and depressive symptoms. *Journal of Substance Abuse Treatment, 39*(4), 378–383. doi:10.1016/j.jsat.2010.06.012.

Van Tulder, M. W., Touray, T., Furlan, A. D., Solway, S., & Bouter, L. M. (2003). Muscle relaxants for non-specific low back pain. *Cochrane Database of Systematic Reviews, 2*, CD004252. doi:10.1002/14651858.CD004252.

Van Zee, A. (2009). The promotion and marketing of oxycontin: Commercial triumph, public health tragedy. *American Journal of Public Health, 99*(2), 221–227. doi:10.2105/AJPH.2007.131714.

Venkat, A., Fromm, C., Isaacs, E., Ibarra, J., & Committee, S. E. (2013). An ethical framework for the management of pain in the emergency department. *Academic Emergency Medicine, 20*(7), 716–723. doi:10.1111/acem.12158.

Vickers, A. P., & Jolly, A. (2006). Naltrexone and problems in pain management. *BMJ: British Medical Journal, 332*(7534), 132–133. doi:10.1136/bmj.332.7534.132.

Volkow, N. D., Frieden, T. R., Hyde, P. S., & Cha, S. S. (2014). Medication-assisted therapies—Tackling the opioid-overdose epidemic. *New England Journal of Medicine, 370*(22), 2063–2066. doi:10.1056/NEJMp1402780.

Walley, A. Y., Doe-Simkins, M., Quinn, E., Pierce, C., Xuan, Z., & Ozonoff, A. (2013). Opioid overdose prevention with intranasal naloxone among people who take methadone. *Journal of Substance Abuse Treatment, 44*(2), 241–247. doi:10.1016/j.jsat.2012.07.004.

Walley, A. Y., Xuan, Z., Hackman, H. H., Quinn, E., Doe-Simkins, M., Sorensen-Alawad, A., . . . Ozonoff, A. (2013). Opioid overdose rates and implementation of overdose education and nasal naloxone distribution in Massachusetts: interrupted time series analysis. *BMJ: British Medical Journal, 346*, f174. doi:10.1136/bmj.f174.

Wang, K. H., Fiellin, D. A., & Becker, W. C. (2014). Source of prescription drugs used nonmedically in rural and urban populations. *American Journal of Drug and Alcohol Abuse, 40*(4), 292–303. doi:10.3109/00952990.2014.907301.

Warner, M., Chen, L. H., Makuc, D. M., Anderson, R. N., & Minino, A. M. (2011). Drug poisoning deaths in the United States, 1980–2008. *NCHS Data Brief* (81), 1–8.

Webster, L. R., Cochella, S., Dasgupta, N., Fakata, K. L., Fine, P. G., Fishman, S. M., . . . Wakeland, W. (2011). An analysis of the root causes for opioid-related overdose deaths in the United States. *Pain Medicine, 12 Suppl 2*, S26–S35. doi:10.1111/j.1526-4637.2011.01134.x.

Webster, L. R., & Webster, R. M. (2005). Predicting aberrant behaviors in opioid-treated patients: Preliminary validation of the Opioid Risk Tool. *Pain Medicine, 6*(6), 432–442. doi:10.1111/j.1526-4637.2005.00072.x.

Weiner, S. G., Griggs, C. A., Mitchell, P. M., Langlois, B. K., Friedman, F. D., Moore, R. L., . . . James A. Feldman, J. A. (2013). Clinician impression versus prescription drug monitoring program criteria in the assessment of drug-seeking behavior in the emergency department. *Annals of Emergency Medicine, 62*(4), 281–289. doi:10.1016/j.annemergmed.2013.05.025.

Weiner, S. G., Horton, L. C., Green, T. C., & Butler, S. F. (2015). Feasibility of tablet computer screening for opioid abuse in the emergency department. *Western Journal of Emergency Medicine, 16*(1), 18–23. doi:10.5811/westjem.2014.11.23316.

Weiner, S. G., Horton, L. C., Green, T. C., & Butler, S. F. (2016). A comparison of an opioid abuse screening tool and prescription drug monitoring data in the emergency department. *Drug and Alcohol Dependence, 159,* 152–157. doi:10.1016/j.drugalcdep.2015.12.007.

Weiner, S. G., Perrone, J., & Nelson, L. S. (2013). Centering the pendulum: The evolution of emergency medicine opioid prescribing guidelines. *Annals of Emergency Medicine, 62*(3), 241–243. doi:10.1016/j.annemergmed.2013.02.028.

Weissman, D. E., & Haddox, J. D. (1989). Opioid pseudoaddiction—An iatrogenic syndrome. *Pain, 36*(3), 363–366.

World Health Organization. (2014). *Community Management of Opioid Overdose.* Geneva, Switzerland: World Health Organization.

Yi, P., & Pryzbylkowski, P. (2015). Opioid induced hyperalgesia. *Pain Medicine, 16 Suppl 1,* S32–S36. doi:10.1111/pme.12914.

Yoburn, B. C. (1988). Opioid antagonist-induced upregulation and functional supersensitivity. *Reviews in Clinical & Basic Pharmacology, 7*(1-4), 109–128.

Yousefshahi, F., Predescu, O., & Francisco Asenjo, J. (2017). The efficacy of systemic lidocaine in the management of chronic pain: A literature review. *Anesthesiology and Pain Medicine, 7*(3), e44732. doi:10.5812/aapm.44732.

CHAPTER ELEVEN

Regulation of Opioid Medications in the United States

Kenneth Kemp Jr. and Martin Grabois

This chapter will review the current state of opioid prescribing in the United States and how federal laws, state laws, and prescribing guidelines influence it. The current guidelines of opioid prescribing will be reviewed; over time, these guidelines have evolved from direction on proper opioid prescribing into stronger regulations, all in an attempt to control the current epidemic of opioid misuse, diversion, and overdose death. For more information on opioid medications themselves, see chapter 2; for more information on the history of opioids, see chapters 9 and 13.

Opioid Problem in the United States

While opioids have been used for pain treatment for centuries, in the 1980s, a group of physicians began treating pain in patients with chronic nonmalignant diagnoses, with chronic pain defined as pain lasting longer than three months (Portenoy & Foley, 1986). The prescribing of opioids for chronic noncancer pain became a widespread practice in the 1990s, with a large number of new opioids produced, including long-acting formulations (Estep, Hjalmarson, & Abdullah, 2011). The growth in opioid prescribing continued into the 2000s, fueled by a Joint Commission on Accreditation of Healthcare Organizations' (JCAHO) proclamation that pain should be considered the "fifth vital sign." Emphasis was placed on proper evaluation and management of pain in patients (Baker, 2017), but some providers erroneously took this emphasis to mean that patients have a right to be pain-free.

Several guidelines exist on appropriate prescribing of opioid medications for nonmalignant chronic pain, including, but not limited to, those from the Federation of State Medical Boards, the American Academy of Pain Medicine, the American Pain Society, and the State of Washington. These guidelines are all similar in their calls for appropriate evaluation of pain, assessing the risk of addiction potential or misuse by a patient, setting functional goals for treatment, and close monitoring of patient response. Physician-patient opioid contracts were suggested to educate and obtain informed consent prior to instituting long-term opioid medication use (Chou et al., 2009; Washington State Agency Medical Directors' Group, 2015). Despite these guidelines, the numbers of opioid prescriptions and opioid overdose deaths have continued to climb. From 2007 to 2012, opioid prescriptions increased by over 7 percent (Paulozzi, Mack, & Hockenberry, 2014), and almost 260 million prescriptions were written for opioids in 2012 (Levy, Paulozzi, Mack, & Jones, 2015).

In some instances, providers ignored guidelines for opioid prescribing, with the most excessive taking the form of practices termed "pill mills"; these practices allowed patients to obtain opioids for cash with little treatment documentation or medical assessment of misuse (i.e., medication use in ways not intended by the prescriber), addiction, or diversion (i.e., intentional removal of a medication from appropriate medically established guidelines for profit, recreational misuse) risk (Katz et al., 2007). No discussion of alternative treatment options or risks of opioids were undertaken, and only opioid treatment was offered (Zuzek, 2013).

The guidelines written for opioid management are not rules or regulations, and they have limited effect on curbing inappropriate opioid prescribing, particularly among (rare) bad actors. In addition to less scrupulous providers, patients can present with fictitious pain conditions, seek out multiple opioid providers, and, ultimately, misuse or divert medications (Katz et al., 2007). The North Carolina Medical Board, in its policy on opioid treatment of pain, lists patient characteristics that are risk factors for patient misuse or diversion, including vague history of illness, "soft diagnosis," a history of taking multiple combinations of controlled substances, multiple pain physicians or doctors, traveling a significant distance to a physician's office, no past medical records, and requests for specific drugs by name. Many patients with at-risk characteristics lack objective physical exam findings or pain-related radiographic findings but have exaggerated pain complaints or inconsistent actions in the medical setting. During reassessments, inconsistent urine drug screening findings (e.g., illicit substances, lack of medication prescribed), frequent calls for early refills, and lost or stolen prescriptions also suggest misuse and diversion (North Carolina Medical Board, 2014).

The increase in opioid prescriptions in the United States has correlated with the increase of opioid misuse, addiction, and opioid-related overdose. From 1999 to 2014, 165,000 people died from opioid-related overdose, and over 400,000 emergency department visits related to opioid misuse occurred in 2011 alone (Dowell, Haegerich, & Chou, 2016). Despite the increase in opioids prescribing over this time period, only half of chronic pain sufferers stated that their pain was being adequately treated (Langer, 2005), with over 11 percent of U.S. adults reporting daily pain in 2012 (Nahin, 2015). Therefore, physicians are responsible for appropriately treating pain in their patients and limiting the potential societal impact of opioid use and misuse.

Government Regulations

One of the first steps in the United States to regulate opioids occurred in 1909 through the Opium Exclusion Act, which aimed to prevent opium importation. In 1914, the Harrison Tax Act legally required pharmacies and physicians to register to prescribe or dispense opioids (Brownstein, 1993). The 1924 Heroin Act made heroin, which had been developed by Bayer as a less addictive substitute for morphine, illegal. The Food, Drug and Cosmetic Act of 1938, allowed the U.S. Food and Drug Administration (FDA) to regulate the use of all drugs based on their level of safety. The FDA remains responsible for standards of safety and efficacy of drugs, the approval process for new drugs, and public and provider education regarding the safe use and risks of drugs (Brownstein, 1993).

In 1970, the United States passed the Controlled Substances Act (CSA), which placed drugs and potentially addictive medications on a schedule corresponding to the level of abuse potential, treatment effectiveness, and potential of harm. Lower numbers denote greater potential harm and greater control; thus, controlled substances are placed on Schedule I (most dangerous) to Schedule V (least dangerous). Schedule I medications are for research but have no accepted medical benefits, and Schedule II medications have appropriate medical uses with a high potential for physical and psychological dependence leading to a substance use disorder (U.S. Department of Justice, 2006a). In 1973, President Richard Nixon created the Drug Enforcement Administration (DEA) by executive order, and the DEA is charged with enforcing the CSA (Brownstein, 1993). It is responsible for prevention, detection, and investigations into the diversion of opioids, and it controls the dispensing, manufacturing, and distribution of all controlled substances. The DEA also makes the final decision on scheduling medications (U.S. Department of Justice, 2014a), using input from the FDA and U.S. Department of Health and Human Services.

Because of the strict regulation of opioids in the United States, many physicians in the 1980s were hesitant to prescribe them, but there were physician groups proclaiming their safety for treating pain. As noted above, a consensus eventually emerged that pain was being undertreated by many physicians during this time. The DEA policy states that a prescription for a controlled substance is legal if there is a legitimate medical reason for its use, it is given by a physician in the usual course of medical practice, and the prescriber is taking reasonable steps to prevent its misuse and diversion. This policy was meant to give prescribers of opioids some confidence after the DEA withdrew its approval of a consensus statement published in 2004 (delineating appropriate opioid-prescribing practices) without a clear explanation. This lack of a consensus statement still leaves appropriate prescribing of opioids in a significant gray area (U.S. Department of Justice, 2006b).

The current backlash against opioid medications and a general lack of direction on prescribing has caused some physicians to stop prescribing them. Consequences for inappropriate opioid prescribing have included sanctions against a physician's license, revoking that license, or criminal prosecution, with potential incarceration from 20 years to life if a person is injured related to a Schedule II medication prescription (Yeh, 2015).

Regulatory Response to the Current Opioid Problem in the United States

In a recent response to the growing opioid problem in the United States, the DEA changed the classification of hydrocodone from Schedule III to the more regulated Schedule II level (U.S. Department of Justice, 2014b). Schedule II medications are more strictly controlled than those on Schedule III, with the following restrictions (some specific to the state of Texas) on Schedule II medications: a patient has to see a physician to obtain a prescription; the medication cannot be prescribed or refilled by a phone call or fax; a special paper prescription (triplicate) is required to fill the opioid medication; a 90-day supply requires a physician to write three separate 30-day prescriptions; lost or stolen prescriptions are not to be replaced or rewritten; voided prescription are returned to the state so that accounting for control numbers can occur; and no postdating of prescriptions is allowed (Legislature of the State of Texas, 1989; U.S. Department of Justice, 2006a).

The ability to electronically prescribe Schedule II medications is now available in Texas and in other states, and such procedures are accepted by many pharmacies (Legislature of the State of Texas, 1989). Electronic prescriptions should help to curtail the forgery of written prescriptions, but, at this time, electronic prescribing of Schedule II medications is not common. There are regulations on the refill of opioid medications, but there is no cap on the amount or dose that a physician can prescribe for a patient. Despite generally very strict regulations, it is explicitly noted in the CSA that these medications are legitimate medical treatments for intractable pain (U.S. Department of Justice, 2006a). The regulation of these medications was not meant to interfere with the proper treatment of patients truly in need of pain management, but they do require a significant time commitment for the physician just to physically write out the prescription. Also, the restrictions require that the patient make frequent trips (i.e., at least every 30 days) to the doctor, even with no change to the medication regimen, fulfilling the expectation of a face-to-face meeting and scheduled reevaluation of a patient on opioids (U.S. Department of Justice, 2014b). The Schedule II requirements in Texas may be a major reason why many physicians do not carry the necessary triplicate prescription pads.

The intent of such regulation is to limit the amount of opioid medication in circulation, but it has also negatively impacted the trust necessary for positive doctor-patient relationships and medication availability for legitimate patients with chronic pain (Chambers et al., 2016). The DEA has also mandated a 34 percent reduction in hydrocodone manufacture and at least a 25 percent reduction in production of other opioids in 2017 (Drug Enforcement Administration Public Affairs, 2016). The tighter control over hydrocodone and the calls to decrease opioid production have interfered with the ability of pharmacies to maintain adequate stocks of opioid medication. In most states, including Texas, the physician-patient opioid contract requires the use of only a pharmacy for the filling of medications (Texas Medical Board, 1989). If the medication is not in stock, the patient will have to wait or find a pharmacy that carries the prescribed opioid, without penalty—though this is not always the case. When reviewed, the prescription drug monitoring program (PDMP) revealed one physician prescriber but multiple pharmacies; the ability to better monitor opioid prescriptions received by an individual should render the requirement to receive prescriptions from one pharmacy obsolete. Nonetheless, while reduced opioid availability and greater regulation of use may decrease opioid diversion, it will likely increase the cost and decrease the availability of opioids for patients being appropriately treated for chronic pain. The increase in cost of mainstream pain medications has resulted in the increased use of cheaper forms of street opioids, mainly heroin and synthetic fentanyl, and the rate of overdose linked to these two substances has increased in recent years (O'Donnell, Gladden, & Seth, 2017).

In 2012, the FDA began to require opioid manufacturers to educate physicians and prescribers regarding the risks and appropriate management of extended-release or long-acting opioid medications. Such risk evaluation and mitigation strategies (REMS) included education regarding the safe use of opioids, evaluation of the risk of addiction or opioid misuse, and the use of opioid contracts to delineate the rights and responsibilities of the physician and patient in regard to the long-term opioid prescribing and use. REMS are basically a reiteration of opioid prescription guidelines that have been in place for years. Also, warnings about opioid use during pregnancy, including risk to the newborn infant, possibility of addiction, respiratory depression, and opioid misuse were mandated. The FDA has also encouraged continued development of opioids with abuse-deterrent technology and the public availability of naloxone to treat opioid overdose (see chapter 13 for more on opioids). A greater number of states are increasing naloxone availability and even allowing over-the-counter sales. The hope is that naloxone availability will prevent overdose-related death from both opioid medications and illicit opioids, such as heroin (Brownstein, 1993; Califf, Woodcock, & Ostroff, 2016; U.S. Food and Drug Administration, 2017).

Recently, the Centers for Disease Control and Prevention (CDC) has published guidelines for physicians when prescribing opioid medications for patients with nonmalignant pain on a chronic basis (Dowell et al., 2016). We will review these guidelines and discuss the state of current prescribing guidelines and how they evolved into regulations.

The efficacy of chronic (i.e., long-term) opioid use is poorly supported scientifically (Dowell et al., 2016); conversely, the potential harm associated with opioid use is well established and is illustrated by the U.S. opioid epidemic. The risk of medication misuse is higher in patients taking psychiatric medications, with concomitant depression or a history of substance use disorder and of a younger age (Banta-Green, Merrill, Doyle, Boudreau, & Calsyn, 2009; Reid et al., 2002). A subset of patients does benefit from long-term opioid use, but these patients do not represent the entire population exposed to opioids. Current CDC guidelines recommend that opioids not be the first line of treatment for chronic pain, with efficacious nonopioid medications (e.g., nonsteroidal anti-inflammatory medications, tricyclic antidepressants, SSRIs, SNRIs, and topical agents) prioritized. A patient should not be started on an opioid without first establishing treatment goals for pain and, more importantly, functional outcomes. The goals should include both physical and psychosocial ones, and they should be reviewed at every visit and revised as needed (Dowell et al., 2016).

Before starting an opioid for long-term use, the risks and lack of known long-term benefits of opioids should be discussed with the patient. The idea that total pain relief will be the goal of treatment should be discouraged, as it is unrealistic for many patients. The necessity of regular follow-up assessment of treatment, including the use of urine drug screening and PDMP review, needs to be emphasized. The benefits and possible side effects of opioids should be followed closely in the beginning and then at least every three months or sooner based on the patient's risk of misuse or side effects of the opioid medication (Dowell et al., 2016). While these are well-supported and useful steps, none of them are novel. These guidelines follow a format consistent with the pain treatment or opioid contracts that have existed for years (Dowell et al., 2016).

Physicians are also told to begin opioid treatment of chronic pain with the lowest dose of short-acting medication possible. Careful titration of opioids is acceptable, but caution needs to be used when the dose reaches 50 morphine milligram equivalents (MME). The MME is a standardized value based on the potency of morphine, and any opioid medication can be converted to an MME total. An opioid dose above 90 MME should be avoided or, if considered necessary, supported by proper documentation. Also, concomitant use of benzodiazepines and opioids should be avoided, given the elevated risk for overdose in those using both. Any patient taking greater than 90 MME or 50 MME in combination with benzodiazepines should be offered naloxone, and naloxone should also be discussed with patients with an overdose or substance use disorder history.

Once a patient is started on chronic opioid therapy, regular follow-up visits should reevaluate the risks of opioid use in each patient individually. This includes regular PDMP review (at least every three months) and the regular use of urine drug testing to assess for the presence of prescribed medications, illicit substances, and other controlled substances (Dowell et al., 2016).

At any sign of opioid misuse, a physician should not discharge a patient from care but should assist in the provision of appropriate treatment by referring for medication-assisted addiction treatment, including buprenorphine or methadone (Dowell et al., 2016).

Prescription Drug Monitoring Programs (PDMPs)

While described in much greater detail in chapter 12 of this volume, we will briefly address PDMPs here. As of October 2016, every state except for Missouri had enacted a PDMP and had an operational website. PDMP use reduces both doctor shopping and the amount of opioids available for misuse (Reifler et al., 2012), and it is an effective way to monitor a patient's medication history and current prescribing physicians. In the CDC guidelines on opioid prescribing, the danger of concomitant use of opioids and benzodiazepines is stressed, and a PDMP allows physicians to prevent such concomitant use when the prescriptions come from different providers. Ultimately, PDMP use helps physicians recognize early signs of opioid misuse, prevent drug interactions, and learn of prescriptions not disclosed by a patient.

Urine Drug Screening

Urine drug screening (UDS) is now a common component of opioid treatment of chronic nonmalignant pain. While there is no consensus on how often UDS testing should be done, one recommendation suggests UDS at an initial visit, with follow-up testing every year for low-risk patients, every 6 months for moderate-risk patients, and every visit for high-risk or problematic patients. Also, patients should know that UDS is possible at any visit, as the potential for UDS can improve adherence and prevent misuse (Peppin et al., 2012). UDS are helpful in confirming the presence of known medications prescribed and in divulging the presence of illicit substances and medications not known by the treating physician. Inconsistent results on UDS should lead to a discussion of the dangers of not taking medications as prescribed, of illegal substances, and of mixing of medications without the knowledge the treating physician. As with other signs of opioid misuse, concerning UDS results should not lead to patient discharge, but rather a plan to address misuse, addiction, or proper tapering of opioids (Dowell et al., 2016).

To combat the indiscriminate opioid prescribing, the Texas State Legislature (in 167.001 of the Texas Medical Practice Act) required privately or publicly owned clinics that routinely prescribe opioids to register as pain management clinics. The owners had to be practicing physicians with an unrestricted medical license, holding a certificate of pain management clinic registration. Clinics associated with medical schools, hospitals, or private physician practices that use multiple treatment options are not required to register. This regulation is consistent with the CDC guidelines, which state that all treatment options need to be utilized and that opioid prescriptions paid for in cash without proper evaluation or continued assessment are illegal (Berlin, 2016). Other states take different approaches: for instance, in its regulatory code, Rhode Island suggests, but does not require, a multidisciplinary approach to the treatment of chronic pain (State of Rhode Island Department of Health, 2017).

Current Texas Administrative Code sets minimum requirements for chronic pain treatment in the state. Such treatment includes an appropriate history and a physical examination (including past and current treatment), the effect of pain on function, a history or potential of substance abuse or diversion, and an appropriate diagnosis. Before starting an opioid medication, a physician is required to obtain a baseline UDS and review the state PDMP. Documentation is required when a physician decides not to review the PDMP or obtain UDS; thus, the code is basically a law requiring the use of UDS and PDMP. This code also requires the documentation of treatment goals and informed consent by way of a pain contract. The contract must include the provision for future UDS, prescriptions from the named or covering physician only, use of one pharmacy for filling the medication, and reasons why the opioid prescription may be terminated. Close and regular follow-up is suggested by the code, including the PDMP review and repeat UDS or documentation of why this is not necessary (Texas Medical Board, 1989).

Rhode Island has similar rules and regulations for the prescribing of opioids. The Rhode Island Code requires PDMP review prior to initiating an opioid prescription, even for acute pain. Rhode Island also restricts the treatment for acute pain to no more than 30 MME per day and a maximum prescription of 20 doses (State of Rhode Island Department of Health, 2017). Furthermore, the code states that only short-acting medications should be used due to the elevated risk of death from respiratory depression in opioid-naive patients taking stronger and long-acting opioids (Dowell et al., 2016). The State of New York recently moved to limit acute pain prescribing to seven days after surgery (New York State Department of Health, 2016), and New Jersey limits prescriptions for postoperative opioids and opioids for acute pain to five days (King, 2017). These limited prescriptions are designed to limit opioid tolerance and physical dependence as well as unused opioid pills available for diversion. Conversely, such restrictions can lead to inadequate pain treatment for certain patients in acute pain, including patients after a traumatic injury or surgical intervention where pain duration can exceed the time-limited prescription. Such regulatory actions rarely take into account individual patient pharmacokinetics or dynamics (Hill, 1996) and can leave some patients in ongoing pain.

The CDC guidelines discuss the risk of opioid overdose or misuse in terms of MME. The 50 and 90 MME cut points in the guidelines (noted above) are based on data showing risk of overdose death is almost nine times greater if the daily MME is greater than 100, as compared to doses below 20 (Dowell et al., 2016). This 90 MME threshold in the CDC guidelines is now a rule in Rhode Island, with such a prescription requiring a pain management consultation or documentation in cases where one was not completed (State of Rhode Island Department of Health, 2017). The State of Washington requires a pain management consultation prior to implementing an opioid dose above 120 MME per day (Washington State Agency Medical Directors' Group, 2015), and the Maine has mandated that all noncancer or nonpalliative care patients to be at or below 100 MME per day by July 1, 2017. For patients with chronic nonmalignant pain, such a dose ceiling will likely have negative effects on their ability to function (St. Amour, 2017).

Transitions of Care in Chronic Opioid Management

One gap in the medical treatment guidelines is evident in the transition of a patient already on chronic opioids to another physician. The Rhode Island regulations call for the referring physician to "facilitate a safe transition of care," which includes a documented physician-to-physician interaction to avoid patient care lapses (State of Rhode Island Department of Health, 2017). There is little guidance for transitioning the care of a patient on chronic opioid management from one physician to another when the patient initiates the transition without consulting the treating physician. The new physician encounters a new patient who might claim a need to transition care because of insurance changes, geographic distances, or a poor patient-physician relationship. This kind of transition places the new treating physician in a difficult situation, especially if the patient does not bring adequate documentation from the previous treating physician.

A new physician should follow the guidelines for starting a patient on chronic opioid therapy, even when the patient claims to have been on the same medications for years. The patient could be a valid patient with a valid need. It is best not to accept a patient requesting the continuation of chronic opioid treatment without first getting full records from the previous treating physician. A patient's own medical and treatment history can be erroneous, whether innocently or intentionally, as in the case of a patient who goes to multiple providers looking for opioid medication to misuse or divert. Furthermore, improper dosing based on a patient's history can lead to overdose and death. Thus, proper documentation of previous treatment, diagnostic testing, opioid risk, PDMP review, and UDS should be done before starting a patient new to a physician practice on chronic opioids (Dowell et al., 2016). Unfortunately, requiring full documentation from the previous physician can have the unintended effect of angering the patient, undermining the physician-patient relationship and preventing patients in pain from receiving timely treatment. Finally, patients may claim that the new physician must prescribe the medication requested to prevent opioid withdrawal, but federal regulations state that it is illegal to write an opioid prescription for the sole purpose of preventing withdrawal (U.S. Department of Justice, 2017).

Conclusion

As stated before, pain has always been a part of the human condition. In the 1980s, efforts were made to improve the treatment of pain, including a call for all patients to receive appropriate pain evaluation and management. When the use of opioid medication was initially indicated for nonmalignant pain management, physician groups and organizations developed guidelines for appropriate evaluation, management, and treatment. Unfortunately, many health care professionals did not adequately follow these guidelines. When combined with the marketing efforts of pharmaceutical companies to increase opioid prescribing, a shift in health care goals to try to achieve freedom from pain for patients and a belief that opioids are the key treatment for pain, evolving attitudes about opioid use by physicians led to a rise in opioid prescriptions and, eventually, deaths due to opioid overdose. In response, both the U.S. government and states have increased the number and scope of regulations about the use, distribution, prescription, and manufacturing of opioid medications.

As the U.S. and state law and regulations continue to limit the quantity, strength, and length of opioid prescriptions, the physician-patient relationship will sometimes be strained. To limit this, physicians need to educate their patients regarding opioid medications, and physicians need to be compassionate when treating patients who are suffering. The right to be pain-free can no more be guaranteed than the right to be cancer-free, but appropriate pain evaluation and management is paramount. Unfortunately, both patients and health professionals in the United States have been trained to believe that opioid medication is the only way to treat pain. As such, increasing regulation of opioid prescribing will not stop the current epidemic; the change to a more compassionate and patient-centered approach in the treatment of pain and suffering holds greater promise.

References

Baker, D. W. (2017). History of the joint commission's pain standards: Lessons for today's prescription opioid epidemic. *JAMA, 317*(11), 1117–1118. doi:10.1001/jama.2017.0935.

Banta-Green, C. J., Merrill, J. O., Doyle, S. R., Boudreau, D. M., & Calsyn, D. A. (2009). Opioid use behaviors, mental health and pain—Development of a typology of chronic pain patients. *Drug and Alcohol Dependence, 104*(1-2), 34–42. doi:10.1016/j.drugalcdep.2009.03.021.

Berlin, J. (2016). Revised TMG rules target nefarious prescribers, but physicians say the rules are a burden. *Texas Medicine, 112*(1), 28–35.

Brownstein, M. J. (1993). A brief history of opiates, opioid peptides, and opioid receptors. *Proceedings of the National Academy of Sciences, 90*(12), 5391–5393.

Califf, R. M., Woodcock, J., & Ostroff, S. (2016). A proactive response to prescription opioid abuse. *New England Journal of Medicine, 374*(15), 1480–1485. doi:10.1056/NEJMsr1601307.

Chambers, J., Gleason, R. M., Kirsh, K. L., Twillman, R., Webster, L., Berner, J., . . . Passik, S. D. (2016). An online survey of patients' experiences since the rescheduling of hydrocodone: The first 100 days. *Pain Medicine, 17*(9), 1686–1693. doi:10.1093/pm/pnv064.

Chou, R., Fanciullo, G. J., Fine, P. G., Adler, J. A., Ballantyne, J. C., Davies, P., . . . Miaskowski, C. (2009). Clinical guidelines for the use of chronic opioid therapy in chronic noncancer pain. *Journal of Pain, 10*(2), 113–130. doi:10.1016/j.jpain.2008.10.008.

Dowell, D., Haegerich, T. M., & Chou, R. (2016). CDC Guideline for prescribing opioids for chronic pain—United States, 2016. *JAMA, 315*(15), 1624–1645. doi:10.1001/jama.2016.1464.

Drug Enforcement Administration Public Affairs. (2016). DEA reduces amount of opioid controlled substances to be manufactured in 2017. Press release, October 4. https://www.dea.gov/divisions/hq/2016/hq100416.shtml.

Estep, B., Hjalmarson, D., & Abdullah, H. (2011). OxyContin abuse spreads from U.S. Appalachia across US. http://www.mcclatchydc.com/2011/03/13/110243/oxycontin-abuse-spreads-from-appalachia.html.

Hill, C. S., Jr. (1996). Government regulatory influences on opioid prescribing and their impact on the treatment of pain of nonmalignant origin. *Journal of Pain and Symptom Management, 11*(5), 287–298.

Katz, N. P., Adams, E. H., Chilcoat, H., Colucci, R. D., Comer, S. D., Goliber, P., . . . Weiss, R. (2007). Challenges in the development of prescription opioid abuse-deterrent formulations. *Clinical Journal of Pain, 23*(8), 648–660. doi:10.1097/AJP.0b013e318125c5e8.

King, K. (2017). New Jersey to limit amount of opioid pills in prescriptions. *Wall Street Journal*, February 15, https://www.wsj.com/articles/new-jersey -to-limit-amount-of-opioid-pills-in-prescriptions-1487198253.

Langer, G. (2005). Poll: Americans searching for pain relief. ABC News, May 9. http://abcnews.go.com/Health/PainManagement/story?id=732395&singl ePage=true.

Legislature of the State of Texas. (1989). *Texas Controlled Substances Act*. http:// www.statutes.legis.state.tx.us/Docs/HS/htm/HS.481.htm.

Levy, B., Paulozzi, L., Mack, K. A., & Jones, C. M. (2015). Trends in opioid analgesic-prescribing rates by specialty, U.S., 2007–2012. *American Journal of Preventive Medicine, 49*(3), 409–413. doi:10.1016/j.amepre.2015.02.020.

Nahin, R. L. (2015). Estimates of pain prevalence and severity in adults: United States, 2012. *Journal of Pain, 16*(8), 769–780. doi:10.1016/j.jpain. 2015.05.002.

New York State Department of Health. (2016). Narcotic enforcement: Laws and regulations. https://www.health.ny.gov/professionals/narcotic/laws_ and_regulations.

North Carolina Medical Board. (2014). *North Carolina Medical Board Policy for the Use of Opiates for the Treatment of Pain*. Raleigh, NC: North Carolina Medical Board.

O'Donnell, J. K., Gladden, R. M., & Seth, P. (2017). Trends in deaths involving heroin and synthetic opioids excluding methadone, and law enforcement drug product reports, by census region—United States, 2006–2015. *MMWR: Morbidity and Mortality Weekly Report, 66*(34), 897–903. doi:10.15585/mmwr.mm6634a2.

Paulozzi, L. J., Mack, K. A., & Hockenberry, J. M. (2014). Vital signs: Variation among states in prescribing of opioid pain relievers and benzodiazepines—United States, 2012. *MMWR: Morbidity and Mortality Weekly Report, 63*(26), 563–568.

Peppin, J. F., Passik, S. D., Couto, J. E., Fine, P. G., Christo, P. J., Argoff, C., . . . Goldfarb, N. I. (2012). Recommendations for urine drug monitoring as a component of opioid therapy in the treatment of chronic pain. *Pain Medicine, 13*(7), 886–896. doi:10.1111/j.1526-4637.2012.01414.x.

Portenoy, R. K., & Foley, K. M. (1986). Chronic use of opioid analgesics in nonmalignant pain: Report of 38 cases. *Pain, 25*(2), 171–186.

Reid, M. C., Engles-Horton, L. L., Weber, M. A. B., Kerns, R. D., Rogers, E. L., & O'Connor, P. G. (2002). Use of opioid medications for chronic noncancer pain syndromes in primary care. *Journal of General Internal Medicine,* 17(3), 173–179. doi:10.1046/j.1525-1497.2002.10435.x.

Reifler, L. M., Droz, D., Bailey, J. E., Schnoll, S. H., Fant, R., Dart, R. C., & Bucher Bartelson, B. (2012). Do prescription monitoring programs impact state trends in opioid abuse/misuse? *Pain Medicine, 13*(3), 434–442. doi: 10.1111/j.1526-4637.2012.01327.x.

St. Amour, M. (2017). Pain patients brace for Maine law cutting opiate prescriptions. *Portland Press Herald,* January 21, https://www.pressherald.com/2017/01/21/pain-patients-brace-for-maine-law-cutting-opiate-prescriptions/.

State of Rhode Island Department of Health. (2017). *Rules and Regulations for Pain Management, Opioid Use and the Registration of Distributors of Controlled Substances in Rhode Island.* Providence, RI: State of Rhode Island Department of Health.

Texas Medical Board. (1989). *Pain Management, Texas Administrative Code, Title 22, Part 9, Chapter 170, Rule 3.* Austin, TX: Texas Medical Board.

U.S. Department of Justice. (2006a). *21 Code of Federal Regulations, Part 1306.* Washington, D.C.: U.S. Department of Justice.

U.S. Department of Justice. (2006b). Purpose of issue of prescription: Dispensing controlled substances for the treatment of pain, DEA policy statement. *Federal Register, 71*(172).

U.S. Department of Justice. (2014a). Organization, mission and functions manual: Drug Enforcement Administration. September 9. https://www.justice.gov/jmd/organization-mission-and-functions-manual-drug-enforcement-administration.

U.S. Department of Justice. (2014b). Schedules of controlled substances: Rescheduling of hydrocodone combination products from Schedule III to Schedule II. *Federal Register, 79*(163).

U.S. Department of Justice. (2017). *21 Code of Federal Regulations, Part 1306.07, Administering or Dispensing of Narcotic Drugs.* Washington, D.C.: U.S. Department of Justice.

U.S. Food and Drug Administration. (2017). New safety measures announced for extended-release and long-acting opioids. Press release, May 11.

Washington State Agency Medical Directors' Group. (2015). *Washington State Agency Medical Directors' Group. AMDG 2015 Interagency Guideline on Prescribing Opioids for Pain.* Olympia, WA: Washington State Agency Medical Directors' Group.

Yeh, B. T. (2015). *Drug Offenses: Maximum Fines and Terms of Imprisonment for Violation of the Federal Controlled Substances Act and Related Laws.* Washington, D.C.: Congressional Research Service.

Zuzek, C. (2013). Pill mills: Feds and state crackdown. *Texas Medicine, 109*(4), 18–24.

CHAPTER TWELVE

Promoting Prescription Drug Monitoring Programs for Population Health: Research and Policy Implications

*David S. Fink, Julia P. Schleimer, Aaron Sarvet,
Kiran K. Grover, Chris Delcher, June H. Kim, Alvaro
Castillo-Carniglia, Ariadne E. Rivera-Aguirre, Stephen
G. Henry, Magdalena Cerdá, and Silvia S. Martins*

The volume of prescription opioids prescribed in the United States nearly quadrupled from less than two kilograms per 10,000 people in 1999 to more than seven kilograms per 10,000 people in 2009 (Centers for Disease Control and Prevention, 2011). Absent any evidence for an overall change in the amount of pain reported by Americans (Chang, Daubresse, Kruszewski, & Alexander, 2014; Daubresse et al., 2013), this change in the supply of prescription opioids is concerning and came with attendant population health consequences. For example, during this same 10-year period from 1999 to 2009, the United States observed a three-fold increase in both the rate of prescription opioid-induced deaths (Rudd, Aleshire, Zibbell, & Matthew Gladden, 2016) and the rate of neonatal abstinence syndrome (Patrick et al., 2012). The age-adjusted rate of drug overdose deaths involving prescription opioids increased from 3.1 per 100,000 in 1999 to 10.7 per 100,000 in 2015 (Centers for Disease Control and Prevention, National Center for Health Statistics, 2016), and the incidence of neonatal abstinence syndrome among newborns increased from 1.2 per 1,000 hospital births per year in 2000 to 3.4 per 1,000 hospital births per year in 2009 (Patrick et al., 2012)

And while heroin-induced overdose deaths held steady during this same 10-year period from 1999 to 2009, rates of heroin-induced deaths have since quadrupled in the five years from 2010 to 2015 (Hedegaard, Warner, & Minino, 2017). As rates of opioid prescriptions and opioid-induced deaths have increased, prescribers increasingly face pressures to adapt prescribing behaviors to reduce diversion of opioid pain relievers for nonmedical use without limiting access to these medications among persons with a genuine medical need. State prescription drug monitoring programs (PDMPs) have been advanced as a critical tool to better inform clinical care and address overprescribing and its consequences (National Center for Injury Prevention and Control, 2013; Office of National Drug Control Policy, 2011).

PDMPs are statewide electronic databases that collect data on medications dispensed within the state. This information is transmitted to a central repository and can be accessed by authorized users to inform clinical decisions, identify potentially illegal behaviors, and track changing pharma-coepidemiologic trends. For example, prescribers and dispensers might use PDMP data to identify dangerous drug interactions or patients exhibiting drug-seeking behaviors (e.g., interacting with multiple providers and pharmacies with the presumed intent of obtaining controlled drugs for misuse or diversion), whereas law enforcement agencies might use PDMP data to identify prescribers or clinics involved in illegal prescribing practices (i.e., "pill mills"). In 2018, all 50 states and Washington, D.C., have passed legislation authorizing the development of a PDMP. However, the evidence for their effect on reducing the nonmedical use of prescription drugs and the consequences to population health that follow from nonmedical use remains contested.

In this chapter, we consider the potential for PDMPs to address the current prescription opioid epidemic and its attendant consequences on population health. This chapter consists of three sections: (1) historical overview and development of the modern PDMP in the United States; (2) evidence on the effect of PDMPs on prescriber behaviors and population health; and (3) challenges in the existing literature and directions for future research.

Development of the Modern PDMP

Although PDMPs originated as a tool to assist law enforcement in detecting inappropriate or illegal prescribing, dispensing, or use of controlled substances, recently these databases have increasingly been called on to reduce opioid-related harm and improve population health (Deyo et al., 2013). In an evolution since the middle of the 20th century, PDMPs have become a key tool in control efforts to address inappropriate and illegal opioid prescribing and its health consequences.

The potential for PDMPs to both inform clinical care and improve law enforcement efforts to address the growing misuse and diversion of prescription drugs has led to a substantial federal investment in these programs. Prescription drug monitoring programs have become ubiquitous over the past 25 years. Since Oklahoma introduced the first electronic PDMP in 1990, every state except for Missouri has implemented, or enacted legislation to implement (Missouri), an electronic PDMP. This widespread adoption of PDMPs among nearly all the states has received substantial support from a wide array of federal agencies. Specifically, PDMPs are recommended by the Centers for Disease Control and Prevention (CDC) as an overdose prevention tool and have been advanced as a key component of the president's Prescription Drug Abuse Prevention Plan, which recommends that all states operate PDMPs and require prescribers to be trained in their use. Furthermore, the U.S. Department of Justice (DOJ) and U.S. Department of Health and Human Services (DHHS) offer grant funding to support states in planning, implementing, and enhancing the capacity of their PDMPs. Through these grants, the Harold Rogers Prescription Drug Monitoring Program (HRPDMP) grant program and the National All Schedules Prescription Electronic Reporting Act (NASPER), the DOJ and DHHS have awarded over a combined $100 million to 47 states and one U.S. territory (Guam).

Early Prescription Drug Monitoring Programs

Programs to monitor and control the distribution of controlled substances have become both more common and more sophisticated over time. This history of prescription drug monitoring programs consists of two eras: a paper era (1939–1990) and the more modern digital era (1990 to today (2018)). Dating back to the first half of the 20th century, the earliest PDMPs used special state-issued prescription forms that allowed law enforcement and professional agencies to monitor the prescription and distribution of certain controlled substances. Whether using individually serialized prescription forms or triplicate prescription pads, early PDMPs were burdensome and time-consuming for prescribers and pharmacies to supply data to, for states to maintain, and for providers to use.

To illustrate, a provider using a triplicate prescription pad would write a patient a prescription for a controlled substance, and the provider would retain a copy of that prescription for his or her office records. Next, the patient would take the original prescription and one copy to the pharmacist for dispensing. Upon dispensing the medication to the patient, the pharmacist would retain the copy for the pharmacy's records and send the original prescription to a central data repository where representatives from the state operating agency would enter the information into the agency's computer system. To obtain a history of the controlled substances dispensed to a patient, a prescriber or pharmacist was required to complete a patient activity form that would be faxed or mailed to the operating agency for processing. Burdened by time and access issues, only nine U.S. states ever adopted these early paper-based prescription monitoring programs from 1939 to 1989: California (1939), Hawaii (1943), Illinois (1961), Idaho (1967), Pennsylvania (1972), New York (1972), Rhode Island (1978), Texas (1981) and Michigan (1988). A more widespread adoption of PDMPs was not realized until the advancement of more sophisticated electronic systems in the 1990s, systems that could address many of the impediments and time constraints associated with these early paper-based PDMPs. For the remainder of this chapter, unless otherwise specified, the term PDMP refers to these more modern electronic PDMPs.

PDMPs in the Digital Age

Prescription drug monitoring programs have been reshaped in the digital age. Once a time-consuming and labor-intensive process, PDMPs have become increasingly valuable, easy to use, real-time digital resources for law enforcement and prescribers alike. Data collected by PDMPs can vary substantially by state. In general, however, U.S. states require that the dispensing pharmacist or provider enter all information about the prescription of controlled substances into the electronic database. Most often this includes data about the patient, prescriber, dispenser, drug, dose, and amount dispensed. After these data are submitted to the PDMP, an authorized user can log in to a computer and access a patient's history of controlled substances dispensed. Before further discussing PDMPs, a brief explanation of controlled substances and scheduling is needed.

Controlled prescription drugs are scheduled by two federal agencies, the Food and Drug Administration (FDA) and Drug Enforcement Administration (DEA), according to their abuse liability and accepted medical uses. The schedules range from Schedule I to Schedule V, with higher numbers denoting lesser abuse liability. Schedule I substances are reserved for illicit drugs that have no currently accepted medical use in treatment (e.g., heroin, LSD, psilocybin mushrooms). Schedule II prescription drugs are those with medical use but the greatest potential for abuse and dependence; examples of Schedule II prescription opioids include fentanyl (Sublimaze, Duragesic); hydrocodone (Zohydro, Vicodin); hydromorphone (Dilaudid); methadone (Dolophine); meperidine (Demerol); and oxycodone (OxyContin, Percocet). Common Schedule III prescription opioids include buprenorphine (Subutex,

Suboxone) and combination products containing either less than 15 milligrams of hydrocodone per dosage unit (Vicodin), less than 90 milligrams of codeine per dosage unit (Tylenol with Codeine), or less than 50 milligrams of morphine per dosage unit. Examples of Schedule IV and Schedule V prescriptions include tramadol (Ultram) and low-dose codeine cough suppressants.

While state PDMPs have commonalities in terms of centralized statewide data systems and basic elements of electronically transmitted prescription data, state law allows them to adapt their programs to fit their particular priorities. One way that PDMPs vary is how rapidly the pharmacists must enter these data into the system. In 2014, for example, about half of the states (55%) required pharmacists to enter data within seven days of dispensing a controlled substance, whereas about a fifth of the remaining states required pharmacists to enter these data more quickly (20%) and a quarter less quickly (25%). Other differences among PDMPs include whether providers must register for or use the system to prescribe drugs, the types of drugs that are monitored (Schedule II to Schedule V), the type of operating agency (e.g., law enforcement agency, professional licensing board, public health department), and whether the system is reactive or proactive; in contrast to a reactive system that requires a provider to query a patient's prescription history, a proactive system can automatically notify providers about any patient's or prescriber's unusual prescribing behaviors.

By tracking patient, prescriber, and dispenser information, PDMPs make it easier for law enforcement to detect drug diversion within the state. Diversion of controlled substances can occur at either the patient or provider level. At the patient level, diversion activity might occur through forged prescriptions or "doctor shopping." Doctor shopping describes the behavior of patients who seek out prescriptions from multiple providers to either supply their personal use or sell (divert) to others engaged in nonmedical use. At the provider level, health care providers or clinics might prescribe controlled substances with little consideration of patient need or outside the scope of standard medical practices (i.e., "pill mills").

To improve legitimate prescribing and patient care and to reduce prescription drug-related harm, health care professionals who prescribe or dispense prescription drugs can access PDMPs. PDMPs can provide prescribers with important information about a patient's prescription medication history that can help inform clinical decisions. For example, data indicating multiple prescribers, multiple pharmacies, early refills, high doses, multiple controlled substances, or high-risk coprescriptions (e.g., opioid pain relievers and benzodiazepines) can prompt medical providers to avoid prescribing a controlled drug, to discuss overdose risk with a patient, or to refer patients to substance abuse treatment services. In the next section, we will explore the value of PDMPs to population health.

Prescription Drug Monitoring Programs and Population Health

While pain places a substantial burden on the U.S. population, with approximately 126.1 million Americans (55%) reporting some pain in the previous three months and 25.5 reporting pain every day (Nahin, 2015). The clinical management of pain is difficult, and the level of personal pain experienced can only be assessed indirectly using self-reported pain ratings, often by using a unidimensional pain rating scale. Pain and pain management are very subjective and idiosyncratic experiences (Lembke, 2013). Therefore, two different people might report different levels of pain from the same condition, and the same symptom might require different doses of medication in these different people to alleviate the pain. This lack of an objective measure for pain and its relief, places the burden on the prescriber to discern a clinically appropriate prescription to address legitimate suffering while limiting the risk for misuse and unintended dependence. And although PDMPs cannot help a prescriber measure a patient's pain relief needs, a PDMP might identify high-risk situations (e.g., drug-drug interactions, high number of existing prescriptions for opioids) or drug-seeking behaviors.

A large body of literature has investigated the effect of PDMPs on prescribing practices and drug-induced deaths (e.g., Deyo et al., 2013; Haegerich, Paulozzi, Manns, & Jones, 2014; Worley, 2012). In the next section, we will focus on a plausible mechanism for how PDMPs can shape prescribing behavior and, ultimately, population health.

Effect of PDMPs on Prescribing Behavior

The medical community is currently grappling with a number of difficult questions related to opioids: How can the medical community maximize the use of opioids when appropriate and minimize their overuse? How does one develop an effective prescribing protocol for prescription opioids without a good measure for pain? Pain's subjective nature is complicating, and prescribers must rely on patient feedback to determine the best course of action. This decision is particularly difficult in an emergency room setting where decisions need to be made quickly, often with no or very little information on prior medical records. Unlike most other areas of medicine, a patient enters an emergency room without an existing health record or referral for care. Prescription drug monitoring programs can be a tool to inform clinical care in such settings. A 2010 study of emergency department physicians from the state of Ohio found that prescribers, after reviewing PDMP data, altered their opioid prescribing in 41 percent of cases (Baehren et al., 2010). The reasons for physicians altering their opioid prescribing ranged in frequency from the number of addresses a patient had listed in the system (16%) to the number of previous prescriptions filled (41%). Although this study was limited to the behaviors of 17 physicians from a single emergency department, a growing body of literature supports this study's findings, documenting a substantial decrease in opioid prescribing after states have implemented PDMPs.

Research has documented that states experience a significant reduction in opioid prescribing following the implementation of a PDMP (Bao et al., 2016; Paulozzi, Kilbourne, & Desai, 2011; Reisman, Shenoy, Atherly, & Flowers, 2009; Simeone & Holland, 2006; Simoni-Wastila & Qian, 2012). For example, Bao and colleagues (2016) found a 30 percent reduction in the probability of being prescribed a Schedule II prescription opioid following the implementation of a PDMP. Furthermore, this change in the prescribing of Schedule II opioids was not offset by increases in Schedule III opioids (i.e., opioid pain relievers with lower potential for abuse and dependence than Schedule II). This observation that prescribing of Schedule III opioids remained unchanged post-PDMP implementation reduced previous concerns of a substitution effect, whereby the less stringently monitored Schedule III drugs would be prescribed more often in lieu of reductions to Schedule II prescriptions (Wastila & Bishop, 1996). Furthermore, the potential for a substitution effect has become substantially less likely following the rescheduling of hydrocodone in 2014 from a less restrictive Schedule III to a more restrictive Schedule II drug.

The effectiveness of PDMPs to reduce unnecessary or inappropriate prescribing is contingent upon providers' awareness and use of these programs. While prescribers' overall awareness of PDMPs has increased in recent years, with data from a 2014 survey indicating that 72 percent of prescribers were aware of their state's PDMP (Rutkow, Turner, Lucas, Hwang, & Alexander, 2015), PDMP use remains low. A recent DOJ report found that only about one in five licensed prescribers in states that had a PDMP were registered to use the system in 2013, whereas over one in three licensed pharmacists were registered to do so (Brenwald, 2014). States' increasing adoption of policies and practices governing the use of PDMPs, such as their mandatory registration or use and the delegating of access authority, could increase take-up and regular PDMP use among prescribers (Clark, Eadie, Knue, Kreiner, & Strickler, 2012).

Currently, about half of states require prescribers to register with their state's PDMP; however, registration is not sufficient to ensure that physicians use the system. Consequently, 30 of the 49 states with PDMPs now mandate prescribers to access a patient's prescription drug history in the PDMP system prior to writing any prescription for a controlled substance. Early adopters of prescriber mandates, such as Kentucky, Ohio, Tennessee, and New York, have documented significant increases in system queries and reductions in opioid prescribing after the implementation of such mandates (Kreiner, Nikitin, & Shields, 2013). Furthermore, provider mandates have been found to reduce drug overdose in general and opioid-related overdose specifically (Dowell, Zhang, Noonan, & Hockenberry, 2016). As such, provider mandates are increasingly being recognized as a best practice for PDMPs to affect prescription drug diversion and population health (Prescription Drug Monitoring Program Center of Excellence, 2016).

Attenuated Effect of PDMPs on Opioid Prescribing

Since implementation, the effect of PDMPs on physician prescribing has been found to vary with time. Bao and colleagues (2016), for example, found PDMP implementation to be associated with an immediate reduction in the prescribing of all opioids in general and Schedule II opioids in particular, the effect on the prescribing of all opioids attenuated after the first six months, and the effect on the prescribing of Schedule II opioids became small or non-significant at other times over the two years after implementation. There are a variety of legitimate reasons why the effect of PDMP implementation on prescribing behaviors might vary over time. First, the effect of PDMP implementation on prescriber behavior might be confounded by other co-occurring public health strategies. Prescription drug monitoring programs are often implemented in response to rapid changes in opioid overdose within a state (Paulozzi et al., 2011). As such, a state might implement a PDMP as part of a more comprehensive public health campaign to address a growing opioid epidemic.

There are a number of evidence-based public health strategies that can address opioid overdose deaths, including, for example, expanding availability of naloxone (Rees, Sabia, Argys, Latshaw, & Dave, 2017; Walley et al., 2013); expanding access to treatment, particularly medication-assisted treatment (McLellan, Lewis, O'Brien, & Kleber, 2000; Volkow, Frieden, Hyde, & Cha, 2014); and establishing guidelines for safe opioid prescribing (Franklin et al., 2012; Gellad, Good, & Shulkin, 2017). If these other public health strategies are implemented at a similar time to PDMPs, the estimated effect of PDMP implementation would be difficult to disentangle from the effect of the other co-occurring public health strategies. As such, the attenuating effect of PDMPs on prescribing behavior over time might reflect the shorter duration of other public health programs (e.g., limited duration social marketing campaign).

For example, in response to a four-fold increase in the rate of prescription opioid overdose deaths on Staten Island, the State of New York advanced a multipronged public health strategy that targeted prescribers and the population alike. This strategy included the distribution of opioid prescribing guidelines to all providers in New York City, the introduction of two public service campaigns to highlight the risk of overdose from prescription drug misuse, the assembly of several town hall meetings in highly affected areas to improve relations with key stakeholders, and the implementation of a law requiring prescribers to review the state's PDMP before prescribing a controlled substance (Paone et al., 2015). Although New York City observed a substantial decrease in the rate of prescription opioid overdose deaths following this systematic public health approach to the epidemic, it is difficult to isolate the effect of mandating prescriber review of PDMPs from the other co-occurring programs that targeted this epidemic. Furthermore, as several of these programs ran over a short interval, it would be likely that, absent consideration of these other co-occurring programs during analysis, we would observe a large effect early on (while all these programs were active) that attenuates over time (as the other non-PDMP programs ceased).

Three other possible explanations exist for the attenuating effect of PDMP implementation over time. First, it is possible that a state's decision to implement a PDMP increased prescribers' awareness about controlled substance misuse in their state, altering prescriber behavior for a period of time before providers returned to normal prescribing practices. Second, it is possible that the implementation of a PDMP might deter drug-seeking behaviors in the short term, but, over time, drug seekers might learn new methods to circumvent the system. Finally, the attenuating effect of PDMP implementation might arise from the challenges with using administrative data on clinical encounters for law enforcement purposes. Specifically, in the immediate months following PDMP implementation, law enforcement might be able to use the system to easily identify the prescribers and patients exhibiting the most egregious behaviors. However, after identifying the most egregious prescribers and patients, the appropriateness of any given prescriber's or patient's pattern of behavior will become more subjective and make it more challenging for law enforcement to discern what qualifies as appropriate behavior, reducing the rate of legal interventions over time.

Effect of PDMPs on Population Health

The increased rates of drug-related overdose in the United States reflect the changing patterns of prescription drug misuse in the population. Although much literature has demonstrated the utility of PDMPs at changing physician prescribing, the effectiveness of PDMPs at reducing nonfatal and fatal drug-related overdose remains inconclusive. To the best of our knowledge, to date, 10 studies have examined the effect of PDMPs on nonfatal and fatal drug overdoses, including one study, reported in two manuscripts, that examined the association between PDMP implementation and emergency department visits involving either benzodiazepines (Bachhuber, Hennessy, Cunningham, & Starrels, 2016) or prescription opioids (Maughan, Bachhuber, Mitra, & Starrels, 2015), and 9 studies that examined the association between PDMP implementation and drug-related overdose deaths (Delcher, Wagenaar, Goldberger, Cook, & Maldonado-Molina, 2015; Dowell et al.,

2016; Kim, 2013; Li et al., 2014; Pardo, 2016; Patrick, Fry, Jones, & Buntin, 2016; Paulozzi et al., 2011; Radakrishnan, 2015). From these studies, there is no evidence that PDMPs are associated with nonfatal drug overdose events; however, the association between PDMPs and drug-related overdose deaths is more complicated.

Nonfatal Drug-Related Overdose

Although no study, to our knowledge, has documented an association between PDMP implementation and changes in nonfatal drug overdose events, the current evidence comes from a single study that examined emergency department visits from a limited geographic area and time period (Bachhuber et al., 2016; Maughan et al., 2015). Published in two reports from the same research group, this study examined the association between PDMP implementation and emergency department visits involving either opioid analgesics (Maughan et al., 2015) or benzodiazepines (Bachhuber et al., 2016). And while this study found no association between PDMP implementation and emergency department visits involving either opioids (incident rate difference (IRD) of 0.08 visits (95% CI: –3.7, 5.2) per 100,000 residents per quarter) or benzodiazepines (IRD of 0.08 visits (95% CI: –0.1, 1.8) per 100,000 residents per quarter), results from this study are likely to have limited generalizability to the United States in general for a few reasons.

First, data for this study came from the Drug Abuse Warning Network (DAWN) for just 11 geographically dispersed metropolitan areas in the United States (Boston, Chicago, Denver, Detroit, Houston, Miami-Dade County, Minneapolis–St. Paul, New York City, Phoenix, San Francisco, Seattle) from 2004 to 2011. Furthermore, the 11 metropolitan areas included in this study did not include data from several of the most populated areas (e.g., San Diego, San Antonio, Dallas, Houston, Philadelphia) nor the areas most affected by the current opioid overdose epidemic (e.g., West Virginia, Pennsylvania, Ohio, Kentucky, Tennessee). Thus, it is unlikely that these results can be generalized to the rural areas that have been most directly affected by the opioid epidemic. The limited generalizability of these findings, and the paucity of research into nonfatal drug overdose events in general, suggest that this area of research is in desperate need of further study.

Fatal Drug-Related Overdose

Studies of the association between PDMPs and drug-related overdose deaths have found mixed results. Data from seven of the eight studies on drug-related overdose deaths came from the National Vital Statistics System Multiple Causes of Death mortality file reported by CDC Wide-ranging Online Data for Epidemiologic Research (CDC WONDER). Studies used the multiple cause of death data available on CDC WONDER to calculate state-level mortality and population data. The remaining study on drug-related overdose deaths came from the Florida Medical Examiners Commission (Delcher et al., 2015). The years analyzed by these studies ranged from 1999 to 2014 and examined 10 years of data on average. Although all 50 states and Washington, D.C., now have enacted PDMPs, only a median of 31 PDMP states (with a range 1 to 47) contributed to overall estimates of PDMP effects among these studies.

Estimating pre- versus post-PDMP implementation changes in drug-related overdose deaths was the most basic target of these studies (four of eight). Of these four studies, one study did not find significant ($p > 0.05$) changes in drug-related overdose deaths (Paulozzi et al., 2011), and two studies reported a significant decrease in drug-related overdose deaths (Dowell et al., 2016; Patrick et al., 2016). The remaining single study (Li et al., 2014) reported a significant increase in drug-related overdose deaths, but the analysis conducted in this study failed to account for pre-PDMP differences in drug-related overdose death rates among states. Because states implementing a PDMP tend to have higher preimplementation death rates than states that do not implement a PDMP (Paulozzi et al., 2011), it is likely that confounding by indication led to biased estimates in the Li and colleagues (2014) study.

The studies on fatal substance-related overdose otherwise examined one or more of four different outcomes (in order of frequency): opioid-related overdose deaths (six of eight), drug-related overdose deaths (four of eight), heroin overdose deaths (three of eight), and benzodiazepine overdose deaths (one of eight). Of these six studies that examined opioid-related overdose deaths, three studies did not find significant changes in opioid-related overdose deaths (Kim, 2013; Paulozzi et al., 2011; Radakrishnan, 2015), whereas the other three studies found a significant decrease in opioid-related overdose deaths (Delcher et al., 2015; Dowell et al., 2016; Pardo, 2016). Finally, three studies testing whether PDMPs induced substitution away from prescription opioids to affect heroin-related overdose deaths found nonsignificant results (Delcher et al., 2015; Dowell et al., 2016; Radakrishnan, 2015); however, heroin-related overdose deaths, and opioid-related overdose deaths in general, are relatively rare events, limiting the power of such studies to detect a true effect.

The mixed results among the studies on drug- and opioid-related overdose deaths is likely explained by studies not accounting for differences in PDMP operational characteristics across states. For example, Paulozzi and colleagues (2011) found no association between PDMP implementation and drug- or opioid-related overdose; however, this study used data from earlier years (1999 to 2005) and examined fewer PDMPs (19 state PDMPs, compared to the median 31 state PDMPs in other studies) than later studies that found significant decreases in these outcomes. Because early PDMPs tended to have less restrictive policies than later PDMPs, it is possible that certain more restrictive operational characteristics that were common in later PDMPs (e.g., mandatory prescriber registration and review of the system before writing for a controlled substance) are driving the reductions in overdose deaths that were observed in later studies (Delcher et al., 2015; Dowell et al., 2016; Pardo, 2016; Patrick et al., 2016). In the following section, we summarize how variations in PDMP characteristics might affect prescriber behavior and attendant health consequences.

Prescription Drug Monitoring Programs: Operational Characteristics

The operational characteristics of PDMPs have varied substantially over time. While state PDMPs have substantial commonalities in terms of centralized statewide data systems and basic elements of electronically transmitted prescription data, they also differ in key ways that may affect their effectiveness. A key reason for the inconsistent findings in terms of prescription opioid-related harm may be that most studies treat the presence of a PDMP as a binary variable without considering the influence that implementation of specific PDMP characteristics can have on prescribing behavior and health. Two models are proposed here to explain the differential effect of PDMPs on health outcomes. First, there is evidence that specific operational characteristics exist that have a greater influence on prescribing behavior and subsequent health outcomes. For example, several operational characteristics have been found to decrease drug-related overdose and opioid-related overdose deaths, including the monitoring of noncontrolled substances (Kim, 2013; Patrick et al., 2016); data updated at least weekly to the PDMP (Patrick et al., 2016); mandatory provider review (Dowell et al., 2016); and data sharing with other states (Kim, 2013). Under this model, the specific operational characteristic drives the change in prescribing behavior and subsequent health outcomes.

Second, a "robustness" hypothesis emphasizes the critical role that multiple diverse operational characteristics play in changing prescriber behavior and subsequent health. The robustness hypothesis is grounded in an appreciation of a multifactorial characterization of PDMPs. To test this hypothesis, a recent study by Pardo (2016) developed a measure of PDMP robustness, informed by Brandeis University's PDMP Center of Excellence 2012 report on best practices, to estimate the relationship of PDMP robustness with opioid-related overdose deaths. Pardo assigned different weights to operational characteristics that have an empirical or analytical basis in changing prescriber behavior or reducing overdose deaths. For example, access to PDMP for law enforcement and prosecutors was assigned a weight of one, whereas requiring that prescribers check PDMPs before prescribing to a patient was assigned a weight of four. Next, Pardo calculated scores by summing the total weights for each state by year, with scores ranging from 0 to 23, and found a 1.5 percent (95% confidence interval: 0.3, 30.0%) reduction in the opioid-related overdose death rate for each point assigned to a state's PDMP score. This one-point reduction is associated with preventing approximately 300 overdose deaths nationwide per year. The linear relationship between the robustness of PDMPs and opioid-related overdose deaths raises the question of whether it is the specific operational characteristics, the overall robustness of programs, or some combination of certain characteristics that matter most. While recent adoption of best practices, such as mandates for prescribers to use PDMP data, could lead to reductions in inappropriate prescribing and decreases in opioid-related deaths, this has not been objectively and systematically examined to date.

Can PDMPs Have Unintended Negative Consequences?

Existing research has largely failed to examine possible unintended negative effects of PDMPs. Prescription drug monitoring programs that have adopted such best practices as real-time reporting and proactive provision of unsolicited patient reports to prescribers may reduce the feasibility of doctor shopping as well as the overall supply of prescription opioids available from the illicit market. This reduction in the supply of prescription opioids in the illicit market, although generally viewed as positive, may also generate unanticipated outcomes, such as replacement of the preferred prescription opioid with heroin or nonpharmaceutical fentanyl.

Heroin use and heroin-related overdose deaths have increased dramatically in the United States. From 2001–2002 to 2012–2013, the prevalence of lifetime heroin use increased almost five-fold, from 0.33 percent to 1.61 percent, and prevalence of past-year heroin use increased approximately seven-fold, from 0.03 percent to 0.21 percent (Martins et al., 2017). Moreover, the rates of heroin-induced deaths have quadrupled in the five years from 2010 to 2015 (Hedegaard et al., 2017). This increase may be partly driven by the transition to heroin use among the growing population of people with a history of prescription opioid misuse. The National Survey on Drug Use and Health (NSDUH) found that past-year heroin initiation was 19 times higher among adults who reported prior nonmedical prescription opioid use compared to those who did not report past nonmedical prescription opioid use (Muhuri, Gfroerer, & Davies, 2013). Moreover, initiation patterns of heroin and prescription opioids have changed in more recent birth cohorts, such that persons born after 1980 are more likely than persons born before 1980 to initiate opioids through nonmedical use of prescription opioids than heroin (Novak, Bluthenthal, Wenger, Chu, & Kral, 2016).

Qualitative studies of those who use heroin illustrates the dynamic behind the transition from prescription opioids to heroin (Cicero, Ellis & Surratt, 2012; Cicero & Kuehn, 2014; Lankenau, Schrager et al., 2012; Lankenau, Teti et al., 2012; Mars, Bourgois, Karandinos, Montero, & Ciccarone, 2014). An ethnographic study of those at high risk for development of heroin use in Philadelphia and San Francisco, for example, found that key drivers of the progression from prescription opioid misuse to heroin use were the rising cost of prescription opioid use and the easy availability and comparatively lower cost of heroin (Mars et al., 2014). As such, changes to either the supply or cost of prescription opioids following the implementation of a PDMP might reasonably drive opioid-dependent persons to try heroin. And while increases in heroin overdoses have been observed following the implementation of Florida's PDMP in 2011(Delcher et al., 2015; Delcher et al., 2016), a recent study found no association between the combined implementation of mandatory provider review of PDMP data and pain clinic laws and changes in heroin-related overdose deaths. Future research is needed in this area (Dowell et al., 2016).

Prescription Drug Monitoring Programs and Health Disparities

Prescription drug monitoring programs may affect low- and high-income populations in different ways, widening existing health disparities (King, Fraser, Boikos, Richardson, & Harper, 2014). Prescription drug monitoring programs that reduce the supply of prescription opioids may potentially generate any number of outcomes on opioid-dependent persons, including the replacement of the preferred prescription opioid with alternative opioid medications or heroin use or the decision to seek out treatment for opioid dependence. Differences in the probability of transitioning to heroin use versus treatment might differ between low- and high-income populations.

High-income populations might be more likely to benefit from PDMP implementation than low-income populations. Whereas low-income populations are more likely to access prescription opioids through informal networks such as friends, family, and drug markets than through medical providers, high-income populations are more likely to access prescription opioids through medical providers than through illegal drug markets (Joynt et al., 2013). Medical providers, notified of a patient exhibiting drug-seeking behaviors, may be more likely to refer that patient to treatment and other medical professionals in more affluent populations (Joynt et al., 2013; McGuire & Miranda, 2008; Saloner & Le Cook, 2013). A study of drug and alcohol treatment completion rates in a national sample of outpatient and residential treatment discharges found that higher socioeconomic status was associated with better treatment outcomes (Saloner & Le Cook, 2013). Furthermore, prior studies have found that access to high-quality mental health treatment is more likely among higher socioeconomic status groups (McGuire & Miranda, 2008).

In contrast, those with low incomes who also misused prescription opioids identified in health care settings may be more likely to be dismissed from their health care provider without a referral to another provider or a referral to a treatment option the patient can afford. Without access to affordable treatment, someone with a low income who was engaged in misuse might be particularly vulnerable to transition to heroin. Understanding whether PDMPs might exacerbate socioeconomic disparities in prescription opioid and heroin overdose is critical to developing public health interventions to target groups that may be most vulnerable to transition into heroin use as prescription opioid availability decreases.

Challenges in Existing Research and Directions for Future Research

The complexity of using observational data to evaluate the effects of policies on health outcomes is particularly true for programs that act within complex and dynamic policy environments. Responding to the current opioid epidemic has required collaboration among stakeholders from diverse sectors and policy areas, and each stakeholder will tend to focus efforts on one part of the crisis. For example, medical boards and law enforcement bodies might concentrate efforts to reduce overprescribing and black market opioid availability, whereas public health groups might focus their efforts on reducing high-risk use of prescription opioids and overdose prevention. And while this epidemic necessitates a multifaceted prevention strategy, it becomes difficult to isolate the effect of a single intervention within such dynamic policy environments (Fink & Keyes, 2017).

Prescription drug monitoring programs exist within a wide battery of drug use prevention tools. However, extant studies have largely focused on isolating the effect of PDMPs on prescribing behaviors or health outcomes while statistically adjusting for complementary drug prevention programs (e.g., naloxone distribution programs, pill mill laws) as time-varying covariates in a multivariable model. From these models, studies tend to report how either prescribing behaviors or some health outcome changed after PDMP implementation, as compared to states without a PDMP. This method of isolating the effect of PDMPs from the effect of other drug prevention programs and comparing changes in prescriber behaviors or a health outcome, pre- and post-PDMP implementation, to states without a PDMP is likely to have limited utility to decision makers who require information about the health consequences of various policy options during the policy development process. To inform about the health consequences of various policy options, a systems science approach is useful to understand and compare the action and interaction of complementary policies (Fink & Keyes, 2017; Fink, Keyes, & Cerdá, 2016).

Furthermore, a systems science approach can be used to understand and avoid unintended consequences that might arise from policy interventions.

Conclusions

Although PDMPs originated as a tool to assist law enforcement in detecting the inappropriate or illegal prescribing, dispensing, or use of controlled substances, recently these databases are increasingly being expected to reduce opioid-related harm and improve population health. While early evidence has demonstrated the utility of these programs on changing physician prescribing and attendant health consequences, empirically based identification of PDMP best practices is needed to maximize population health benefits and reduce unintended consequences. Future studies will need to account for how the operational characteristics of PDMPs have varied both across states and over time. Finally, studies will need to evaluate the effect of PDMPs within a suite of potential drug prevention programs to inform future policy decisions.

Acknowledgments

The work in this chapter was supported in part by research grants from the U.S. National Institute on Drug Abuse of the National Institute of Health (grant numbers T32DA031099 and R01DA039962) and the Bureau of Justice Assistance (grant number 2016-PM-BX-K005).

References

Bachhuber, M. A., Hennessy, S., Cunningham, C. O., & Starrels, J. L. (2016). Increasing benzodiazepine prescriptions and overdose mortality in the United States, 1996–2013. *American Journal of Public Health, 106*(4), 686–688. doi:10.2105/ajph.2016.303061.

Baehren, D. F., Marco, C. A., Droz, D. E., Sinha, S., Callan, E. M., & Akpunonu, P. (2010). A statewide prescription monitoring program affects emergency department prescribing behaviors. *Annals of Emergency Medicine, 56*(1), 19–23. e13.

Bao, Y., Pan, Y., Taylor, A., Radakrishnan, S., Luo, F., Pincus, H. A., & Schackman, B. R. (2016). Prescription drug monitoring programs are associated with sustained reductions in opioid prescribing by physicians. *Health Affairs, 35*(6), 1045–1051. doi:10.1377/hlthaff.2015.1673.

Brenwald, S. (2014). *Program Performance Report: Prescription Drug Monitoring Program (PDMP): January–December 2013.* Washington, D.C.: U.S. Department of Justice, Bureau of Justice Assistance. https://www.bja.gov/Publications/PDMP_PPR_Jan-Dec13.pdf.

Centers for Disease Control and Prevention. (2011). Vital signs: Overdoses of prescription opioid pain relievers—United States, 1999–2008. *MMWR: Morbidity and Mortality Weekly Report, 60*, 1487–1492.

Centers for Disease Control and Prevention, National Center for Health Statistics. (2016). Multiple cause of death 1999–2015 on CDC WONDER online database. https://wonder.cdc.gov/mcd-icd10.html.

Chang, H. Y., Daubresse, M., Kruszewski, S. P., & Alexander, G. C. (2014). Prevalence and treatment of pain in EDs in the United States, 2000 to 2010. *American Journal of Emergency Medicine, 32*(5), 421–431. doi:10.1016/j.ajem.2014.01.015.

Cicero, T. J., Ellis, M. S., & Surratt, H. L. (2012). Effect of abuse-deterrent formulation of OxyContin. *New England Journal of Medicine, 367*(2), 187–189.

Cicero, T. J., & Kuehn, B. M. (2014). Driven by prescription drug abuse, heroin use increases among suburban and rural whites. *JAMA, 312*(2), 118–119. doi:10.1001/jama.2014.7404.

Clark, T., Eadie, J., Knue, P., Kreiner, P., & Strickler, G. (2012). *Prescription Drug Monitoring Programs: An Assessment of the Evidence for Best Practices.* Waltham, MA: Heller School for Social Policy and Management, Brandeis University. http://www.pdmpexcellence.org/sites/all/pdfs/BrandeisPDMP_Report.pdf.

Daubresse, M., Chang, H. Y., Yu, Y., Viswanathan, S., Shah, N. D., Stafford, R. S., . . . Alexander, G. C. (2013). Ambulatory diagnosis and treatment of nonmalignant pain in the United States, 2000–2010. *Medical Care, 51*(10), 870–878. doi:10.1097/MLR.0b013e3182a95d86.

Delcher, C., Wagenaar, A. C., Goldberger, B. A., Cook, R. L., & Maldonado-Molina, M. M. (2015). Abrupt decline in oxycodone-caused mortality after implementation of Florida's prescription drug monitoring program. *Drug and Alcohol Dependence, 150*, 63–68. doi:10.1016/j.drugalcdep.2015.02.010.

Delcher, C., Wang, Y., Wagenaar, A. C., Goldberger, B. A., Cook, R. L., & Maldonado-Molina, M. M. (2016). Prescription and illicit opioid deaths and the prescription drug monitoring program in Florida. *American Journal of Public Health, 106*(6), e10–11. doi:10.2105/ajph.2016.303104.

Deyo, R. A., Irvine, J. M., Millet, L. M., Beran, T., O'Kane, N., Wright, D. A., & McCarty, D. (2013). Measures such as interstate cooperation would improve the efficacy of programs to track controlled drug prescriptions. *Health Affairs,* 10.1377/hlthaff. 2012.0945.

Dowell, D., Zhang, K., Noonan, R. K., & Hockenberry, J. M. (2016). Mandatory provider review and pain clinic laws reduce the amounts of opioids prescribed and overdose death rates. *Health Affairs, 35*(10), 1876–1883. doi:10.1377/hlthaff.2016.0448.

Fink, D. S., & Keyes, K. (2017). Wrong answers: When simple interpretations create complex problems. In A. M. El-Sayed & S. Galea (Eds.), *Systems Science and Population Health,* 25–35. New York: Oxford University Press.

Fink, D. S., Keyes, K. M., & Cerdá, M. (2016). Social determinants of population health: A systems sciences approach. *Current Epidemiology Reports, 3*(1), 98–105. doi:10.1007/s40471-016-0066-8.

Franklin, G. M., Mai, J., Turner, J., Sullivan, M., Wickizer, T., & Fulton-Kehoe, D. (2012). Bending the prescription opioid dosing and mortality curves: Impact of the Washington State opioid dosing guideline. *American Journal of Indian Medicine, 55*(4), 325–331. doi:10.1002/ajim.21998.

Gellad, W. F., Good, C. B., & Shulkin, D. J. (2017). Addressing the opioid epidemic in the United States: Lessons from the Department of Veterans Affairs. *JAMA Internal Medicine, 177*(5), 611–612. doi:10.1001/jamainternmed.2017.0147.

Haegerich, T. M., Paulozzi, L. J., Manns, B. J., & Jones, C. M. (2014). What we know, and don't know, about the impact of state policy and systems-level interventions on prescription drug overdose. *Drug and Alcohol Dependence, 145*, 34–47. doi:10.1016/j.drugalcdep.2014.10.001.

Hedegaard, H., Warner, M., & Minino, A. M. (2017). Drug overdose deaths in the United States, 1999–2015. *NCHS Data Brief, 173*, 1–7.

Joynt, M., Train, M. K., Robbins, B. W., Halterman, J. S., Caiola, E., & Fortuna, R. J. (2013). The impact of neighborhood socioeconomic status and race on the prescribing of opioids in emergency departments throughout the United States. *Journal of General Internal Medicine, 28*(12), 1604–1610. doi:10.1007/s11606-013-2516-z.

Kim, M. (2013). *The Impact of Prescription Drug Monitoring Programs on Opioid-related Poisoning Deaths.* (Unpublished doctoral dissertation), Johns Hopkins University, Baltimore, MD.

King, N. B., Fraser, V., Boikos, C., Richardson, R., & Harper, S. (2014). Determinants of increased opioid-related mortality in the United States and Canada, 1990–2013: A systematic review. *American Journal of Public Health, 104*(8), e32–42. doi:10.2105/ajph.2014.301966.

Kreiner, P., Nikitin, R., & Shields, T. (2013). *Bureau of Justice Assistance: Prescription Drug Monitoring Program Performance Measures Reports: January 2009 through June 2012.* http://www.pdmpassist.org/pdf/COE_documents/Add_to_TTAC/BJA%20PDMP%20Performance%20Measures%20Report%20Jan%202009%20to%20June%202012%20FInal_with%20feedback.pdf.

Lankenau, S. E., Schrager, S. M., Silva, K., Kecojevic, A., Bloom, J. J., Wong, C., & Iverson, E. (2012). Misuse of prescription and illicit drugs among high-risk young adults in Los Angeles and New York. *Journal of Public Health Research, 1*(1), 22–30. doi:10.4081/jphr.2012.e6.

Lankenau, S. E., Teti, M., Silva, K., Jackson Bloom, J., Harocopos, A., & Treese, M. (2012). Initiation into prescription opioid misuse amongst young injection drug users. *International Journal of Drug Policy, 23*(1), 37–44. doi:10.1016/j.drugpo.2011.05.014.

Lembke, A. (2013). Why doctors prescribe opioids to known opioid abusers. *New England Journal of Medicine, 368*(5), 485. doi:10.1056/NEJMc1214553.

Li, G., Brady, J. E., Lang, B. H., Giglio, J., Wunsch, H., & DiMaggio, C. (2014). Prescription drug monitoring and drug overdose mortality. *Injury Epidemiology, 1*(1), 1–8.

Mars, S. G., Bourgois, P., Karandinos, G., Montero, F., & Ciccarone, D. (2014). "Every 'never' I ever said came true": Transitions from opioid pills to heroin injecting. *International Journal of Drug Policy, 25*(2), 257–266.

Martins, S. S., Sarvet, A., Santaella-Tenorio, J., Saha, T., Grant, B. F., & Hasin, D. S. (2017). Changes in US lifetime heroin use and heroin use disorder: Prevalence from the 2001–2002 to 2012–2013 national epidemiologic survey on alcohol and related conditions. *JAMA Psychiatry.* doi:10.1001/jamapsychiatry.2017.0113.

Maughan, B. C., Bachhuber, M. A., Mitra, N., & Starrels, J. L. (2015). Prescription monitoring programs and emergency department visits involving opioids, 2004–2011. *Drug and Alcohol Dependence, 156*, 282–288. doi:10.1016/j.drugalcdep.2015.09.024.

McGuire, T. G., & Miranda, J. (2008). New evidence regarding racial and ethnic disparities in mental health: Policy implications. *Health Affairs, 27*(2), 393–403. doi:10.1377/hlthaff.27.2.393.

McLellan, A. T., Lewis, D. C., O'Brien, C. P., & Kleber, H. D. (2000). Drug dependence, a chronic medical illness: Implications for treatment, insurance, and outcomes evaluation. *JAMA, 284*(13), 1689–1695.

Muhuri, P. K., Gfroerer, J. C., & Davies, M. C. (2013). Associations of nonmedical pain reliever use and initiation of heroin use in the United States. *CBHSQ Data Review.* https://www.samhsa.gov/data/sites/default/files/DR006/DR006/nonmedical-pain-reliever-use-2013.htm.

Nahin, R. L. (2015). Estimates of pain prevalence and severity in adults: United States, 2012. *Journal of Pain, 16*(8), 769–780. doi:10.1016/j.jpain.2015.05.002.

National Center for Injury Prevention and Control. (2013). *From Epi to Policy: Prescription Drug Overdose. State Health Department Training and Technical Assistance Meeting.* Atlanta, GA: Centers for Disease Control and Prevention. http://www.cdc.gov/drugoverdose/pdf/pdo_epi_to_policy_meeting-a.pdf.

Novak, S. P., Bluthenthal, R., Wenger, L., Chu, D., & Kral, A. H. (2016). Initiation of heroin and prescription opioid pain relievers by birth cohort. *American Journal of Public Health, 106*(2), 298–300. doi:10.2105/ajph.2015.302972.

Office of National Drug Control Policy. (2011). Epidemic: Responding to America's prescription drug abuse crisis. Washington, D.C.: Office of National Drug Control Policy.

Paone, D., Tuazon, E., Kattan, J., Nolan, M. L., O'Brien, D. B., Dowell, D., . . . Kunins, H. V. (2015). Decrease in rate of opioid analgesic overdose deaths—Staten Island, New York City, 2011–2013. *MMWR: Morbidity and Mortality Weekly Report, 64*(18), 491–494.

Pardo, B. (2016). Do more robust prescription drug monitoring programs reduce prescription opioid overdose? *Addiction.* doi:10.1111/add.13741.

Patrick, S. W., Fry, C. E., Jones, T. F., & Buntin, M. B. (2016). Implementation of prescription drug monitoring programs associated with reductions in opioid-related death rates. *Health Affairs, 35*(7), 1324–1332. doi:10.1377/hlthaff.2015.1496.

Patrick, S. W., Schumacher, R. E., Benneyworth, B. D., Krans, E. E., McAllister, J. M., & Davis, M. M. (2012). Neonatal abstinence syndrome and associated health care expenditures: United States, 2000–2009. *JAMA, 307*(18), 1934–1940. doi:10.1001/jama.2012.3951.

Paulozzi, L. J., Kilbourne, E. M., & Desai, H. A. (2011). Prescription drug monitoring programs and death rates from drug overdose. *Pain Medicine, 12*(5), 747–754.

Prescription Drug Monitoring Program Center of Excellence. (2016). *PDMP Prescriber Use Mandates: Characteristics, Current Status, and Outcomes in Selected States.* Waltham, MA: Heller School for Social Policy and Management, Brandeis University. http://www.pdmpassist.org/pdf/COE_documents/Add_to_TTAC/COE%20briefing%20on%20mandates%203rd%20revision.pdf.

Radakrishnan, S. (2015). *Essays in the Economics of Risky Health Behaviors.* (Unpublished doctoral dissertation), Cornell University, Ithaca, NY.

Rees, D. I., Sabia, J. J., Argys, L. M., Latshaw, J., & Dave, D. (2017). *With a Little Help from My Friends: The Effects of Naloxone Access and Good Samaritan Laws on Opioid-related Deaths.* Cambridge, MA: National Bureau of Economic Research.

Reisman, R. M., Shenoy, P. J., Atherly, A. J., & Flowers, C. R. (2009). Prescription opioid usage and abuse relationships: an evaluation of state prescription drug monitoring program efficacy. *Substance Abuse, 3*, 41–51.

Rudd, R. A., Aleshire, N., Zibbell, J. E., & Matthew Gladden, R. (2016). Increases in drug and opioid overdose deaths—United States, 2000–2014. *American Journal of Transplantation, 16*(4), 1323–1327. doi:10.1111/ajt.13776.

Rutkow, L., Turner, L., Lucas, E., Hwang, C., & Alexander, G. C. (2015). Most primary care physicians are aware of prescription drug monitoring programs, but many find the data difficult to access. *Health Affairs, 34*(3), 484–492. doi:10.1377/hlthaff.2014.1085.

Saloner, B., & Le Cook, B. (2013). Blacks and Hispanics are less likely than whites to complete addiction treatment, largely due to socioeconomic factors. *Health Affairs, 32*(1), 135–145. doi:10.1377/hlthaff.2011.0983.

Simeone, R., & Holland, L. (2006). *An Evaluation of Prescription Drug Monitoring Programs.* Albany, NY: Simeone Associates, Inc. http://www.simeoneassociates.com/simeone3.pdf.

Simoni-Wastila, L., & Qian, J. (2012). Influence of prescription monitoring programs on analgesic utilization by an insured retiree population. *Pharmacoepidemiology and Drug Safety, 21*(12), 1261–1268.

Volkow, N. D., Frieden, T. R., Hyde, P. S., & Cha, S. S. (2014). Medication-assisted therapies—Tackling the opioid-overdose epidemic. *New England Journal of Medicine, 370*(22), 2063–2066. doi:10.1056/NEJMp1402780.

Walley, A. Y., Xuan, Z., Hackman, H. H., Quinn, E., Doe-Simkins, M., Sorensen-Alawad, A., . . . Ozonoff, A. (2013). Opioid overdose rates and implementation of overdose education and nasal naloxone distribution in Massachusetts: Interrupted time series analysis. *BMJ: British Medical Journal, 346*, f174. doi:10.1136/bmj.f174.

Wastila, L. J., & Bishop, C. (1996). The influence of multiple copy prescription programs on analgesic utilization. *Journal of Pharmaceutical Care in Pain & Symptom Control, 4*(3), 3–19.

Worley, J. (2012). Prescription drug monitoring programs, a response to doctor shopping: Purpose, effectiveness, and directions for future research. *Issues in Mental Health Nursing, 33*(5), 319–328. doi:10.3109/01612840.2011.654046.

CHAPTER THIRTEEN

Harm Reduction Approaches to Opioids

Lucas Hill

Opioid History

Humans have utilized opioids for medicinal and recreational purposes for more than 5,000 years (Brownstein, 1993). Initially, this use existed in the botanical realm with consumption of opium poppies. When scored, poppies produce a white fluid sap that can be ingested orally or allowed to dry for subsequent smoking. Oral use of a tincture of opium, also referred to as laudanum, is still occasionally prescribed by conventional medical professionals in the United States (Brownstein, 1993). Inhalational use of opium is uncommon in the United State. and is not generally accepted for medicinal purposes. Opium and related compounds (collectively referred to as *opioids*) have been deployed medically for a broad range of symptoms that include, but are not limited to, pain reduction, cough suppression, and antidiarrheal effects. The effects of opium are primarily related to one active molecule, morphine, which was isolated in 1806. This is generally believed to be the first instance of a specific compound being isolated from a plant for therapeutic application (Brownstein, 1993).

Morphine quickly became a mainstay of conventional medicine in the United States and abroad (Ferrari, Capraro, & Visentin, 2012). It was especially popular for use by soldiers for acute physical pain. The term "soldier's disease" was later coined to describe the physical and psychological dependence that some individuals developed after being exposed to morphine (Casey, 1978). The introduction of the hypodermic needle in 1853 expanded the use of morphine to include perioperative pain management and sedation (Brownstein, 1993). As the burden of morphine addiction grew, there was a clear need for a safer alternative. To address this need, the Bayer pharmaceutical company developed a closely related molecule named dihydromorphine in 1898 (Brownstein, 1993). This drug is now more commonly known as *heroin*. The structural modifications that transformed morphine into heroin made it more lipophilic, allowing it to cross the blood-brain barrier more rapidly and exert a more potent effect in the central nervous system. In addition to the medicinal uses that were common for morphine, heroin was marketed as a treatment for morphine addiction. At one point, free samples of heroin were even mailed to the homes of individuals suffering from opioid use disorder (PBS Frontline, 1998).

Mass production of heroin by Bayer ceased in the early 1900s and was followed by an opposite strategy of decreasing opioid potency. This has largely continued through the modern era. Oxycodone, one of the most commonly prescribed opioids in the United States today, was synthesized in 1916 at the initiation of this movement (Understanding Addictions, 2010). A number of structurally related molecules have been studied and approved by the Food and Drug Administration (FDA) since that time. Access to these medications is generally limited through the requirement of a prescription from a physician or other authorized medical professional. The Controlled Substances Act of 1970 established guidelines for stratifying regulatory barriers for various medications based on their accepted medical use and potential for misuse or addiction. These restrictions, combined with a general wariness toward opioid prescribing in the medical community, kept discussions of opioid misuse out of the mainstream while fear of more commonly misused drugs like cocaine raged in the public sphere.

In the early 1990s, a groundswell of popular sentiment grew to counter the perceived undertreatment of physical pain. Patient advocacy groups and medical professional organizations lobbied to increase the frequency of pain assessment and accessibility to effective pain treatment (Catan & Perez, 2012). This advocacy culminated in a concept known as "pain as the fifth vital sign," which was ultimately incorporated into accreditation policies for health care institutions and clinical practice guidelines for health care professionals in the late 1990s (Geriatrics and Extended Care Strategic Healthcare Group, 2000). Two simple truths mark the subsequent period of extreme opioid overprescribing: (1) pain is remarkably difficult to assess, and (2) busy health care providers typically default to the easiest treatment option.

The most common method for assessing a patient's pain is to ask them to self-rate on a scale of 1 to 10. An alternative scale with cartoon faces demonstrating various levels of pain is also frequently utilized. The institutionalized process of assessing pain in this manner and documenting the pain score in a patient's health record is fraught with potential inaccuracies. Thus, the treating health care provider is entrusted with the responsibility to reconcile this score with a more comprehensive assessment of physical function, emotional well-being, and susceptibility for opioid use disorder. Based on this comprehensive assessment, the health care provider is expected to implement a treatment plan that will result in maximum efficacy with minimal adverse effects. Unfortunately, the ideal implementation of this procedure did not take place. As we can understand in retrospect, simple pain scores were easy to address pharmacologically and may have created a feeling of pressure on health care providers to do so. Additionally, perceived incentives to reduce pain scores rapidly during a hospitalization or between outpatient clinic visits appear to have pushed providers away from long-term solutions (e.g., weight loss, exercise, physical therapy) and toward rapid-acting medications (e.g. opioids).

The Prescription Epidemic

While the exact dynamics of the revolution in pain management of the 1990s are debatable, objective data tells a clear story regarding its outcomes. From 1999 to 2008, opioid prescribing quadrupled. In that same time frame, opioid overdose deaths also quadrupled, and admission to treatment programs for opioid dependence increased six-fold (Paulozzi, Jones, Mack, & Rudd, 2011). Overdose deaths as a result of use of any drug, which began climbing steadily around 1990, surpassed motor vehicle crashes as the leading cause of injury death in the United States in 2009 (Behavioral Health Coordinating Committee, 2013). Those lines have been diverging ever since, as motor vehicles have become safer and drug use has seemingly become more dangerous.

In 2014, 61 percent of all drug overdose deaths involved an opioid (Rudd, Aleshire, Zibbell, & Gladden, 2016). The majority of these deaths resulted from commonly-prescribed opioid analgesics produced by pharmaceutical companies, such as morphine, oxycodone, and hydrocodone. However, rates of overdose due to these opioid analgesics plateaued in 2011 and was holding steady through 2014 while rates of overdose due to heroin and other illicit opioids (e.g., fentanyl) continued to rise in parallel with all drug overdoses (Rudd et al., 2016). From 2005 to 2014, opioid-related emergency department (ED) visits increased 99 percent, and opioid-related inpatient stays increased 64 percent (Weiss et al., 2016). From 2009 to 2014, opioid-related inpatient stays increased in most states, with the greatest increase seen in Georgia. Opioid-related ED visits, meanwhile, rose in nearly every state, with the greatest increase noted in Ohio (Weiss et al., 2016).

In 2016, the Centers for Disease Control and Prevention (CDC) published a controversial guideline for primary care clinicians regarding opioid prescribing (Dowell, Haegerich, & Chou, 2016). The guideline was developed using a systematic review methodology, but analyses were limited due to the low quality and high heterogeneity of the included studies. Twelve broad recommendations were provided to steer prescribers away from routine long-term opioid therapy. This guideline built on a foundation of previous shifts in institutional policy and governmental regulation that have profoundly impacted patients and providers. Chief among these shifts was the creation and implementation of prescription drug monitoring programs (PDMPs).

PDMPs are state-level databases that provide controlled substance dispensing data to prescribers and pharmacists. A brief consideration of PDMPs and their utility in opioid harm reduction is warranted here. For a more detailed discussion of PDMPs, see chapter 12. Authorized professionals can search for a patient in these databases by name and find every controlled substance that has been dispensed to them. The goal of these databases is to prevent patients from visiting several clinics and hospitals to obtain multiple opioid prescriptions at once without prescriber knowledge. Additionally, analyzing the databases can assist the DEA in identifying truly prolific opioid prescribers for closer scrutiny.

PDMP specifics vary greatly by state. Some PDMPs only track Schedule II drugs; others include all controlled substances. A small number of states require health care providers to review their PDMP prior to prescribing or dispensing a controlled substance. A number of other details may vary, and a recent analysis demonstrated that stronger PDMPs were associated with greater reductions in overdose death rates due to opioid analgesics (Pardo, 2017). However, a separate analysis of Medicare beneficiaries suggested that PDMP implementation in 10 states was not associated with a significant decrease in morphine milligram equivalents (MME) or total quantity of opioid prescriptions (Moyo et al., 2017).

In states where provider review of the PDMP is voluntary, the proportion of health care providers who utilize them is often quite low. An analysis from Ohio five years after PDMP implementation found that 84 percent of physicians were aware of its existence, but fewer than 59 percent had accessed it even once (Feldman, Williams, Coates, & Knox, 2011). Since that time, a growing number of states have passed legislation to enact mandatory review of PDMPs by health care providers. Mandating provider review of PDMPs has been associated with an 8 percent decrease in opioid prescribing and 12 percent decrease in overdose death rates due to opioid analgesics (Dowell, Zhang, Noonan, & Hockenberry, 2016). However, states that have implemented mandatory review tend to do so in response to severe crises. These states have much higher rates of opioid prescribing and overdose death due to opioid analgesics than voluntary review states, making a conclusive comparison impossible.

Harm-reduction experts have been quick to point out that analyses of PDMP impacts have been too focused on opioid analgesic harms without thorough consideration of their effects on illicit opioid harms (Davis, 2017). Additionally, PDMP studies generally do not control sufficiently for the impact of co-occurring interventions. To highlight this problem with available research, a PDMP analysis in Florida demonstrated a rapid decrease in oxycodone-related mortality after the PDMP was implemented despite the fact that only 5 percent of Florida prescribers had registered to access it (Delcher, Wagenaar, Goldberger, Cook, & Maldonado-Molina, 2015). It is likely reasonable to conclude that interventions to reduce the available supply of prescribed opioids have had a modest impact to arrest the growth in overdose death for these agents. After increasing dramatically from 1999 to 2006, overdose death rates due to opioid analgesics grew more slowly from 2006 to 2011 (Chen, Hedegaard, & Warner, 2014). From 2010 to 2013, overdose death rates for opioid analgesics actually decreased very slightly (Hedegaard, Chen, & Warner, 2015). However, this perceived improvement has distracted many health care providers from the unintended public health consequences of supply-side interventions for the opioid crisis.

The Illicit Epidemic

From 2000 to 2013, the rate of overdose deaths due to heroin nearly quadrupled (Hedegaard et al., 2015). At the beginning of this time frame, non-Hispanic black persons were the most common victims of heroin overdose. By 2013, non-Hispanic white persons had skyrocketed into the lead. Many harm-reduction advocates believe that increased public attention on the opioid crisis is a result of this escalating impact on white Americans, prompting renowned expert Mark Kinzly to state, "Thank God white people started dying!" At the end of the studied time frame, as supply-side interventions began to have a significant impact on opioid analgesic availability, heroin-related overdoses nearly tripled in just four years (Hedegaard et al., 2015). This unexpected harm is easily understood in retrospect. Predatory pain clinics, often referred to as "pill mills," provided easy access to escalating opioid doses for thousands of vulnerable patients. Since 2010, federal and state authorities have partnered to shutter many of these clinics. When this occurred, patients were left without access to opioid medications to which they had developed significant dependence. The reemergence of underlying pain and symptoms of opioid withdrawal drove many to the illicit opioid market for relief (Gotbaum, 2015). Proven medications for opioid use disorder, often referred to as *medication-assisted treatment*, could be lifesaving for these patients. However, federal actions to increase the availability of these medications (i.e., buprenorphine and methadone) have consistently followed a too little, too late pattern.

Coupled with the decrease in the available supply of opioid analgesics has been a remarkable increase in the available supply of cheap and potent illicit opioids. Sudden increases in novel opioid supplies have led to devastation in the past, as described in a recent article by Ciccarone (2017). The first such shocks in the United State. were seen with the introduction of morphine and heroin for medical purposes. In the 1970s and 1990s, new sources of refined heroin from Southeast Asia and Colombia led to decreased prices, increased use, and widespread consequences. Similar fluctuations in supply and cost have been seen since 2000, with Mexican drug cartels sourcing new forms of heroin and expanding their reach into the eastern United States. Adulteration of heroin supplies with illicitly manufactured fentanyl and fentanyl derivatives (illicitly manufactured fentanyls (IMF)) has further driven the current crisis. The Drug Enforcement Administration (DEA) reported a 1400 percent increase in fentanyl seizures from 2013 to 2015. Fentanyl is a synthetic opioid that is approximately 40 times stronger than heroin by milligram, and it is not the only ultra-potent opioid entering the U.S. heroin supply (Ciccarone, 2017).

Experts agree IMFs have only begun wreaking havoc. Beletsky and Davis (2017) note this transition from heroin to IMF is not incidental, but rather a result of the "iron law of prohibition," or that aggressive enforcement of prohibitive drug laws frequently leads to increasingly risky drug use. The implementation of PDMPs, tamper-resistant opioid formulations, and other interventions to minimize opioid analgesic misuse ultimately encouraged heroin use. Escalating heroin use and related harms garnered public attention, and aggressive law enforcement activities quickly followed. To elude law enforcement officers, the illicit opioid supply had to become easier to transport and conceal. IMF perfectly addresses this need and, like any successful consumer-directed product, was produced in response to market forces.

No U.S. subpopulation is immune from the opioid crisis. From 1999 to 2007, the drug overdose death rate among adolescents increased sharply alongside the rate for adults (Curtin, Tejada-Vera, & Warner, 2017). However, in stark contrast to adult data, adolescent overdose rates fell slightly from 2007 to 2014. Preliminary data from 2015 indicates the rate has begun to climb once more. Through the entire time frame from 1999 to 2015, opioids were involved in a large majority of all adolescent drug overdose deaths. Similar to adults, adolescent overdose deaths due to heroin and IMF have been trending upward and jumped dramatically from 2013 to 2015. Texas is suffering from a related crisis of maternal mortality due to opioids (Maternal Mortality and Morbidity Task Force and Department of State Health Services, 2016). Maternal mortality is generally defined as the death of a mother during pregnancy, childbirth, or in the year following delivery. Maternal mortality rates in Texas are the highest of any state in the United States. From 2000 to 2014, Texas saw an 86 percent increase in maternal mortality (from 18.6 to

34.0 per 100,000 live births), while the rest of the country experienced a much smaller 26 percent increase (from 18.8 to 23.8). Drug overdose is the second leading cause of maternal mortality in Texas, with limited toxicology records indicating a majority of these fatalities involved opioids.

Overdose Prevention

Opioids can cause fatal overdose by activating opioid receptors in the brain (Boyer, 2012). A specific subset of opioid receptors on the brainstem are responsible for this, as excessive activation suppresses the human body's intrinsic respiratory drive. Naloxone, a potent blocker of mu-opioid receptors (including those on the brainstem), is the drug of choice for reversing an acute opioid overdose. Naloxone is a prescription medication, but it is not a controlled substance and cannot be misused, as it produces no opioid-like effects. Several naloxone formulations are available with a broad spectrum of cost and ease of use (Lim, Bratberg, Davis, Green, & Walley, 2016). Harm-reduction organizations in the United States have been the primary source of naloxone access for nonmedical personnel over the past several decades, as these organizations worked to prevent overdose deaths in numerous communities. From 1996 to 2010, these programs distributed naloxone to more than 150,000 individuals, with nearly 27,000 overdose reversals reported (Wheeler, Jones, Gilbert, & Davidson, 2015). Based on the success of this approach, a movement has been growing to also provide naloxone access through the conventional health care system.

At least 47 states have enacted naloxone access laws to prevent opioid overdose deaths (Davis & Carr, 2017). Naloxone access laws vary, but they tend to include three core components. The first core component is an allowance for standing orders that enable pharmacists to dispense naloxone, under the delegated authority of a physician, without a prescription. The second core component is legal recognition of third-party prescribing, which allows naloxone to be prescribed or dispensed to someone other than the individual at risk for overdose. The third core component is broad liability protection for anyone who prescribes, dispenses, or administers naloxone. In states that have enacted naloxone access laws with these core components, a concerned friend or family member should be able to obtain naloxone from a pharmacy without a prescription. If they then administer it to an overdose victim but fail to successfully reverse the overdose, neither they nor the pharmacist need to fear liability for that failure. Adoption of naloxone access laws has been associated with a 9–11 percent reduction in opioid-related deaths (Rees, Sabia, Argys, Latshaw, & Dave, 2017).

The San Francisco Department of Public Health (SFDPH) has been at the leading edge of researching overdose prevention and naloxone prescribing in primary care. One key study, funded by the National Institute for Drug

Abuse, evaluated the impact of naloxone coprescribing for patients prescribed opioids for chronic pain (Coffin et al., 2016). Six primary care clinics that had previously implemented robust naloxone coprescribing programs were included in the analysis. These programs provided initial education to primary care clinicians regarding overdose risk, patient communication, and naloxone formulations. Rates of opioid-related emergency department (ED) visits were compared between patients who did and did not receive naloxone prescriptions. Nearly 2,000 patients taking opioids daily were included, with the majority receiving fewer than 60 MME daily.

Naloxone recipients experienced 47 percent fewer opioid-related ED visits per month in the six months after receiving a prescription and 63 percent fewer visits after one year, as compared to subjects who did not receive naloxone. This was a landmark study in the history of naloxone research, particularly in the context of a health care setting. However, there is still widespread disagreement about the threshold at which opioid overdose risk becomes worthy of naloxone prescribing. Additionally, many providers are hesitant to initiate a naloxone program for fear that it will alienate patients. A subsequent study from SFDPH published the results of surveys conducted to assess patient perceptions of naloxone coprescribing (Behar, Rowe, Santos, Murphy, & Coffin, 2016). They demonstrated that most patients had a positive response to being offered naloxone, and nearly all patients believed naloxone coprescribing for patients taking opioids should be standard. This data is consistent with a similar project conducted at the University of Pittsburgh Medical Center that also demonstrated that family medicine physician residents feel more comfortable caring for patients who request opioids when they are equipped with naloxone counseling tools (Han, Hill, Koenig, & Das, 2017).

In addition to the epidemic of opioid overdoses, the United States is experiencing a resurgence of human immunodeficiency virus (HIV) and an unprecedented spike in hepatitis C virus (HCV) among people who inject drugs (PWID) (Foundation for AIDS Research, 2017). PWID experience severe stigma and isolation, and they are often forced to inject in public spaces. This can lead to inappropriate disposal of used syringes, putting the public at risk for infectious disease transmission. When PWID are able to access a private space to inject, it is likely to be secluded and nonhygienic (e.g., a fast food restroom). Injecting alone in these spaces and often reusing syringes due to difficulty accessing sterile injection equipment put PWID at dramatically increased risk for HIV, HCV, and fatal overdose.

The United States is far behind in this domain, but a number of other countries have demonstrated a progressive approach to this problem through the implementation of supervised injection facilities (SIFs). SIFs allow PWID to inject drugs they have obtained independently in a hygienic space using sterile injection equipment with monitoring from trained staff. The goal of these facilities is to prevent overdose death and infectious disease transmission while demonstrating respect and compassion for PWID. Many SIFs provide further support to connect patients with addiction treatment and other social services. Research demonstrates that SIF implementation is associated with reductions in public drug use, enhanced access to medical and social services, and no increase in overall drug use or drug-related crimes (Foundation for AIDS Research, 2017). SIFs remain explicitly illegal in the United States under the "Crack House Statute," which criminalizes the opening or maintenance of any place for the purpose of unlawfully using a controlled substance. Despite this legal issue, several U.S. cities have discussed piloting SIFs in the near future. In the meantime, drop-in centers in Boston and other cities offer monitoring after drug use but do not allow drug use inside their facilities to conform with federal law (Wakeman, 2017).

Operation Naloxone

In March 2015, Texas enacted Senate Bill (SB) 1462 to combat opioid overdoses (Texas Legislature, 2015). This legislation increases access to naloxone and removes barriers to its use by implementing the three core components previously mentioned, including an allowance for pharmacists to enter into standing orders with physicians and dispense naloxone at their discretion. The Texas Pharmacy Association has a standing order that can be obtained by completing an online one-hour continuing education program. Several retail pharmacy chains have their own standing orders, although naloxone availability is dependent on the individual store and pharmacist. As is true in most states, the push for naloxone and other harm-reduction measures has been led by community organizations and advocates rather than health care professionals. The Texas Overdose Naloxone Initiative (TONI) and Austin Harm Reduction Coalition (AHRC) are essential leaders in Texas who built public support for SB 1462. They continue to fight an uphill battle against a Texas law that prevents syringe service programs (SSPs), also known as syringe or needle exchange programs, from operating by criminalizing the provision of drug paraphernalia (Smith, 2017).

The University of Texas at Austin (UT) has cultivated a proactive recovery-oriented campus environment that is prepared for potential opioid overdoses (Steiker, 2016). The development of this progressive model was spurred by students in the form of a unanimously-passed student government resolution that naloxone should be available in the campus pharmacy without a prescription. In response, UT University Health Services and the UT College of Pharmacy collaborated to implement a standing order for naloxone that has increased access for students, faculty, and staff. An interprofessional group that included a variety of campus stakeholders was convened with input from TONI and AHRC to form the UT Wellness Network Committee on Substance Safety and Overdose Prevention. Several novel initiatives have spun out of this committee's work. Faculty from the UT College of Pharmacy now provide annual training to all resident advisers to prepare them for overdose response, and naloxone is stocked at centrally located desks that are accessible to every residence hall. Additionally, every UT Police Department officer has received overdose response training and a supply of naloxone. To expand the reach of overdose prevention efforts into off-campus housing, UT College of Pharmacy students created a service-learning program through which they provide peer education to other UT students and furnish free naloxone to training attendees (Saksena, 2016).

Faculty leaders from Operation Naloxone have received funding from the Texas Health and Human Services Commission for multiple statewide overdose prevention projects. An initiative targeting health care professionals included the development of a continuing education course on opioid harm reduction for prescribers, pharmacists, and social workers. Supporting educational materials are available at OperationNaloxone.org to guide discussions of opioid risks and naloxone with patients. Another initiative targeting people who use illicit drugs focuses on the distribution of overdose prevention kits with training for community organizations. Each overdose prevention kit contains naloxone vials, intramuscular syringes, a fentanyl test strip, a rescue breathing barrier, latex gloves, and user-friendly instructions with colorful illustrations. These kits are distributed to community organizations that work with people who use illicit drugs for secondary distribution. Staff and affiliates of the community organizations are invited to attend live seminars from leading harm-reduction experts at TONI and AHRC.

Policy Recommendations

Federal, state, and local governments should promote harm reduction through legislative policy. First, variable state legislation regarding naloxone access should be standardized to ensure consistent access to every available formulation. As of 2017, most states do not have statewide standing orders for naloxone. Of those that do, many restrict access to only certain formulations. For example, the statewide naloxone standing order in Pennsylvania does not allow pharmacists to provide naloxone vials and intramuscular syringes. As this is the cheapest version of naloxone, it is likely that many Pennsylvanians at risk for opioid overdose are unable to access naloxone due to this state policy. Second, to further reduce harm by preventing severe infections such as HCV and HIV, federal or state action should be taken to ensure SSPs are legally allowed to operate throughout the United States. In many states, including Texas, harm-reduction groups must operate in relative secrecy due to the fear of prosecution for providing sterile injection equipment. Negative attitudes about SSPs are often based on the thoroughly debunked belief that SSPs enable drug use; overwhelming evidence demonstrates they reduce drug use and increase entry into substance use disorder treatment.

Third, the "Crack House Statute" should be repealed or amended to allow for domestic implementation of SIFs. PWID are among the most marginalized individuals in contemporary American society, and it is illogical to believe those with the most severe substance use disorders will be able to achieve recovery from their disorder with currently available treatments. Many of these potential patients justifiably see the health care system as an enemy rather than a friend. Showing respect for PWID as autonomous individuals worthy of compassion might just be the missing link to increase their engagement in treatment and prevent overdose death. Finally, the U.S. government should declare the opioid crisis a national emergency. Such a declaration was suggested by the President's Commission on Combating Drug Addiction and the Opioid Crisis, and President Trump signaled that he may do so in August 2017. However, as of October 2017, no such declaration has been issued. Experts believe the primary benefit of declaring a national emergency would be to attract attention and promote coordination between federal agencies (Fitzpatrick, 2017). The majority of ongoing national emergencies are related to terrorism, but the number of Americans who die each year due to opioid overdose is exponentially larger than the number who die due to terrorism. A national emergency declaration would complement recent increases in opioid-related treatment and research funding from the Substance Abuse and Mental Health Services Administration (SAMHSA). Recognizing the acuity of this emergency, the funding primarily supports interventions that can have an immediate impact, such as increasing access to naloxone and training for overdose prevention and response.

Health care professionals and institutions should reallocate resources to invest in staff education that bolsters harm reduction. First, every hospital and clinic should be prepared to prescribe naloxone to patients at risk for opioid overdose and individuals who may witness an opioid overdose. In hospitals around the country, many patients who are admitted to EDs for opioid overdose are treated and discharged without receiving naloxone or a prescription to obtain it from a pharmacy. If this were true for a less stigmatized disease, the treating health care providers would almost certainly face professional liability for subsequent outcomes. Second, every pharmacy should have a standing order to dispense any formulation of naloxone the pharmacist deems appropriate. Pharmacies should honor these standing orders by maintaining a supply of naloxone so that no patient is turned away when they request it. Even in states that have issued statewide standing orders, many patients report facing interrogation from pharmacists regarding their need for naloxone. When pharmacists are knowledgeable and willing to dispense naloxone, patients may still have to wait for it to be ordered from a supplier. In Texas and some other states, pharmacists are authorized to administer naloxone for an acute opioid overdose. Knowledge of this fact could lead a bystander to transport a patient to a pharmacy for overdose reversal, and the time wasted traveling to a pharmacy that didn't have naloxone in stock could result in the overdose victim's death.

In addition, all health care providers should become proficient in harm-reduction counseling. This should include education about safe use practices, such as never using alone, always having naloxone available, and consistently using sterile injection equipment. With the rise of IMF, people who use drugs should also be counseled to start with a much lower dose than they typically use to avoid overdose. Testing drug products for fentanyl using nonapproved urine test strips could also be recommended to increase awareness of the fentanyl epidemic. Furthermore, all health care providers should consider it their professional responsibility to facilitate access to sterile injection equipment for PWID. This should include prescribing or dispensing of appropriate syringes, alcohol, and gauze as well as professional advocacy for the implementation of SIFs. Finally, all primary care clinicians should complete the required training to obtain a buprenorphine waiver and subsequently integrate opioid use disorder treatment in their practice. Until opioid use disorder treatment is available in every community, supply-side interventions for the opioid crisis will continue to have negative short-term public health consequences.

References

Behar, E., Rowe, C., Santos, G. M., Murphy, S., & Coffin, P. O. (2016). Primary care patient experience with naloxone prescription. *Annals of Family Medicine, 14*(5), 431–436. doi:10.1370/afm.1972.

Behavioral Health Coordinating Committee. (2013). *Addressing Prescription Drug Abuse in the United States.* Washington, D.C.: U.S. Department of Health and Human Services.

Beletsky, L., & Davis, C. S. (2017). Today's fentanyl crisis: Prohibition's Iron Law, revisited. *International Journal of Drug Policy, 46,* 156–159. doi:10.1016/j .drugpo.2017.05.050.

Boyer, E. W. (2012). Management of opioid analgesic overdose. *New England Journal of Medicine, 367*(2), 146–155. doi:10.1056/NEJMra1202561.

Brownstein, M. J. (1993). A brief history of opiates, opioid peptides, and opioid receptors. *Proceedings of the National Academy of Sciences, 90*(12), 5391–5393.

Casey, E. (1978). History of drug use and drug users in the United States. www .druglibrary.org/schaffer/history/casey1.htm.

Catan, T., & Perez, E. (2012). A pain drug champion has second thoughts. http:// online.wsj.com/news/articles/SB10001424127887324478304578173342657044604.

Chen, L. H., Hedegaard, H., & Warner, M. (2014). *Drug-poisoning Deaths Involving Opioid Analgesics: United States, 1999–2011*. NCHS data brief, no 166. Hyattsville, MD: National Center for Health Statistics.

Ciccarone, D. (2017). Fentanyl in the US heroin supply: A rapidly changing risk environment. *International Journal of Drug Policy, 46*, 107–111. doi: 10.1016/j.drugpo.2017.06.010.

Coffin, P. O., Behar, E., Rowe, C., Santos, G. M., Coffa, D., Bald, M., & Vittinghoff, E. (2016). Nonrandomized intervention study of naloxone coprescription for primary care patients receiving long-term opioid therapy for pain. *Annals of Internal Medicine, 165*(4), 245–252. doi:10.7326/m15-2771.

Curtin, S. C., Tejada-Vera, B., & Warner, M. (2017). *Drug Overdose Deaths among Adolescents Aged 15–19 in the United States: 1999–2015*. NCHS Data Brief, no. 282. Hyattsville, MD: National Center for Health Statistics.

Davis, C., & Carr, D. (2017). State legal innovations to encourage naloxone dispensing. *Journal of the American Pharmacists Association, 57*(2s), S180–S184. doi:10.1016/j.japh.2016.11.007.

Davis, C. S. (2017). Commentary on Pardo (2017) and Moyo et al. (2017): Much still unknown about prescription drug monitoring programs. *Addiction, 112*(10), 1797–1798. doi:10.1111/add.13936.

Delcher, C., Wagenaar, A. C., Goldberger, B. A., Cook, R. L., & Maldonado-Molina, M. M. (2015). Abrupt decline in oxycodone-caused mortality after implementation of Florida's prescription drug monitoring program. *Drug and Alcohol Dependence, 150*, 63–68. doi:10.1016/j.drugalcdep .2015.02.010.

Dowell, D., Haegerich, T. M., & Chou, R. (2016). CDC guideline for prescribing opioids for chronic pain—United States, 2016. *JAMA, 315*(15), 1624–1645. doi:10.1001/jama.2016.1464.

Dowell, D., Zhang, K., Noonan, R. K., & Hockenberry, J. M. (2016). Mandatory provider review and pain clinic laws reduce the amounts of opioids prescribed and overdose death rates. *Health Affairs, 35*(10), 1876–1883. doi:10.1377/hlthaff.2016.0448.

Feldman, L., Williams, K. S., Coates, J., & Knox, M. (2011). Awareness and utilization of a prescription monitoring program among physicians. *Journal of Pain and Palliative Care Pharmacotherapy, 25*(4), 313–317. doi:10.3109/1 5360288.2011.606292.

Ferrari, R., Capraro, M., & Visentin, M. (2012). Risk factors in opioid treatment of chronic non-cancer pain: A multidisciplinary assessment. In G. B. Racz & C. E. Noe (Eds.), *Pain Management—Current Issues and Opinions*, 419–458. London, England: InTech.

Fitzpatrick, K. (2017). This is why the opioid crisis is as dangerous as a terrorist attack. https://news.utexas.edu/2017/09/26/why-the-opioid-crisis-is-as -dangerous-as-a-terrorist-attack.

Foundation for AIDS Research. (2017). *The Case for Supervised Consumption Services*. Washington, D.C.: Foundation for AIDS Research.

Geriatrics and Extended Care Strategic Healthcare Group. (2000). *Pain as the 5th Vital Sign Toolkit*. Washington, D.C.: Veterans Health Administration.

Gotbaum, R. (2015). DEA "pill mill" crackdown may be causing an unintended consequence. http://www.wbur.org/hereandnow/2015/08/04/pill-mill -crackdown.

Han, J. K., Hill, L. G., Koenig, M. E., & Das, N. (2017). Naloxone counseling for harm reduction and patient engagement. *Family Medicine, 49*(9), 730–733.

Hedegaard, H., Chen, L. H., & Warner, M. (2015). *Drug-poisoning Deaths Involving Heroin: United States, 2000–2013*. NCHS data brief, no 190. Hyattsville, MD: National Center for Health Statistics.

Lim, J. K., Bratberg, J. P., Davis, C. S., Green, T. C., & Walley, A. Y. (2016). Prescribe to prevent: Overdose prevention and naloxone rescue kits for prescribers and pharmacists. *Journal of Addiction Medicine, 10*(5), 300–308. doi:10.1097/adm.0000000000000223.

Maternal Mortality and Morbidity Task Force and Department of State Health Services. (2016). *Joint Biennial Report*. Austin, TX: Department of State Health Services.

Moyo, P., Simoni-Wastila, L., Griffin, B. A., Onukwugha, E., Harrington, D., Alexander, G. C., & Palumbo, F. (2017). Impact of prescription drug monitoring programs (PDMPs) on opioid utilization among Medicare beneficiaries in 10 US states. *Addiction, 112*(10), 1784–1796. doi:10.1111/add.13860.

Pardo, B. (2017). Do more robust prescription drug monitoring programs reduce prescription opioid overdose? *Addiction, 112*(10), 1773–1783. doi:10.1111 /add.13741.

Paulozzi, L. J., Jones, C. M., Mack, K. A., & Rudd, R. A. (2011). Vital signs: Overdoses of prescription opioid pain relievers—United States, 1999–2008. *MMWR: Morbidity and Mortal Weekly Report, 60*(43), 1487–1492.

PBS Frontline. (1998). Opium throughout history. http://www.pbs.org/wgbh /pages/frontline/shows/heroin/etc/history.html.

Rees, D. I., Sabia, J. J., Argys, L. M., Latshaw, J., & Dave, D. (2017). *With a Little Help from My Friends: The Effects of Naloxone Access and Good Samaritan Laws on Opioid-related Deaths* (NBER Working Paper No. 16026). Cambridge, MA: National Bureau of Economic Research.

Rudd, R. A., Aleshire, N., Zibbell, J. E., & Gladden, R. M. (2016). Increases in drug and opioid overdose deaths—United States, 2000–2014. MMWR: *Morbidity and Mortality Weekly Report, 64*(50-51), 1378–1382. doi:10.15585 /mmwr.mm6450a3.

Saksena, S. (2016). College of pharmacy combats opioid overdoses with campus campaign. *Daily Texan*, October 4. http://dailytexanonline.com/2016 /10/04/college-of-pharmacy-combats-opioid-overdoses-with-campus -campaign.

S.B.1462. An act relating to the prescription, administration, and possession of certain antagonists for the treatment of suspected opioid overdoses (2015).

Smith, M. (2017). syringe exchange for drug users hopes to emerge from the shadows. http://reportingtexas.com/needle-exchange-for-drug-users-hopes-to-emerge-from-the-shadows.

Steiker, L. H. (2016). Opioid overdose prevention initiatives on the college campus: Critical partnerships between academe and community experts. *Journal of Drug Abuse, 2,* 2.

Understanding Addictions. (2010). Prescription painkiller abuse still rising. http://www.understandingaddictions.com/2010/06/prescription-painkiller-abuse-still.html.

Wakeman, S. E. (2017). Another senseless death—The case for supervised injection facilities. *New England Journal of Medicine, 376*(11), 1011–1013. doi:10.1056/NEJMp1613651.

Weiss, A. J., Elixhauser, A., Barrett, M. L., Steiner, C. A., Bailey, M. K., & O'Malley, L. (2016). *Opioid-related Inpatients Stays and Emergency Department Visits by State, 2009–2014.* HCUP Statistical Brief #219. Rockville, MD: Agency for Healthcare Research and Quality.

Wheeler, E., Jones, T. S., Gilbert, M. K., & Davidson, P. J. (2015). Opioid overdose prevention programs providing naloxone to laypersons—United States, 2014. *MMWR: Morbidity and Mortality Weekly Report, 64*(23), 631–635.

CHAPTER FOURTEEN

A Comparison of Recent Trends in Prescription Drug Misuse in the United States and the United Kingdom

Trevor Bennett, Katy Holloway, and Tom May

Until recently, it was widely believed that the nonmedical use of prescription medications is much less of a problem in the United Kingdom than in the United States (Giraudon, Lowitz, Dargan, Wood, & Dart, 2013; Strang, Drummond, McNeill, Lader, & Marsden, 2014). More recent publications have suggested that this may now be changing, and diversion of prescription medications in the United Kingdom might be increasing (Advisory Council on the Misuse of Drugs, 2016; European Monitoring Centre for Drugs and Drug Addiction, 2016). However, the authors of these reports have also drawn attention to the relative lack of evidence to support these views.

It should be noted from the outset, that the definition of *nonmedical use* of prescription medications is unclear, both conceptually and in practice. Non-medical use, along with the associated concept of prescription drug misuse (PDM), can refer to the use of drugs not prescribed to the individual or inappropriate use of medications prescribed to them. In practice, it is hard to identify either form of misuse, as the source of the medication or the precise method of its use are rarely known. Hence, some assumptions have to be made to measure nonmedical use or PDM.

Trends in PDM have been investigated in the research literature using six main sources of information:

1. national surveys of PDM among the general population
2. data on individuals presenting to treatment agencies with problems relating to prescription drugs
3. information on prescription drug use among prisoners
4. data on the number of drug-related deaths involving prescription drugs
5. data on the number of prescriptions dispensed as part of general prescribing
6. records of seizures involving prescription drugs

Each of these data sources has advantages and disadvantages. Not everyone responds to national surveys. Trends in the number of people who use a drug and present for treatment only provide evidence on individuals who use at problematic levels. Information on PDM in prisons refers only to drug-using offenders. Drug-related deaths identify trends in drug overdose rather than use. Records on the number of prescriptions dispensed per year cover both use and PDM. And drug seizures reflect police activity and effectiveness as much as the quantity of drugs in circulation.

Despite these limitations, these are the main sources of evidence available to investigate trends in PDM. One of the aims of the current chapter is to compare the evidence from the United States and the United Kingdom to find out whether the two countries are following similar or different paths.

The main data sources rarely refer to a general category of PDM. Instead, they tend to provide data on specific types of prescription medications that are frequently misused. As the selection of these drugs is variable, it is necessary to standardize the selection of comparison medications as much as possible. We have done this by identifying five categories of commonly misused prescription drugs and selecting, when possible, one example of each of these categories from each data source. The five categories used are opiates; sedatives (e.g., tranquilizers); sedative-hypnotics; stimulants; and antidepressants. On occasions when more than one medication per category was mentioned, we chose the one most frequently misused as identified in the data sources and in the research literature. Common examples of these categories in the United Kingdom are opiates (tramadol); tranquilizers (diazepam and other benzodiazepines); hypnotics ("Z" drugs, such as zopiclone, and non-"Z" drug hypnotics, such as ketamine); stimulants (amphetamine); and antidepressants (citalopram). We will then estimate trends in PDM across each data source by comparing similar packages of prescription drugs across the United Kingdom and United States.

Trends in the United Kingdom

Trends in the General Population

The main source of information on PDM in the United Kingdom's general population is the annual Crime Survey for England and Wales (Office for National Statistics, 2016a). This is a general household survey of a representative sample of the population. Questions on taking prescription-only painkillers not prescribed to the user were first included in the 2014–2015 survey. However, information on a small number of frequently misused prescription drugs have been included in the surveys since 1996. These include "amphetamines," "tranquilizers," and "ketamine" (added in 2005–2006).

Figure 14.1 shows that trends in the use of amphetamines and tranquilizers declined over the period 1996 to 2015–2016. Information on ketamine use has only recently been recorded, and after an early increase during the period 2005–2006 to 2010–2011, it has also since declined. The percentage of reduction in the proportion of the population using amphetamines over this period was 82 percent and 67 percent in relation to tranquilizers. Hence, we conclude that U.K. trends in the use of the selected prescription drugs (which may or may not have been prescribed to anyone) *decreased.*

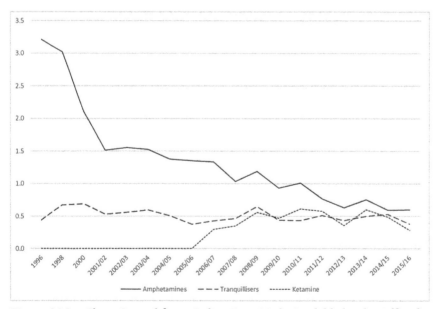

Figure 14.1   Chart Created from Online Data Made Available by the Office for National Statistics (2016a).

Trends in Individuals Presenting to Treatment Agencies

National-level information on the numbers of individuals presenting to treatment agencies were obtained from the National Drug Treatment Monitoring System (NDTMS) published by the Department of Health (Public Health England, 2016). The annual reports provide information on all clients aged 18 and older who were receiving help for problems with drugs or alcohol in structured treatment agencies during the previous year. The drug types included in the data cover tranquilizers (benzodiazepines), stimulants (amphetamine), and hypnotics (ketamine). Each client can register several problematic drug types.

Trends in the number of adults engaged in use presenting to treatment agencies over the period 2005–2006 to 2015–2016 are shown in Figure 14.2. The number of individuals seeking treatment over this period reduced for benzodiazepine use (–24%) but marginally increased for amphetamine (+1%) and notably for ketamine use (+374%). We conclude that the number of individuals presenting to U.K. treatment agencies mentioning PDM *increased* for two of the three drugs investigated.

Trends among Prisoners

There are currently no routinely collected data on prescription drug misuse among prisoners. However, there are regular annual reports prepared by Her Majesty's (HM) Chief Inspector of Prisons for England and Wales, which

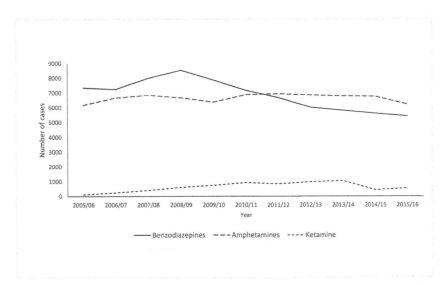

Figure 14.2 Trends in Reported Drug Use Among New Adult Presentations for Treatment for Substance-Related Problems (Chart created from online data made available by Public Health England [2016])

Table 14.1   Selected Comments Made in HM Chief Inspector Annual Reports Showing Trends in Prescribed Medication Misuse in Prisons 2010–2011 to 2015–2016

Date	Annual Report Comment on Prescribed Medications in Prisons
2010–2011	A major issue in high security and vulnerable prisoner populations.
2011–2012	This problem is spreading to mainstream populations.
2012–2013	A growing problem.
2013–2014	A dangerous new trend.
2014–2015	Too many prisoners were prescribed highly tradeable medications.
2015–2016	Inadequate officer supervision in medication queues all too often continue to contribute to bullying and diversion.

include commentary on diversion of prescription medications in prisons (e.g., Her Majesty's Inspectorate of Prisons, 2016). This method of using qualitative data to measure trends was employed in the 2016 report of the Advisory Council on the Misuse of Drugs (ACMD) on diversion of prescription medications (Advisory Council on the Misuse of Drugs, 2016). The report concluded that the issue of diverted medications in prisons was first mentioned in 2011. By the time of the 2015–2016 report, diverted medications were viewed as a serious problem across most prisons. To examine this progression in more detail, we analyzed the history of prescription drug misuse as described in the six annual HM Inspectorate reports covering the periods 2010–2011 to 2015–2016. A summary of the main points is shown in Table 14.1.

Prior to 2010, there was no indication in the annual inspection reports that PDM in prisons was a problem. During the period from 2010–2011 to 2015–2016, there is evidence that misuse of prescription medications in prisons was increasing. Hence, we conclude that PDM in U.K. prisons over the period 2010–2011 *increased*.

Trends in Drug-Related Deaths

One of the most commonly used measures of changes in drug use and misuse of prescription medications over time is through the analysis of drug-related deaths. Data on drug-related deaths in England and Wales are routinely collected by the Office for National Statistics and made available through annual reports and online databases (e.g., Office for National Statistics, 2016b).

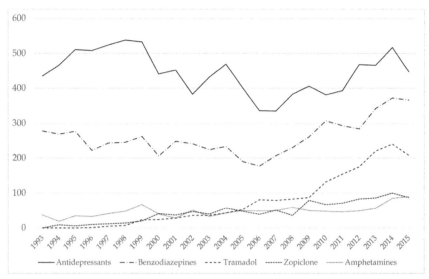

Figure 14.3 Drug-Related Deaths Involving Selected Prescription Medications, England and Wales (Chart created from online data made available by the Office for National statistics [2016b])

A death related to drug misuse is defined as either (a) a death where the underlying cause is drug abuse or drug dependence or (b) a death where the underlying cause is drug poisoning and where any of the substances controlled under the Misuse of Drugs Act 1971 (U.K. Parliament, 2000) are involved. Substances associated with the death are obtained from the death certificate. When a number of drugs are mentioned, it is usually not possible to tell which specific drug was responsible for the death.

As before, examples of the five main prescription drug categories were extracted from the data, including opiates (tramadol), tranquilizers (benzodiazepines), stimulants (amphetamine), hypnotics (zopiclone), and antidepressants (identified only as "antidepressants"). Trends in the involvement of these selected prescription medications in U.K. drug-related deaths are shown in Figure 14.3. Over the period 1993–2015, the trend increased for all drugs: tramadol (+767%), benzodiazepines (+78%), amphetamines (+125%), zopiclone (+112%), and antidepressants (+1%). Hence, we conclude that U.K. drug-related deaths *increased* over the period shown.

Trends in the Number of Prescriptions Dispensed in the Community

Data on the number of medications prescribed in the U.K. community are held by National Health Service (NHS) Prescription Services. The data system is based on all prescriptions dispensed in the community by pharmacists and

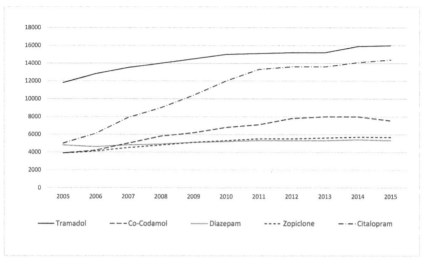

Figure 14.4 UK Trends in Number of Selected Prescription Medications Dispensed in the Community 2005–2015 (Chart created by combining charts published by National Statistics [2016])

dispensing doctors. The majority of prescriptions in England are written by medical practitioners, and the remainder are written by nurses, dentists, other nonmedical prescribers, and hospital doctors.

Trends in the number of commonly misused prescription drugs are presented in chart form in a recent report by National Statistics (2016). Figure 14.4 shows the 10-year trend for selected prescription medications, comprising examples of four of the five main drug categories mentioned earlier: opiates (tramadol and co-codamol), sedatives-tranquilizers (diazepam), sedatives-hypnotics (zopiclone), and antidepressants (citalopram). The trend in the number of prescriptions dispensed increased for all prescription drugs: tramadol (+93%), co-codamol (+36%), diazepam (+11%), zopiclone (+45%), and citalopram (+188%). We conclude that the number of prescriptions dispensed in the U.K. community *increased* over the period studied.

Trends in Seizures of Prescription Drugs

Trends in seizures of prescription drugs in the United Kingdom are provided by the Office for National Statistics in an annual report titled *Seizures of Drugs in England and Wales* and also through online data available on the government website (Office for National Statistics, 2016c). The publication presents figures for drug seizures over the previous financial year by police,

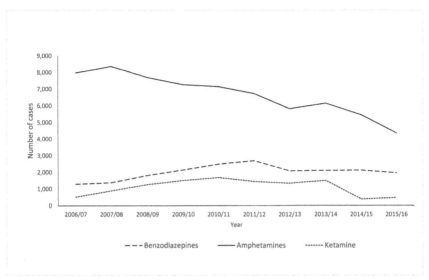

Figure 14.5 Number of Police Seizures of Selected Prescription Medications in England and Wales, 2006 to 2016 (Chart created from online data made available by the Office for National Statistics [2016c])

including the British Transport Police and Border Force, a law enforcement command within the Home Office that controls people and goods entering the United Kingdom. The data relate to all drugs controlled under the Misuse of Drugs Act 1971, including selected prescription drugs.

The number of seizures for benzodiazepines over the period (2006–2007 to 2015–2016) increased by 52 percent (see Figure 14.5). Over the same period, amphetamine seizures decreased by 45 percent, and ketamine seizures decreased by 36 percent. Hence, the overall conclusion is that seizures for selected prescription drugs in the United Kingdom on average *decreased* over the period shown.

Summary of PDM Trends in the United Kingdom

Overall, there are two data sources that show that PDM has decreased over the study period: drug use in the general population and seizures of prescription drugs. Conversely, there are four data sources that show that PDM has increased: prisons, prescriptions dispensed in the community, drug-related deaths, and individuals presenting for drug treatment. The main factor that differentiates these two data sources is that the former two address the general population or the country as a whole and the latter four focus on the criminal and drug-using population.

Trends in the United States

Trends in the General Population

The National Survey on Drug Use and Health (NSUDH; Center for Behavioral Health Statistics and Quality, 2015) provides national- and state-level data on the use of tobacco, alcohol, illicit drugs (including the nonmedical use of prescription drugs), and mental health in the United States. The NSDUH is sponsored by the Substance Abuse and Mental Health Services Administration (SAMHSA), and it examines the use of four main categories of psychotherapeutics: pain relievers, tranquilizers, stimulants, and sedatives. Over the 2002–2014 period, the use of pain relievers decreased from 1.9 percent in the general population to 1.6 percent (see Figure 14.6). Similarly, tranquilizer use reduced from 0.8 percent to 0.7 percent and sedatives from 0.2 percent to 0.1 percent. Stimulants remained stable over this period, with 0.6 percent of the population reporting use of these drugs in 2002 and the same proportion using these drugs in 2014. Over the last five years (2010–2014) of available data, the proportion of those using analgesics reduced by 0.4 percent, tranquilizers reduced by 0.2 percent, sedatives stayed constant at 0.1 percent, and stimulants increased by 0.2 percent. Apart from one or two increases over the period, the dominant trend of prescription drug misuse among the general population in the United States is a *decreasing* one.

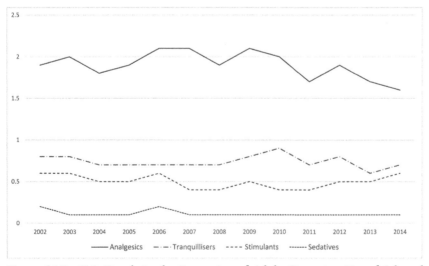

Figure 14.6   U.S. Trends in the Proportion of Adults Reporting Use of Selected Prescription Drugs 1996 to 2015/16 (Chart created from data published by SAMSHA [Substance Abuse and Mental Health Services Administration] [SAMSHA, 2016].)

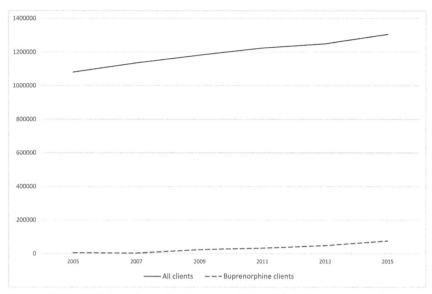

Figure 14.7 U.S. Trends in the Number of New Adult Presentations for Treatment for Problems Relating to Selected Prescription Drugs 2005/06 to 2015/16. (Chart created from data provided by the National Survey of Substance Abuse Treatment Services [N-SSATS, 2017].)

Trends in Individuals Presenting to Treatment Agencies

Trends in the number of people attending treatment agencies can be viewed from data provided by the National Survey of Substance Abuse Treatment Services (N-SSATS, 2017). The data showed that over the 2005–2015 period, the number of clients attending treatment services increased from 1.1 million to 1.3 million (see Figure 14.7). Unfortunately, no data were available on use of prescription drugs. Overall, the general trend was an *increase*.

Trends among Prisoners

There is no national database that provides trend data on prescription drug use or misuse in U.S. prisons. However, a special report written by the Bureau of Justice (2006) based on the Survey of Inmates in State and Federal Correctional Facilities during 1997 and 2004 reported on the use of depressants and stimulants by prisoners. This showed that, between 1997 and 2004, the percentage of federal prisoners who used stimulants at the time of the offense for which they had been imprisoned increased from 4.1 percent to 7.4 percent (see Figure 14.8). Over the same period, the proportion of

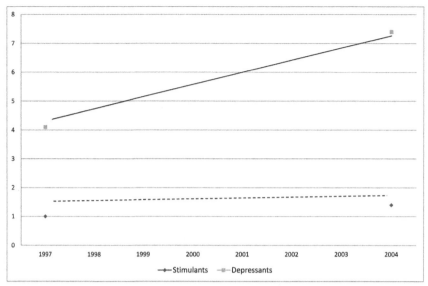

Figure 14.8 U.S. Trends in the Number of Federal Prisoners Who Reported Use of Prescription of Drugs at the Time of the Offence for Which They Were Currently Convicted 1997 to 2004. (Chart created from data published by the Bureau of Justice Statistics [2006].)

federal prisoners who reported use of depressants at the time of the offense increased from 1.0 percent to 1.4 percent. Overall, these (albeit limited) findings suggest that the use of prescription medications among U.S. prisoners has *increased* since the late 1990s.

Trends in Drug-Related Deaths

Data on drug-related deaths are collected by the National Vital Statistics System (NVSS) in their "multiple cause-of-death mortality files" that are used to identify, among other things, drug overdose deaths. The data have been analyzed and published in several papers, including recent studies by Warner and colleagues (2016) and Hedegaard and colleagues (2015). Together, they provide information on drug-related deaths involving several prescription drugs over the 1999–2014 period, including oxycodone and diazepam. The study showed that, during this period, drug-related deaths involving opioid analgesics increased by 400 percent, from 4,000 to 16,000 deaths, and between 2010 and 2014, deaths involving diazepam increased by 19 percent (see Figure 14.9). Despite the small number of drugs available for comparison, the trend suggests that U.S. deaths involving prescription drugs have *increased*.

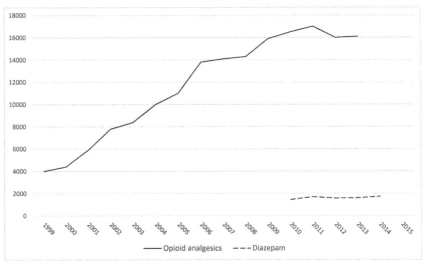

Figure 14.9 U.S. Trends in Drug-Related Deaths Involving Prescription Medications 1999–2015. (Chart created by combining graphs produced by Warner [2016] and Hedegaard et al. [2015] based on data from the National Vital Statistics System multiple cause-of-death mortality files.)

Trends in the Number of Prescriptions Dispensed in the Community

The main data source on the number of prescriptions dispensed in the community is the IMS Health National Prescription Audit. Several articles have analyzed the IMS data, including Pezalla and colleagues (2017) and Levy and colleagues (2015). The former provided a graph of the number of opioid prescriptions filled over the period of 1992–2016 (see Figure 14.10). The figure clearly shows that, between 1992 and 2010, the number of opioid prescriptions increased. However, after 2011, the number of prescriptions for opioid analgesics declined. Hence, the number of U.S. prescriptions dispensed for opioid-based painkillers over most of the period studied *increased*.

Trends in Seizures of Prescription Drugs

Details of drug seizures by the police and by border control are collected by the U.S. Drug Enforcement Administration (DEA). However, we were unable to find any reference to seizures of prescription drugs. The closest evidence that we could find was a report by the DEA that showed a mixed pattern, depending on the type of illicit drug. Heroin seizures, for example, continued to increase over the 1986–2014 period, while marijuana seizures continued to fall.

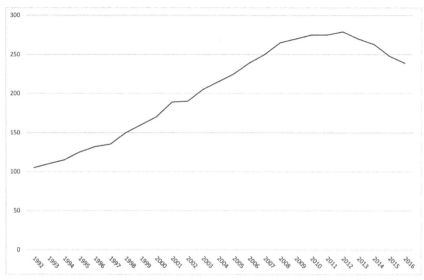

Figure 14.10   U.S. Trends in Number of Prescription Medications Dispensed in the Community 1992–2016 (Chart created from data published by IMS Health National Prescription Audit (Pezalla, et al., 2017).)

Summary of PDM Trends in the United States

The conclusions drawn from the analysis of the six U.S. data sources was that one of them, prescription drug use in the general population, had decreased over recent years; four of them showed that various measures of prescription drug involvement had increased over time, treatment, prisons, drug-related deaths, and prescriptions; and one of them, seizures, could not be evaluated because of lack of data. This pattern of change closely matches the trends found in the United Kingdom. As was the case in the United Kingdom, U.S. data relating to the general population tended to show a decrease in PDM, and data related to offender or drug-using populations showed an increase.

PDM Trends in the United States and United Kingdom Compared

We will now compare what is known about PDM in the United States and in the United Kingdom and consider whether the rate of change is higher or lower in one country or another. We will do this by summarizing the results of the quantitative analysis and by drawing on summaries and commentaries from recent reviews of the literature. There are several studies that have conducted similar investigations of trends in the United States and in the

United Kingdom (Advisory Council on the Misuse of Drugs, 2016; Giraudon et al., 2013; Weisberg, Becker, Fiellin, & Stannard, 2014), and we will include these findings in our overview. The reviews have tended to focus on four main areas: PDM in the general population, the availability of prescription drugs in prisons, drug-related deaths, and prescribing in the community. These are also the topic areas where the best quantitative data can be found. Hence, we will base our comparison of PDM in the United States and the United Kingdom on these four topic areas.

Trends in the General Population

PDM trends in the general population were measured by change in use of amphetamines and tranquilizers in the United Kingdom and by changes in use of analgesics, stimulants, and tranquilizers in the United States. The available evidence suggests that, over the last decade, the use of these drugs tended to decrease in both countries. The reviews of the literature on trends in PDM in the general population were more variable. One study, for example, concluded that, between 1999 and 2006, the proportion of individuals over age 20 in the United States using prescription opioids increased (Frenk, Porter, & Paulozzi, 2015). Another suggested that, during the period 2003 and 2013, nonmedical use of prescription opioids among the adult population decreased (Han, Compton, Jones, & Cai, 2015). Comparing the comments with the charts discussed earlier shows that the differences in the conclusions are, in part, a result of the period of the trend curve under discussion. When the same years are compared, the conclusions are more consistent with our own findings. Hence, on the basis of these comparisons of quantitative data and commentaries in reviews, we conclude that reported misuse of prescription medications decreased in both countries over the last decade, with a greater reduction in the United Kingdom than in the United States.

Trends in PDM among Prisoners

There were no quantitative data available on PDM among prisoners in the United Kingdom and only limited data in the United States. Trends in PDM in the prison population were estimated from qualitative statements made in annual reports from the prison inspectorate in the United Kingdom over the 2010–2015 period and statements arising from a survey of inmates in correctional facilities in the United States during the 1997–2004 period. The conclusions drawn from each of the reports was that PDM in prison populations was increasing.

The main review of drug use in U.K. prisons is a report by the Centre for Social Justice (2015). The authors reported that the number of maintenance prescriptions for opioids increased over the period 2007–2008 to 2012–2013 by 137 percent, suggesting that the number of prisoners dependent on opioids had also increased. However, information provided in response to a parliamentary question showed that the number of positive tests for opiates in prisons declined from 2002 to 2011, as did the number of opiate seizures in prisons (Hansard, 2012). Therefore, the conclusions to be drawn depend on which source of evidence is used. Indeed, these findings are not wholly inconsistent. Drug testing for opiates and seizures of opiates in prisons include heroin. There is some evidence from the prison inspectorate reports that heroin use among prisoners has been decreasing in recent years, in part as a result of prisoners switching to other drugs, such as prescription drugs and new psychoactive substances (NPS), which cannot be detected in tests. Hence, the most plausible conclusion from the information available is that PDM among prisoners in both countries increased over the last decade.

Trends in Drug-Related Deaths

Trends in drug-related deaths were analyzed from quantitative data from the United Kingdom and the United States based on evidence of consumption of tramadol, benzodiazepines, amphetamines, zopiclone, and antidepressants in the United Kingdom and for analgesics and diazepam in the United States. The involvement of prescription drugs in drug-related deaths increased for all drugs investigated over the last decade in the United Kingdom and in the United States. External reviews of the data came to similar conclusions. One study made a distinction between the rate of change and the absolute number of deaths. It was noted that although the number of deaths is proportionately much greater in the United States than in the United Kingdom, the rate of change in the number of deaths is remarkably similar (Giraudon et al., 2013). Overall, the evidence suggests that drug-related deaths involving prescription drugs have been increasing in both countries.

Trends in the Number of Prescriptions Dispensed in the Community

Trends in the number of prescription drugs prescribed in the community were measured in the United States and United Kingdom from records kept by national databases. Data from both the United States and the United Kingdom clearly show that the number of prescriptions for all abusable prescription drugs investigated increased in recent years. Reviews of trends of the number of prescriptions dispensed also suggested recent increases. One U.S. study, for example, reported that, "The total number of opioid pain relievers prescribed in the United States has skyrocketed in the last 25 years" (Volkow, 2014, p. 2). The authors concluded that the United States is now the largest global consumer of hydrocodone and oxycodone (Volkow, 2014, p. 39). Some reviews have made a link between the volume of prescriptions for drugs and misuse of these drugs. As one reviewer noted, "increasingly it is clear that overprescription of these medications over the past two decades has been a major upstream driver of the opioid abuse epidemic" (Compton, Boyle, & Wargo, 2015, p. 1).

Similar trends have been discussed in the U.K. reviews. The ACMD, for example, reported that "rising prescribing opioid medication in the UK are almost wholly attributable to the increase in prescribing for chronic pain" (Advisory Council on the Misuse of Drugs, 2016, p. 27). Overall, the consensus is that the number of prescriptions for abusable medications is increasing in both the United States and the United Kingdom.

Section Summary

Overall, two important findings emerge from the current research. First, from the evidence of both quantitative analysis and the opinions expressed in reviews, it appears that trends in PDM are fairly similar across the United States and the United Kingdom. Second, the research shows that trends in PDM in both the United States and the United Kingdom are declining in the general population and increasing among prisoners, those in drug treatment, and those at risk of drug overdose. These are important findings because these data sources represent *use* better than other measures and more clearly define the *population* involved. Information on number of prescriptions in the community and seizures of drugs are more closely aligned to drug supply rather than use. In the remaining sections, we will attempt to explain these patterns and consider responses to them.

Discussion

The main aim of the chapter is to determine whether PDM has been increasing at a higher rate in the United States than in the United Kingdom and, if so, why. The results of the analysis suggest that there are no major differences in the *rate of change* of PDM in the two countries. However, there is evidence of a difference in the *volume* of use (in terms of prevalence and total numbers). For volume, the amount of use and misuse of prescription medications in the United States is substantially greater than in the United Kingdom.

Explanations

As PDM in the general population has been decreasing in both countries, the main features that need explanation are the current high *volume* of use in the general population of the United States, as compared with the United Kingdom, and the differences in the *rate of use* between the general population and the drug-using and offending populations.

The Volume of PDM in the General Population

One of the most frequently identified causes of PDM mentioned in the reviews is the increasing availability of prescription medications. It is believed that there is a relationship between the levels of prescription drugs in the community and levels of PDM. As one review stated, "First, and perhaps most critically, is the role of total PO [prescription opioid] use volumes dispensed in the population. Growing evidence suggests that both levels of [PDM] as well as PO-related morbidity and mortality correlate strongly with a total of PO volume dispensed in the population" (Fischer, Keates, Bühringer, Reimer, & Rehm, 2014, p. 178).

Why is the volume of dispensed prescription medications higher in the United States than in the United Kingdom? One explanation is recent aggressive marketing to medical professionals and patients (mainly in the United States) by pharmaceutical producers (Fischer et al., 2014). Another is the establishment of private pain clinics, or "pill mills," offering prescriptions for cash (Rigg, March, & Inciardi, 2010). In contrast, it has been suggested that regulations in Europe, including the United Kingdom, have more extensive restrictions and controls, such as authorized prescriber limitations, time limits for repeat prescriptions, and cost limits on the number of prescriptions. This stands in contrast with the lighter regulations in the United States that predominantly rely on prescription drug monitoring programs (see chapter 12 of this volume for more on PDMPs) to detect individual instances of excessive prescribing (Fischer et al., 2014).

It is also speculated that there might be protective factors within the health care system in the United Kingdom that are not shared in the United States that reduce the probability of excessive prescribing (Weisberg et al., 2014). First, there might be features of the U.K. health care system that operate to prevent dependence on prescription medications from developing. Second, there might be provisions within the U.K. system to treat dependence more effectively when it does occur. Weisberg and colleagues (2014), for example, noted that opioid treatment in the two countries is different as a result of their respective cultures and histories and that these differences might guard against heavier levels of prescribing in the United Kingdom.

The Increase in Rate of PDM within Drug-using and Offender Populations

It has been argued that most of the increase in the rate of PDM falls within drug-using and offender populations. Specifically, this refers to increases in use in the prison population, among those using drugs who are vulnerable to fatal overdose, and individuals engaged in problematic drug use in search of treatment. Why has PDM increased within these populations in both the United States and the United Kingdom?

There is some information available in the U.K. report by the Centre for Social Justice about causes of PDM expansion among prisoners (Centre for Social Justice, 2015). The report's authors suggest that, over the last five years, drug use in prison has switched from traditional drugs, such as heroin, to a combination of new psychoactive substances (NPS) and prescription medications. NPS are commonly described as chemical analogs to traditional drugs that have similar effects (e.g., synthetic cannabinoids) but do not contain opioids. NPS are regarded as having benefits over heroin, as they cannot be detected as part of routine drug testing (Centre for Social Justice, 2015). They are also much cheaper to buy or trade than heroin. Prescription medications also have benefits in that they are readily available in prison and easily diverted, either through bullying those in receipt of medications or through trading. In turn, people using NPS benefit from the fact that their supply is virtually constant compared with the more unreliable supply of heroin, which in the United Kingdom has experienced periods of drought in recent years.

There is no hard evidence to explain the increases in prescription drug-related deaths or the increase in the number of those engaged in more severe drug use presenting to treatment agencies reporting misuse of prescription drugs. What little commentary is available links these trends to an increase in the use of and addiction to these drugs within the drug-using population. However, one reviewer suggested a connection relating to the misuse of opioid analgesics. In the United States, there is a tendency for doctors to prescribe oxycodone, and in the United Kingdom, the opioid analgesic of choice is tramadol. These drugs have been described by one reviewer as "highly potent formulations" (Fischer et al., 2014, p. 178). In the United States, oxycodone-related deaths slightly exceed the number of methadone-related deaths, and in the United Kingdom, tramadol-related deaths have more than doubled in recent years (Giraudon et al., 2013).

Prevention

There is some discussion in the literature on what might be done to reduce PDM. The list of proposals can be divided into four main groups: guidelines, surveillance, education, and health care.

Guidelines

In the United States, the primary response to regulating the distribution of abusable medications has been through state legislation. This has included a ceiling on allowable doses of opioids prescribed in general practice and restrictions on purchasing prescriptions over the Internet (Weisberg et al., 2014). In the United Kingdom, there has been a recent recommendation that NHS England issue guidance to local commissioning groups that enables them to collate data on patients visiting multiple practices to obtain specific drugs (Home Affairs Committee, 2013), similar to a PDMP in the United States. There have also been suggestions for new guidelines related to daily dispensing of prescription medications, for more frequent prescriptions for smaller amounts, and for patients to contact the police when tablets are stolen (Advisory Council on the Misuse of Drugs, 2016).

Surveillance

Another proposal mentioned in the reviews is enhancing surveillance and monitoring of the prescription and distribution of abusable medications. In the United Kingdom, the ACMD recommended that medical practices establish data collection systems to identify patients who are, or are suspected of being, dependent on prescription drugs. It has also been suggested that the health care sector monitor repeat prescriptions, particularly with regard to methadone, benzodiazepines, and similar drugs, to identify evidence of diversion (National Institute for Health and Care Excellence, 2016).

Education

The request for education related to PDM is directed at several populations. It has been suggested, for example, that the United Kingdom should implement a universal prescriber education program operated independently of the pharmaceutical industry (Weisberg et al., 2014). In addition, comprehensive educational programs should be provided for practicing physicians to inform them on safe opioid prescribing and the dangers of prescribing methadone for pain relief (Weisberg et al., 2014). Education programs might also be provided for young people and the general public to inform them about the harms of prescription opioid misuse (White & Pitts, 1998).

Health Care

The proposals for prevention through the health care system concern better integration services, sharing of information, and developing strategic approaches to PDM. In the United Kingdom, it has also been recommended that naloxone distribution programs be expanded, opiate use treatment capacity be enhanced, and additional harm-reduction approaches be implemented (Rudd, Aleshire, Zibbell, & Gladden, 2016). There have also been requests that drug treatment should be better linked to mental and physical health care services (Strang et al., 2014).

Conclusions

Overall, the mediators and moderators of PDM in the United States and the United Kingdom are likely to be different, and efforts to reduce PDM might require different approaches. The problem of aggressive sales policies by pharmaceutical companies and overprescribing by doctors in the United States are of special concern. In the state of West Virginia, for example, drug wholesalers distributed 423 million pain-related pills between 2007 and 2012 to the local population. Over the same period, the state experienced 1,728 fatal overdoses linked to hydrocodone and oxycodone medications (Asbury & Dickerson, 2017). In January 2017, the City of Huntington, West Virginia, filed a lawsuit in the circuit court against the distributors of opioid drugs, claiming that pharmaceutical producers had caused an opioid epidemic as a result of "the defendants' illegal, reckless, and malicious actions in flooding the state with highly addictive prescription medications" (City of Huntington, 2017). Previous lawsuits of this kind have typically been resolved in favor of the complainant. Recent settlements have been in the region of $50 million on the grounds of the substantial public funds involved in dealing with the consequences of the defendants' actions (Asbury & Dickerson, 2017).

The main problem related to PDM in the United Kingdom has been the increase in drug use and dependence within the prison population. The main intervention proposed so far is to increase security in the method of distributing and administering opiates within the prison system. For example, it has been suggested that the recent introduction of a new formulation of buprenorphine (Espranor) may help reduce the diversion of prescription drugs as a result of its unique properties. Espranor is a partial agonist and has similar effects as Subutex. However, it also has the potential to reduce diversion, as it disintegrates quickly when placed on the tongue and cannot easily be removed and transferred to other prisoners (Smith, 2017).

Prevention efforts in both the United States and the United Kingdom might also take account of the lessons learned from preventive interventions used in the treatment of traditional drug misuse. There is now a substantial body of research, mainly in the form of systematic reviews, on the effectiveness of measures to reduce drug misuse. There is evidence, for example, that some interventions served to reduce both drug misuse and criminal behavior. Such outcomes would be especially important in tackling PDM in prisoner and criminal populations. A recent systematic review of systematic reviews found that certain interventions performed better than others in reducing drug use and criminal behavior (Holloway & Bennett, 2016). The most consistently successful were naltrexone treatment and therapeutic communities.

Conversely, substitute prescribing programs, such as those based on buprenorphine treatment, were the least effective. This finding is especially worrisome when considering the popularity of buprenorphine treatment in prisons. Not only is buprenorphine a primary source of addiction, but it is also one of the least effective methods of treating it. While substitute prescribing might be viewed as a suitable method of control in prisons, it has to be taken into account that it can also become a double-edged sword in preventing and treating addiction.

References

Advisory Council on the Misuse of Drugs. (2016). *Diversion and Illicit Supply of Medicines.* London, England: Advisory Council on the Misuse of Drugs, Home Office.

Asbury, K., & Dickerson, C. (2017). City of Huntington sues drug wholesalers over opioid epidemic. https://wvrecord.com/stories/511075675-city-of -huntington-sues-drug-wholesalers-over-opioid-epidemic.

Bureau of Justice Statistics. (2006). *Drug Use and Dependence, State and Federal Prisoners, 2004.* Washington, D.C.: U.S. Department of Justice, Bureau of Justice Statistics.

Center for Behavioral Health Statistics and Quality. (2015). Behavioral health trends in the United States: Results from the 2014 National Survey on Drug Use and Health (HHS Publication No. SMA 15-4927, NSDUH Series H-50). http://www.samhsa.gov/data.

Centre for Social Justice. (2015). *Drugs in Prison.* London, England: Centre for Social Justice.

City of Huntington. (2017). City of Huntington files lawsuit against opioid drug distributors. http://www.cityofhuntington.com/news/view/city -of-huntington-files-lawsuit-against-opioid-drug-distributors.

Compton, W. M., Boyle, M., & Wargo, E. (2015). Prescription opioid abuse: Problems and responses. *Preventive Medicine, 80*(Supplement C), 5–9. doi:https:// doi.org/10.1016/j.ypmed.2015.04.003.

European Monitoring Centre for Drugs and Drug Addiction. (2016). *European Drug Report 2016: Trends and Developments.* Luxembourg: Publications Office of the European Union.

Fischer, B., Keates, A., Bühringer, G., Reimer, J., & Rehm, J. (2014). Non-medical use of prescription opioids and prescription opioid-related harms: Why so markedly higher in North America compared to the rest of the world? *Addiction, 109*(2), 177–181. doi:10.1111/add.12224.

Frenk, S. M., Porter, K. S., & Paulozzi, L. J. (2015). *Prescription opioid analgesic use among adults: United States, 1999-2012.* NCHS data brief, No 189. Hyattsville, MD: National Center for Health Statistics.

Giraudon, I., Lowitz, K., Dargan, P. I., Wood, D. M., & Dart, R. C. (2013). Prescription opioid abuse in the UK. *British Journal of Clinical Pharmacology, 76*(5), 823–824. doi:10.1111/bcp.12133.

Han, B., Compton, W. M., Jones, C. M., & Cai, R. (2015). Nonmedical prescription opioid use and use disorders among adults aged 18 through 64 years in the United States, 2003–2013. *JAMA, 314*(14), 1468–1478. doi:10.1001/jama.2015.11859.

Hansard. (2012). Written answers and statements, 3 December 2012. http://www.publications.parliament.uk/pa/cm201213/cmhansrd/cm121203/text/121203w0003.htm.

Hedegaard, H., Chen, L. H., & Warner, M. (2015). *Drug Poisoning Deaths Involving Heroin: United States, 2000–2013* (NCHS data brief, No 190). Hyattsville, MD: National Center for Health Statistics.

Her Majesty's Inspectorate of Prisons. (2016). *Chief Inspector of Prisons for England and Wales Annual Report 2015–16*. London, England: Her Majesty's Inspectorate of Prisons.

Holloway, K., & Bennett, T. H. (2016). Drug interventions. In D. Weisburd, D. P. Farrington, & C. Gill (Eds.), *What Works in Crime Prevention and Rehabilitation: Lessons from Systematic Reviews*. New York: Springer.

Home Affairs Committee. (2013). *Drugs: New Psychoactive Substances and Prescription Drugs*. London, England: The Stationery Office.

Levy, B., Paulozzi, L., Mack, K. A., & Jones, C. M. (2015). Trends in opioid analgesic-prescribing rates by specialty, U.S., 2007–2012. *American Journal of Preventive Medicine, 49*(3), 409–413. doi:10.1016/j.amepre.2015.02.020.

National Institute for Health and Care Excellence. (2016). Guidance and advice list. https://www.nice.org.uk/guidance/published?fromdate=October+2016&todate=October+2016.

National Statistics. (2016). *Prescriptions Dispensed in the Community: England 2005–2015*. Leeds, England: Health and Social Care Information Centre.

Office for National Statistics. (2016a). *Crime in England and Wales: Year Ending March 2016*. Newport, South Wales: Office for National Statistics.

Office for National Statistics. (2016b). *Deaths Related to Drug Poisoning in England and Wales: 2015 Registrations*. Newport, South Wales: Office for National Statistics.

Office for National Statistics. (2016c). *Seizures of Drugs in England and Wales, Year Ending 31 March 2016*. Newport, South Wales: Office for National Statistics.

Pezalla, E. J., Rosen, D., Erensen, J. G., Haddox, J. D., & Mayne, T. J. (2017). Secular trends in opioid prescribing in the USA. *Journal of Pain Research, 10*, 383–387. doi:10.2147/JPR.S129553.

Public Health England. (2016). *Adult Substance Misuse Statistics from the National Drug Treatment Monitoring System (NDTSMS): 1st April 2015 to 31st March 2016*. Manchester, England: Public Health England.

Rigg, K. K., March, S. J., & Inciardi, J. A. (2010). Prescription drug abuse & diversion: Role of the pain clinic. *Journal of Drug Issues, 40*(3), 681–702.

Rudd, R. A., Aleshire, N., Zibbell, J. E., & Gladden, R. M. (2016). Increases in drug and opioid overdose deaths—United States, 2000–2014. *MMWR: Morbidity and Mortality Weekly Report, 64*(50-51), 1378–1382. doi:10.15585/mmwr.mm6450a3.

Smith, K. (2017). Espranor (buprenorphine oral lyophilisate) 2mg and 8mg: Considerations for opioid substitution therapy use in community settings and secure environments. https://www.sps.nhs.uk/articles/espranor-buprenorphine-oral-lyophilisate-2mg-and-8mg.

Strang, J., Drummond, C., McNeill, A., Lader, M., & Marsden, J. (2014). Addictions, dependence and substance abuse. In S. C. Davies (Ed.), *Annual Report of the Chief Medical Officer 2013, Public Mental Health Priorities: Investing in the Evidence*, 251–257. London, England: Department of Health.

Substance Abuse and Mental Health Services Administration. (2017). National Survey of Substance Abuse Treatment Services (N-SSATS). https://wwwdasis.samhsa.gov/dasis2/nssats.htm.

U.K. Parliament. (2000). *Misuse of Drugs Act, 1971*. London, England: The Stationery Office.

Volkow, N. D. (2014). *America's Addiction to Opioids: Heroin and Prescription Drug Abuse*. Testimony before the Senate Caucus on International Narcotics Control, Washington, D.C.: Department of Health and Human Services, National Institutes of Health.

Warner, M., Trinidad, J. P., Bastian, B. A., Minino, A. M., & Hedegaard, H. (2016). Drugs most frequently involved in drug overdose deaths: United States, 2010–2014. *National Vital Statistics Reports, 65*(10), 1–15.

Weisberg, D. F., Becker, W. C., Fiellin, D. A., & Stannard, C. (2014). Prescription opioid misuse in the United States and the United Kingdom: Cautionary lessons. *International Journal of Drug Policy, 25*(6), 1124–1130. doi:https://doi.org/10.1016/j.drugpo.2014.07.009.

White, D., & Pitts, M. (1998). Educating young people about drugs: A systematic review. *Addiction, 93*(10), 1475–1487. doi:10.1046/j.1360-0443.1998.931014754.x.

CHAPTER FIFTEEN

Using Health Behavior Theory to Understand Prescription Drug Misuse

Niloofar Bavarian, Sheena Cruz, and Ty S. Schepis

Health, Health Behavior, and Health Behavior Theory

Health is a concept whose meaning has evolved over time. In its constitution, ratified in 1948, the World Health Organization (WHO) defined *health* as "a state of complete physical, mental, and social well-being and not merely the absence of disease or infirmity" (World Health Organization, 2017). Current definitions of *health* encompass dimensions missing from the WHO definition, such as intellectual, spiritual, and occupational health (McKenzie, Pinger, & Seabert, 2016). *Health behavior* refers to actions than can influence health. Specifically, *health behavior* has been defined as "action taken by a person to maintain, attain, or regain good health and to prevent illness" (Farlex Partner Medical Dictionary, 2012); this definition, however, fails to consider the reality that health behaviors can also be health compromising.

Indeed, prescription drug misuse, the focus of this book, refers to a health behavior that has the potential to compromise health. This behavior, like all health behaviors, is multietiological in nature. The multietiologic nature of prescription drug misuse hinders the ability of a unidimensional effort to prevent the behavior or result in cessation; multifaceted approaches are necessary to attain the greatest, and most sustainable, impact (e.g., Glanz,

Rimer, & Viswanath, 2008). Health behavior theory provides one such lens needed to begin such multifaceted efforts.

According to Glanz and colleagues (2008), health behavior theory is a tool that can be used to explain and predict health behavior by providing a systematic view of the processes that interact to influence decision making. Health behavior theory has been credited with simplifying the complex nature of health behavior. Moreover, interventions guided by a health behavior theory, and that intentionally aim to address constructs within a health behavior theory, have been shown to be more successful at producing behavior change than interventions that are atheoretical in nature (Glanz, et al., 2008). As such, a theoretical understanding of prescription drug misuse is an important first step in developing theory-guided prevention and intervention initiatives.

A multitude of health behavior theories exist, each with their own way of presenting the decision-making process. Intrapersonal (i.e., within-person) theories, such as the theory of planned behavior (Ajzen, 1985), are the narrowest in scope of the health behavior theories. Interpersonal (i.e., between-person) theories, such as social cognitive theory (Bandura, 1986), build upon individual-level theories by incorporating the social dynamic. Ecological theories, such as the theory of triadic influence (Flay & Petraitis, 1994; Flay, Snyder, & Petraitis, 2009), are the broadest in nature, incorporating not only intrapersonal and interpersonal elements, but also broader components of one's environment. This chapter will use these three theories (i.e., theory of planned behavior, social cognitive theory, and theory of triadic influence) to explain the etiology of prescription stimulant, prescription opioid, and prescription benzodiazepine misuse. We will conclude by discussing implications for prevention and intervention.

Intrapersonal Health Behavior Theory—The Theory of Planned Behavior

The theory of planned behavior (TPB; Ajzen, 1985) is an intrapersonal health behavior theory that posits the most important determinant of behavior is behavioral intention. The theory explains that one's intention (i.e., likelihood) of performing a behavior is influenced by one's attitudes toward the behavior, subjective norms, and perceived behavioral control. Moreover, each of these three constructs is shaped by certain beliefs (i.e., behavioral beliefs and evaluation, normative beliefs and motivation to comply, and control beliefs and perceived power). Below, we explain how the theory of planned behavior can be used to explain various forms of prescription drug misuse.

The Theory of Planned Behavior—Applied to Prescription Stimulant Misuse

Attitudes toward a behavior (i.e., whether the behavior is viewed as good or bad) are shaped by the combination of one's behavioral belief and evaluation. A *behavioral belief* refers to outcomes that one believes are or are not likely to occur after performing the actual behavior; an evaluation (positive or negative; good or bad) is placed on each outcome. With respect to prescription stimulants, a college student may believe that using prescription stimulants is likely to improve academic performance (behavioral belief); the belief that improved academic performance will result from using prescription stimulants has been demonstrated in multiple studies (e.g., Bavarian, Flay, Ketcham, & Smit, 2013; Carroll, McLaughlin, & Blake, 2006). Moreover, that same student may view improved academics as a *positive/good* outcome (evaluation). In one campus study, 96.51 percent of students agreed or strongly agreed that they viewed performing well in their courses as important (Bavarian et al., 2013). This combination of constructs (i.e., believing the behavior will improve academic performance and placing a positive value on improved academic performance) would work together to create a positive attitude toward prescription stimulants. A positive attitude toward prescription stimulants has been shown to increase intention to engage in prescription stimulant misuse (Bavarian et al., 2014), and research shows students who have greater intention to misuse are more likely to engage in actual misuse (behavior; Bavarian et al., 2014).

One's *subjective norm*, that is, a belief about others' approval or disapproval toward a behavior, is shaped by *normative beliefs* and *motivation to comply*. Normative beliefs and motivation to comply incorporate key socializing agents (e.g., friends, family, romantic partners) into the decision-making process. Specifically, normative beliefs, which are behavior specific, refer to one's beliefs about whether a socializing agent approves of a behavior. For example, a college student may agree that her friends think they should misuse prescription stimulants. In one college-based study, 44.67 percent of students surveyed reported at least a few of their friends had endorsed stimulant misuse (Bavarian et al., 2017).

Motivation to comply, which is not behavior specific, examines the agreeableness of an individual with a key socializing agent. For example, a college student may agree that she wants to do what her friends think she should do. In the same college-based study, 51.01 percent of students surveyed agreed or strongly agreed with this assertion. This combination of a positive normative belief and a positive motivation to comply would interact to create a positive subjective norm toward prescription stimulant misuse. Moreover, subjective norms have been shown to have a direct relationship with intention to engage in prescription stimulant misuse (Bavarian et al., 2014), and, as previously stated, intention is a strong correlate of actual misuse behavior (Bavarian et al., 2014).

Behavioral intention is also shaped by *perceived behavioral control*. Perceived behavioral control, which refers to whether a student believes a behavior to be easy or difficult to perform, is influenced by a combination of *control beliefs* (i.e., the perceived likelihood of a protective or risk factor occurring) and *perceived power* (i.e., the perceived effect the factor has on the ability to perform the behavior). On a college campus, it is likely that a student will be offered prescription stimulants (control beliefs). The buying or sharing of a prescription drug is known as *diversion* and has been shown to be prevalent on college campuses (e.g., Bavarian et al., 2017). The offering of the prescription stimulant may make engaging in misuse easy (perceived power). Thus, in this situation, a student's perceived behavioral control toward prescription stimulant misuse would be that it is easy; past research has shown that, for female students, being offered prescription stimulants was associated with misuse (Hall, Irwin, Bowman, Frankenberger, & Jewett, 2005). Having a perceived behavioral control that views misuse as an easy behavior to perform may increase intention to engage in misuse, which should increase the likelihood of actually performing the behavior of misuse.

The Theory of Planned Behavior—Applied to Prescription Opioid Misuse

The theory of planned behavior can also be used to understand the misuse of prescription opioids. For example, a college student may believe that using prescription opioids is likely to relieve pain (behavioral belief; McCabe, West, & Boyd, 2013a), and that same student may view pain relief as a good outcome (evaluation; Brandt, Taverna, & Hallock, 2014). This combination of constructs would work together to create a positive attitude toward prescription opioids. A positive attitude toward prescription opioids would lead someone to be more likely to engage in misuse (intention), and those students who have greater intention to misuse will be more likely to engage in actual misuse (behavior). However, there is another common set of beliefs that can lead to positive attitudes toward prescription opioids. Although prescription opioids are most commonly prescribed to treat mild to severe pain (National Institute on Drug Abuse, 2014), college students also report misusing opioids to experience recreational effects of the drug such as euphoria or the feeling of getting high (Kenne et al., 2017; McCabe, Cranford, Boyd, & Teter, 2007; McCabe, West, & Boyd, 2013b). Thus, a college student may believe that using prescription opioids is likely to cause euphoria (behavioral beliefs), that same student may view euphoria as a good outcome (evaluation), and thus a positive attitude is placed toward prescription opioids.

With respect to prescription opioids, a college student may agree that her friends think she should use prescription opioids. In addition, a college student may agree that she wants to do what her friends think she should do (motivation to comply). This combination of a positive normative belief and a positive motivation to comply would interact to create a positive subjective norm toward prescription opioid misuse. Prior research has shown college students may overestimate the number of students who misuse prescription opioids (McCabe, 2008). Moreover, studies have demonstrated that exposure and access to peers misusing prescription opioids increases the likelihood young adults will initiate and engage in opioid use (Eitan, Emery, Bates, & Horrax, 2017; Sanders, Stogner, Seibert, & Miller, 2014). Thus, the creation of a positive subjective norm should increase intention to engage in prescription opioid misuse, and students who have greater intention to misuse will be more likely to engage in actual misuse.

On a college campus, it is likely that a student attends a campus where students will divert their opioid medication (control beliefs); this assertion is supported by prior research. Specifically, one study conducted on a college-aged sample found that 85 percent of participants who engaged in prescription opioid misuse received the medication from friends, and 18 percent reported their parents as the source (Lord, Brevard, & Budman, 2011). The presence of diverters would make using prescription opioids easy (perceived power). Past research has shown high rates of peer-to-peer diversion among young male adults, which ultimately increases the availability of prescription opioids and the risk of nonmedical use (McCabe et al., 2017; Shei et al., 2015). Thus, in this situation, a student's perceived behavioral control toward prescription opioid misuse would be that it is easy; such a belief would increase intention to engage in misuse, which would result in a greater likelihood of behavioral performance.

The Theory of Planned Behavior—Applied to Prescription Benzodiazepine Misuse

Finally, the TPB has utility as applied to the phenomenon of prescription benzodiazepine misuse. Benzodiazepine misuse has multiple, and often unrelated, motives. For instance, Parks et al. (2017) found that college students often engaged in benzodiazepine misuse because they believed that it would be likely to enhance euphoria (behavioral belief); many participants in the study endorsed euphoric enhancement as a good outcome (evaluation). Conversely, other work in college students and adolescents indicated that benzodiazepine misuse was often fueled by the belief that these medications are likely to relieve anxiety or promote sleep, which was seen as a good outcome (evaluation) in those suffering from clinically significant anxiety or insomnia (Boyd, McCabe, Cranford, & Young, 2006; McCabe, Boyd, & Teter, 2009). In both scenarios, the end result is a positive attitude toward benzodiazepines.

Less research has examined subjective norms in prescription benzodiazepine misuse, though Ford and Hill (2012) found that more positive attitudes by peers toward many types of substance use correlated with higher odds of prescription misuse, including benzodiazepine misuse. Similar outcomes were found in college students (Ford & Arrastia, 2008). Thus, depending on one's social circle, an adolescent or young adult may agree that peers believe that she should misuse a prescription benzodiazepine (positive normative belief). This belief may co-occur with a belief that the individual agrees she should do what her peers want (i.e., a positive motivation to comply). Combined, the normative belief that benzodiazepine use and misuse is encouraged and a high motivation to comply lead to a positive subjective norm toward misuse and increased likelihood of such misuse. Nonetheless, given that previous investigations have not looked at specific benzodiazepine norms, this is somewhat speculative.

As noted with opioids, college students often perceive a high degree of availability of benzodiazepines for misuse. Parks and colleagues (2017) found that many college student focus group participants believed that obtaining a benzodiazepine for misuse from a college health center was relatively easy, as clinically significant symptoms of anxiety could be feigned. Furthermore, they noted that availability from friends and family, whether given overtly or stolen covertly from medicine cabinets, was high (Parks et al., 2017). Often, the most common source for benzodiazepines for misuse is from friends or family members in both adolescents (Schepis & Krishnan-Sarin, 2009) and young adults (McCabe & Boyd, 2005). A relatively high level of availability of prescription benzodiazepines for both adolescents and young adults makes misuse of these medications easy, increasing perceived behavioral control for misuse. Increased perceived behavioral control would then increase intention to engage in benzodiazepine misuse, leading to increased likelihood of actual misuse.

Interpersonal Health Behavior Theory—Social Cognitive Theory

Albert Bandura's social cognitive theory (SCT; Bandura, 1986) explains how behavior is acquired and maintained via a reciprocal interaction between constructs at the intrapersonal level (i.e., behavioral capabilities, self-efficacy, expectations and expectancies, and reinforcement); constructs at the interpersonal level (i.e., environment, observational learning); and the behavior itself. Below, we explain how social cognitive theory can be used to explain various forms of prescription drug misuse.

Social Cognitive Theory—Applied to Prescription Stimulant Misuse

Five SCT constructs that occur at the intrapersonal level are behavioral capabilities, self-efficacy, expectations, expectancies, and reinforcement. Behavioral capabilities and self-efficacy are similar constructs in that both refer to skills. *Behavioral capability* relates to the knowledge and skill needed to perform a specific behavior. With respect to prescription stimulants and behavioral capability, college students may lack an understanding of necessary study habits and how to perform such behaviors; in one campus study, 12.91

percent of students reported reading assigned course readings "none of the time" or "a little of the time" (Bavarian et al., 2017). Moreover, poorer study habits have been shown to be associated with an increased probability of prescription stimulant misuse (Bavarian et al., 2013). *Self-efficacy* refers to one's confidence in his or her ability to perform a skill. One important form of self-efficacy, as it relates to prescription stimulant misuse, is avoidance self-efficacy. We define *avoidance self-efficacy* as confidence in one's ability to decline offers to engage in prescription stimulant misuse. Past research has shown avoidance self-efficacy to be an important correlate of prescription stimulant misuse (Bavarian et al., 2017).

Similar to behavioral beliefs and evaluation from TPB, SCT's *expectations* and *expectancies* relate to outcomes one expects to occur from engaging in a behavior (expectations) and the values that the individual places on the outcome (expectancies). As mentioned above, a student may anticipate better academic performance will occur if he or she engages in prescription stimulant misuse, and he or she may also place a positive value on improved academic performance; this thought process, as stated above, has been found to be associated with prescription stimulant misuse.

Reinforcements refer to responses an individual receives after engaging in a behavior that influences reoccurrence. Studies have found that satisfaction with the academic impact of prescription stimulant misuse engagement is associated with the behavior (Rabiner et al., 2009). In a separate study examining 257 students with a lifetime history of prescription stimulant misuse, 48.2 percent of students who engaged in misuse said performing the behavior provided their desired outcome "most" or "all of the time." Moreover, there was a direct relationship between the frequency of receiving one's desired outcome and misuse frequency (Mendez, Yomogida, Figueroa, & Bavarian, in preparation).

Two SCT constructs that occur at the interpersonal level are environment and observational learning. The *environment* construct refers to factors external to the individual (e.g., social, physical environment) that influence the decision-making process. Past research has shown that friends' misuse of prescription stimulants is a correlate of one's own misuse (social environment; Judson & Langdon, 2009). In addition, the college setting (physical environment) has also been shown to be a setting where students often initiate the behavior. For example, in one study, roughly 75 percent of those reporting misuse initiated the behavior after starting college (Bavarian et al., 2013). *Observational learning* is a construct that incorporates reinforcement but instead focuses on observing the behaviors of others and the reinforcements they receive after performing a behavior. For example, observing a friend misusing prescription stimulants, and seeing the fried stay awake to finish writing a paper, may serve as a positive reinforcement of the behavior. According to the concept of *reciprocal determinism*, all of the factors discussed at the personal and environmental levels would interact to increase the likelihood of prescription stimulant misuse.

Social Cognitive Theory—Applied to Prescription Opioid Misuse

With respect to prescription opioids, college students may lack an understanding of proper pain management and how to perform such a behavior (*behavioral capability*), as many young adults never receive comprehensive pain education or coping-skills training for self-care (Stinson et al., 2014). For example, in a study of adult women patients, participants reported misusing prescription opioids because of failed attempts to use alternative pain treatments and the persistence of their untreated pain (McHugh et al., 2013). As a result, a student's *avoidance self-efficacy*, that is, a confidence in his or her ability to not engage in prescription opioid misuse, may be low. Similarly, a student may anticipate pain relief will occur if he or she engages in prescription opioid misuse and may also place a positive value on improved pain relief (*expectations* and *expectancies*). For instance, in a study exploring long-term prescription drug use among 303 college students, 24 percent of participants viewed pain relievers and their ability to mitigate pain symptoms as "rewarding" when asked about perceptions of specific drugs (Brandt et al., 2014).

With respect to *reinforcement*, past research has shown students who experience their desired outcome engage in more frequent opioid misuse as repeated receipt of opioids strengthens the learned associations between drug use and the effects of the drug (whether analgesic or recreational; Volkow & McLellan, 2016). For example, a web-based survey with a sample of 689 college-age students found that those engaged in regular misuse were more likely than those infrequently misusing to endorse improved pain management, depression or anxiety relief, concentration, and energy with prescription opioid use (Lord et al., 2011).

With respect to the interpersonal aspects of the SCT, past research has shown that friends' misuse of prescription opioids is a correlate of one's own misuse (*social environment*). Studies have illustrated that the mere perception of opioid misuse by peers can influence the initiation of drug abuse and that exposure to these deviant behaviors by peers decreases the psychological barrier to engage in illicit substance use (Eitan et al., 2017; Sanders et al., 2014). In addition, the college setting (*physical environment*) is a setting where students often initiate the behavior (Arria et al., 2008; Grossbard et al., 2010). With respect to *observational learning*, observing a friend misusing prescription opioids and seeing the friend experience decreased pain (or increased euphoria), would serve as a positive reinforcement of opioid misuse. According to the concept of *reciprocal determinism*, all of the factors discussed at the personal and environmental levels interact to increase the likelihood of prescription opioid misuse.

Social Cognitive Theory—Applied to Prescription Benzodiazepine Misuse

Qualitative work (Liebrenz et al., 2015; Sirdifield, Chipchase, Owen, & Siriwardena, 2017) in adults who use and misuse benzodiazepines strongly suggests that many individuals taking the medication initiated use following failed attempts to use other therapies, including psychotherapy and herbal supplements. Thus, a subset of those misusing benzodiazepines may initiate use because of a lack of *behavioral capability* to deal with insomnia or anxiety symptoms in other ways. Failed attempts to cope with underlying medical issues may lead to low *avoidance self-efficacy* for benzodiazepine use or misuse; Liebrenz and colleagues (2015) noted the common phenomenon of failure to reduce or cease benzodiazepine use among those regularly using the medication. Work both in college students engaged in benzodiazepine misuse for recreational or euphoric purposes (*expectations* and *expectancies*; Parks, et al., 2017) and in a general adult sample engaged for self-treatment purposes (Liebrenz et al., 2015) found that the medications were highly valued because they consistently produced the desired effects that the person engaged in misuse was seeking; in other words, those who misuse did so to deliver significant *reinforcement*.

No current research has examined the correlation between benzodiazepine misuse by peers and the respondent's likelihood of such misuse; with that said, given the evidence that most adolescents and young adults obtain their medication for misuse from peers (McCabe & Boyd, 2005; Schepis & Krishnan-Sarin, 2009) and that peer attitudes toward substance use covary with benzodiazepine misuse (Ford & Hill, 2012; Rigg & Ford, 2014), it is likely that the *social environment* influences benzodiazepine misuse. Furthermore, the highest rates of initiation and current misuse are found in adolescents and young adults, suggesting that the *physical environment* to which they are exposed influences benzodiazepine misuse as well. *Observational learning* is likely to play a role in benzodiazepine misuse as well, with, for instance, individuals suffering from insomnia noticing peers or family members using a benzodiazepine and receiving enhanced sleep. This positive reinforcement would promote the behavior in the individual. Together, the factors in SCT noted above for benzodiazepine misuse would interact (per *reciprocal determinism*) to promote and entrench misuse.

Ecological Health Behavior Theory—The Theory of Triadic Influence

The theory of triadic influence (TTI; Flay & Petraitis, 1994) is a meta-theory that uses an ecological approach to explain and predict behavior. According to the theory, independent variables are classified by stream of influence as intrapersonal, social, or environmental. Independent variables are further classified by level of causation, with categories including ultimate, distal, proximal, and immediate predictor. The theory posits that variables within and between streams can interact to influence intentions to engage in a behavior, and experiences gained from initial behavior influence the continuation of behavior. The theory can be applied to explain each form of prescription drug misuse. For brevity, we focus on one example per stream per prescription drug misuse behavior.

The Theory of Triadic Influence—Applied to Prescription Stimulant Misuse

Two existing studies (Bavarian et al., 2014; Bavarian et al., 2018) detail the application of the TTI to understanding frequency of prescription stimulant misuse. Multiple causal pathways within and across streams of influence were illustrated and replicated across studies (as noted above, we focus on within stream pathways for brevity). For example, within the intrapersonal stream, students who reported more inattention and hyperactivity (ultimate level) were shown to have poorer study habits (distal level), and students with poorer study habits were shown to have less avoidance self-efficacy (proximal level). Moreover, avoidance self-efficacy had an inverse association with intention to engage in prescription stimulant misuse (immediate precursor).

With respect to the social stream, in the distal level of influence, a friend's endorsement of misuse was found to be significantly and directly associated with perceived prevalence of misuse among friends (proximal level). Moreover, the relationship between perceived prevalence of misuse among friends was significantly and directly associated with intention to engage in misuse (immediate precursor).

In the environment stream, the perception that the campus environment was permissive of drug use (ultimate level) was directly associated with positive expectancies (distal level). Holding more positive expectancies (e.g., that misuse would result in improved academic performance) was associated with holding more positive attitudes toward misuse (proximal level). Moreover, more positive attitudes were associated with greater intention to engage in misuse. As the immediate precursor, intention was directly and significantly associated with frequency of prescription stimulant misuse.

The Theory of Triadic Influence—Applied to Prescription Opioid Misuse

With respect to understanding prescription opioid misuse, the TTI has utility in elucidating risk factors and motives for misuse. Although no one study has tested a full ecological model as it relates to prescription opioids, we can hypothesize a theoretical flow based on prior research. In the intrapersonal stream, students' untreated pain (ultimate level) influences students' ability to manage pain in nonopioid ways (distal level). For example, inadequately addressed chronic pain symptoms result in opioid-seeking behaviors, which in turn increases the risk of prescription opioid misuse

(Garland, 2014). Thus, avoidance self-efficacy in relation to refraining from prescription opioid misuse (proximal level) is low, which may lead to greater intention (immediate precursor), which may influence actual behavior.

In the social stream, residing in a college dorm where prescription opioids are available (ultimate level) will lead to the greater likelihood of being exposed to a friend who may endorse illicit prescription opioid use (distal level). Research has demonstrated that peers' drug abuse behavior has a strong influence on a student's decision to misuse prescription opioids, especially given that the sources of these drugs are commonly students' friends and relatives (Collins, Abadi, Johnson, Shamblen, & Thompson, 2011; Eitan et al., 2017). Thus, the social normative beliefs of prevalent opioid misuse on campus along with the strong desire to comply with friends (proximal level) may increase misuse of prescription opioids (by increasing intention, which is the immediate precursor to behavior).

In the environmental stream, the culture of direct-to-consumer advertising portraying the analgesic efficacy of prescription opioids for stress-related and emotional pain at the ultimate level may be associated with positive expectancies (e.g., that misuse would lead to relief from negative mental or emotional states; Ashrafioun, 2016) at the distal level. Specifically, students may misuse opioids prescribed for pain because they expect to obtain relief from anxiety, depression, insomnia, or distressing memories (Edlund et al., 2015; Martins et al., 2012). Thus, college students may have a positive attitude toward prescription opioids (proximal level) and thus greater intention (immediate precursor) to ultimately engage in the behavior.

The Theory of Triadic Influence—Applied to Prescription Benzodiazepine Misuse

Similar to prescription opioids, no one study has tested a full ecological model as it relates to prescription benzodiazepines. Nonetheless, we can hypothesize a potentially causal chain of influences and events that would lead to prescription benzodiazepine misuse. For the intrapersonal stream, untreated or undertreated anxiety or sleep disorder symptoms (ultimate level), combined with poor coping skills for managing symptoms and seeking appropriate treatment (distal level), could lead to benzodiazepine seeking (Liebrenz et al., 2015). Attempts to obtain benzodiazepines could lead to benzodiazepine seeking for misuse. In such individuals, it is likely that the ability to avoid such misuse (i.e., avoidance self-efficacy; proximal level) is low, and the resultant elevated intention to misuse (immediate precursor) may lead to the actual behavior.

Interpersonally, proximity to those who have used or misused benzodiazepines with positive subjective outcomes (ultimate level) is likely to expose individuals to peers or family who endorse misuse (distal level). This is plausible given that the primary source of benzodiazepines for misuse is a friend or family members (McCabe & Boyd, 2005; Schepis & Krishnan-Sarin, 2009). Whether this student lives in a residence hall, an apartment complex with a high proportion of students, or at home with family members who use benzodiazepines, exposure to others who endorse misuse raises the likelihood of the eventual misuse by the student, resulting from greater endorsement leading to positive subjective norms (proximal level) and the subsequent influence of positive norms on intention (immediate precursor).

Finally, permissive environmental norms (ultimate level), particularly those that see prescription misuse as less harmful than other forms of illicit drug use, can lead to increased risk for benzodiazepine misuse. Norms that allow for misuse as self-treatment, whereby use without a prescription to treat anxiety or sleep disorder symptoms is seen as benign, would further increase risk. Together, these sorts of permissive environmental norms and the positive expectancies they create (distal level) may increase positive attitudes toward benzodiazepine medication and its misuse (proximal level). The positive attitudes could then result in greater intention to misuse (immediate precursor).

Intervention Implications

Prescription Stimulants

Whether examining prescription stimulant misuse through the lens of the TPB, SCT, or TTI, multiple avenues for prevention and intervention exist. In examining the themes and correlates common across theories, a reoccurring risk factor relates to experiencing symptoms of inattention and hyperactivity. Students may be self-medicating to treat these symptoms. Thus, determining the root causes of these symptoms, and alleviating them, may serve as one strategy for prevention. In addition, stimulant use or misuse and endorsement of such behavior by friends was a key determinant across models. Thus, a focus on diversion is necessary, as friends may not only be the main suppliers of these drugs but also key agents whose own misuse may influence initiation among individuals in their social circle. With respect to the environment, a variety of factors lead to positive attitudes toward prescription stimulants (e.g., false beliefs about the ability of these drugs to make one "smarter"). Therefore, correcting positive expectancies may be one potential prevention approach.

Prescription Opioids

Upon exploration of reoccurring themes related to prescription opioid misuse, the implications for prevention and clinical practice to combat the opioid epidemic are multiple. Given the issue of positive norms created via endorsement and diversion by friends and family with a legitimate prescription, implications exist for health care providers. For example, there is a need to advise patients on the importance of proper storage, monitoring, and disposal of prescription opioids (McCabe et al., 2017). Additional strategies include the use of prescription drug monitoring program (PDMP) data to identify doctor shopping and the use of doctor-patient agreements on adherence to ensure patients are aware of the risks of opioid diversion and misuse (see chapter 12 of this volume for more on PDMPs).

Finally, knowledge and skills training for alternative pain management strategies should be available to at-risk populations. For example, an integrative, nonopioid training that incorporates aspects of mindfulness, cognitive behavioral therapy, and positive psychology has shown to decrease pain severity and increase perceived control over pain in a sample of those using opioids (Garland, Froeliger, Zeidan, Partin, & Howard, 2013).

Prescription Benzodiazepines

Preventive and treatment interventions for benzodiazepine misuse will vary according to the demographic group focused on and the motives of that subset of individuals. For adolescents and college students, interventions aimed at changing perceived subjective norms by providing more appropriate estimates of misuse prevalence and through campus-wide campaigns to delegitimize misuse could be effective. Furthermore, on-campus programming and intervention to offer nonpharmacological options (e.g., group behavioral intervention) for anxiety or insomnia could help lower the likelihood of misuse in those self-medicating for these conditions. For young people and adults not attending school, preventive and intervention efforts will likely be most effective in health care settings. Prior to the initiation of benzodiazepine therapy, nonpharmacological interventions should be considered and attempted. For those who receive benzodiazepines, best practice guidelines (Baldwin et al., 2013; Lader, 2011) suggest a time-limited prescription (or nonuse in older adults; Beers Criteria Update Expert Panel, 2015), with other noncontrolled pharmacotherapy (e.g., antidepressant medication) and psychotherapeutic interventions used long-term. Limiting duration of benzodiazepine prescriptions, in addition to benefiting the specific patient, will limit leftover medication, which is a major source for misuse.

Summary and Next Steps

Prescription drug misuse-related behaviors, like all health behaviors, are complex and multietiological in nature. The great value of health behavior theory is in its ability to detangle the complex nature of decision making. Health behavior theory allows for a better understanding of the decision-making process; this enhanced understanding is critical for the development of prevention and intervention efforts. Moreover, using the broader lens afforded by ecological theories has the potential to create more sustainable behavior change. With this foundational understanding (Holder et al., 1999), critical next steps include the development, implementation, and evaluation of theory-guided intervention efforts.

References

Ajzen, I. (1985). From intentions to actions: A theory of planned behavior. In J. Kuhl & J. Beckmann (Eds.), *Action Control: From Cognition to Behavior,* 11–39. Berlin, Germany: Springer.

Arria, A. M., Caldeira, K. M., O'Grady, K. E., Vincent, K. B., Fitzelle, D. B., Johnson, E. P., & Wish, E. D. (2008). Drug exposure opportunities and use patterns among college students: Results of a longitudinal prospective cohort study. *Substance Abuse, 29*(4), 19–38.

Ashrafioun, L. (2016). Prescription opioid craving: Relationship with pain and substance use-related characteristics. *Substance Use & Misuse, 51*(11), 1512–1520. doi:10.1080/10826084.2016.1188948.

Baldwin, D. S., Aitchison, K., Bateson, A., Curran, H. V., Davies, S., Leonard, B., . . . Wilson, S. (2013). Benzodiazepines: Risks and benefits: A reconsideration. *Journal of Psychopharmacology, 27*(11), 967–971. doi:10.1177/0269881113503509.

Bandura, A. (1986). *Social Foundations of Thought and Action: A Social Cognitive Theory.* Englewood Cliffs, NJ: Prentice-Hall.

Bavarian, N., Flay, B. R., Ketcham, P. L., & Smit, E. (2013). Illicit use of prescription stimulants in a college student sample: A theory-guided analysis. *Drug and Alcohol Dependence, 132*(3), 665–673. doi:10.1016/j.drugalcdep.2013.04.024.

Bavarian, N., Flay, B. R., Ketcham, P. L., Smit, E., Kodama, C., Martin, M., & Saltz, R. F. (2014). Using structural equation modeling to understand prescription stimulant misuse: A test of the theory of triadic influence. *Drug and Alcohol Dependence, 138,* 193–201. doi:10.1016/j.drugalcdep.2014.02.700.

Bavarian, N., McMullen, J., Flay, B. R., Kodama, C., Martin, M., & Saltz, R. F. (2017). A mixed-methods approach examining illicit prescription stimulant use: Findings from a Northern California university. *Journal of Primary Prevention, 38*(4), 363–383. doi:10.1007/s10935-017-0465-8.

Bavarian, N., Sumstine, S., Cruz, S., Mendez, J., Schroeder, C., & Takeda, S. (2018). Confirming the prevalence, characteristics and utility of ecological theory in explaining prescription stimulant misuse. *Journal of Drug Issues, 48*(1), 118–133.

Beers Criteria Update Expert Panel. (2015). American Geriatrics Society 2015 updated Beers Criteria for potentially inappropriate medication use in older adults. *Journal of the American Geriatrics Society, 63*(11), 2227–2246. doi:10.1111/jgs.13702.

Boyd, C. J., McCabe, S. E., Cranford, J. A., & Young, A. (2006). Adolescents' motivations to abuse prescription medications. *Pediatrics, 118*(6), 2472–2480. doi:10.1542/peds.2006-1644.

Brandt, S. A., Taverna, E. C., & Hallock, R. M. (2014). A survey of nonmedical use of tranquilizers, stimulants, and pain relievers among college students: Patterns of use among users and factors related to abstinence in non-users. *Drug and Alcohol Dependence, 143*(Supplement C), 272–276. doi:https://doi.org/10.1016/j.drugalcdep.2014.07.034.

Carroll, B. C., McLaughlin, T. J., & Blake, D. R. (2006). Patterns and knowledge of nonmedical use of stimulants among college students. *Archives of Pediatrics & Adolescent Medicine, 160*(5), 481–485. doi:10.1001/archpedi.160.5.481.

Collins, D., Abadi, M. H., Johnson, K., Shamblen, S., & Thompson, K. (2011). Non-medical use of prescription drugs among youth in an Appalachian population: Prevalence, predictors, and implications for prevention. *Journal of Drug Education, 41*(3), 309–326. doi:10.2190/DE.41.3.e.

Edlund, M. J., Forman-Hoffman, V. L., Winder, C. R., Heller, D. C., Kroutil, L. A., Lipari, R. N., & Colpe, L. C. (2015). Opioid abuse and depression in adolescents: Results from the National Survey on Drug Use and Health. *Drug and Alcohol Dependence, 152*, 131–138. doi:10.1016/j.drugalcdep.2015.04.010.

Eitan, S., Emery, M. A., Bates, M. L. S., & Horrax, C. (2017). Opioid addiction: Who are your real friends? *Neuroscience & Biobehavioral Reviews*. doi: https://doi.org/10.1016/j.neubiorev.2017.05.017.

Farlex Partner Medical Dictionary. (2012). Health behavior. http://medical-dictionary.thefreedictionary.com/health+behavior.

Flay, B. R., & Petraitis, J. (1994). The theory of triadic influence: A new theory of health behavior with implications for preventive interventions. *Advances in Medical Sociology, 4*, 19–44.

Flay, B. R., Snyder, F., & Petraitis, J. (2009). The theory of triadic influence. In R. J. DiClemente, M. C. Kegler & R. A. Crosby (Eds.), *Emerging Theories in Health Promotion Practice and Research* (2nd ed.), 451–510). New York: Jossey-Bass.

Ford, J. A., & Arrastia, M. C. (2008). Pill-poppers and dopers: A comparison of non-medical prescription drug use and illicit/street drug use among college students. *Addictive Behaviors, 33*(7), 934–941. doi:10.1016/j.addbeh.2008.02.016.

Ford, J. A., & Hill, T. D. (2012). Religiosity and adolescent substance use: Evidence from the national survey on drug use and health. *Substance Use & Misuse, 47*(7), 787–798. doi:10.3109/10826084.2012.667489.

Garland, E. L. (2014). Treating chronic pain: The need for non-opioid options. *Expert Review of Clinical Pharmacology, 7*(5), 545–550. doi:10.1586/17512433.2014.928587.

Garland, E. L., Froeliger, B., Zeidan, F., Partin, K., & Howard, M. O. (2013). The downward spiral of chronic pain, prescription opioid misuse, and addiction: Cognitive, affective, and neuropsychopharmacologic pathways. *Neuroscience & Biobehavioral Reviews, 37*(10 0 2), 2597–2607. doi:10.1016/j.neubiorev.2013.08.006.

Glanz, K., Rimer, B. K., & Viswanath, K. (Eds.). (2008). *Health Behavior and Health Education: Theory, Research and Practice* (4th ed.). San Francisco, CA: Jossey-Bass.

Grossbard, J. R., Mastroleo, N. R., Kilmer, J. R., Lee, C. M., Turrisi, R., Larimer, M. E., & Ray, A. (2010). Substance use patterns among first-year college students: Secondary effects of a combined alcohol intervention. *Journal of Substance Abuse Treatment, 39*(4), 384–390. doi:10.1016/j.jsat.2010.07.001.

Hall, K. M., Irwin, M. M., Bowman, K. A., Frankenberger, W., & Jewett, D. C. (2005). Illicit use of prescribed stimulant medication among college students. *Journal of American College Health, 53*(4), 167–174. doi:10.3200/JACH.53.4.167-174.

Holder, H., Flay, B., Howard, J., Boyd, G., Voas, R., & Grossman, M. (1999). Phases of alcohol problem prevention research. *Alcoholism: Clinical and Experimental Research, 23*(1), 183–194. doi:10.1111/j.1530-0277.1999.tb04043.x.

Judson, R., & Langdon, S. W. (2009). Illicit use of prescription stimulants among college students: Prescription status, motives, theory of planned behaviour, knowledge and self-diagnostic tendencies. *Psychology, Health & Medicine, 14*(1), 97–104. doi:10.1080/13548500802126723.

Kenne, D. R., Hamilton, K., Birmingham, L., Oglesby, W. H., Fischbein, R. L., & Delahanty, D. L. (2017). Perceptions of harm and reasons for misuse of prescription opioid drugs and reasons for not seeking treatment for physical or emotional pain among a sample of college students. *Substance Use & Misuse, 52*(1), 92–99. doi:10.1080/10826084.2016.1222619.

Lader, M. (2011). Benzodiazepines revisited—Will we ever learn? *Addiction, 106*(12), 2086–2109. doi:10.1111/j.1360-0443.2011.03563.x.

Liebrenz, M., Schneider, M., Buadze, A., Gehring, M. T., Dube, A., & Caflisch, C. (2015). High-dose benzodiazepine dependence: A qualitative study of patients' perceptions on initiation, reasons for use, and obtainment. *PLoS One, 10*(11), e0142057. doi:10.1371/journal.pone.0142057.

Lord, S., Brevard, J., & Budman, S. (2011). Connecting to young adults: An online social network survey of beliefs and attitudes associated with prescription opioid misuse among college students. *Substance Use & Misuse, 46*(1), 66–76. doi:10.3109/10826084.2011.521371.

Martins, S. S., Fenton, M. C., Keyes, K. M., Blanco, C., Zhu, H., & Storr, C. L. (2012). Mood/anxiety disorders and their association with non-medical prescription opioid use and prescription opioid use disorder: Longitudinal evidence from the National Epidemiologic Study on Alcohol and Related Conditions. *Psychological Medicine, 42*(6), 1261–1272. doi:10.1017/S0033291711002145.

McCabe, S. E. (2008). Misperceptions of non-medical prescription drug use: A web survey of college students. *Addictive Behaviors, 33*(5), 713–724. doi:10.1016/j.addbeh.2007.12.008.

McCabe, S. E., & Boyd, C. J. (2005). Sources of prescription drugs for illicit use. *Addictive Behaviors, 30*(7), 1342–1350. doi:10.1016/j.addbeh.2005.01.012.

McCabe, S. E., Boyd, C. J., & Teter, C. J. (2009). Subtypes of nonmedical prescription drug misuse. *Drug and Alcohol Dependence, 102*(1-3), 6370. doi:10.1016/j.drugalcdep.2009.01.007.

McCabe, S. E., Cranford, J. A., Boyd, C. J., & Teter, C. J. (2007). Motives, diversion and routes of administration associated with nonmedical use of prescription opioids. *Addictive Behaviors, 32*(3), 562–575.

McCabe, S. E., West, B. T., & Boyd, C. J. (2013a). Medical use, medical misuse, and nonmedical use of prescription opioids: Results from a longitudinal study. *Pain, 154*(5), 708–713. doi:10.1016/j.pain.2013.01.011.

McCabe, S. E., West, B. T., & Boyd, C. J. (2013b). Motives for medical misuse of prescription opioids among adolescents. *Journal of Pain, 14*(10), 1208–1216. doi:10.1016/j.jpain.2013.05.004.

McCabe, S. E., West, B. T., Veliz, P., McCabe, V. V., Stoddard, S. A., & Boyd, C. J. (2017). Trends in medical and nonmedical use of prescription opioids among US adolescents: 1976–2015. *Pediatrics.* doi:10.1542/peds.2016-2387.

McHugh, R. K., DeVito, E. E., Dodd, D., Carroll, K. M., Potter, J. S., Greenfield, S. F., . . . Weiss, R. D. (2013). Gender differences in a clinical trial for prescription opioid dependence. *Journal of Substance Abuse Treatment, 45*(1), 38–43. doi:10.1016/j.jsat.2012.12.007.

McKenzie, J., Pinger, R. R., & Seabert, D. M. (2016). *An Introduction to Community Health* (9th ed.). Boston, MA: Jones & Bartlett Publishers.

Mendez, J., Yomogida, K., Figueroa, W., & Bavarian, N. (in preparation). High frequency prescription stimulant misuse at two California colleges: Association with cost, routes, sources, and experiences.

National Institute on Drug Abuse. (2014). Abuse of pain medications risks heroin use. http://www.drugabuse.gov/related-topics/trends-statistics/info graphics/abuse-prescription-pain-medications-risks-heroin-use.

Parks, K. A., Levonyan-Radloff, K., Przybyla, S. M., Darrow, S., Muraven, M., & Hequembourg, A. (2017). University student perceptions about the motives for and consequences of nonmedical use of prescription drugs (NMUPD). *Journal of American College Health*, 1–9. doi:10.1080/07448481.2017.1341895.

Rabiner, D. L., Anastopoulos, A. D., Costello, E. J., Hoyle, R. H., McCabe, S. E., & Swartzwelder, H. S. (2009). Motives and perceived consequences of nonmedical ADHD medication use by college students. *Journal of Attention Disorders, 13*(3), 259–270. doi:10.1177/1087054708320399.

Rigg, K. K., & Ford, J. A. (2014). The misuse of benzodiazepines among adolescents: Psychosocial risk factors in a national sample. *Drug and Alcohol Dependence, 137*, 137–142. doi:10.1016/j.drugalcdep.2014.01.026.

Sanders, A., Stogner, J., Seibert, J., & Miller, B. L. (2014). Misperceptions of peer pill-popping: The prevalence, correlates, and effects of inaccurate assumptions about peer pharmaceutical misuse. *Substance Use & Misuse, 49*(7), 813–823. doi:10.3109/10826084.2014.880485.

Schepis, T. S., & Krishnan-Sarin, S. (2009). Sources of prescriptions for misuse by adolescents: Differences in sex, ethnicity, and severity of misuse in a population-based study. *Journal of the American Academy of Child and Adolescent Psychiatry, 48*(8), 828–836. doi:10.1097/CHI.0b013e3181a8130d.

Shei, A., Rice, J. B., Kirson, N. Y., Bodnar, K., Birnbaum, H. G., Holly, P., & Ben-Joseph, R. (2015). Sources of prescription opioids among diagnosed opioid abusers. *Current Medical Research and Opinion, 31*(4), 779–784. doi:10.1185/03007995.2015.1016607.

Sirdifield, C., Chipchase, S. Y., Owen, S., & Siriwardena, A. N. (2017). A systematic review and meta-synthesis of patients' experiences and perceptions of seeking and using benzodiazepines and z-drugs: Towards safer prescribing. *Patient, 10*(1), 1–15. doi:10.1007/s40271-016-0182-z.

Stinson, J. N., Lalloo, C., Harris, L., Isaac, L., Campbell, F., Brown, S., et al. (2014). iCanCope with Pain™: User-centred design of a web- and mobile-based self-management program for youth with chronic pain based on identified health care needs. *Pain Research & Management, 19*(5), 257–265.

Volkow, N. D., & McLellan, A. T. (2016). Opioid abuse in chronic pain— Misconceptions and mitigation strategies. *New England Journal of Medicine, 374*(13), 1253–1263. doi:10.1056/NEJMra1507771.

World Health Organization. (2017). Constitution of WHO: Principles. http://www.who.int/about/mission/en.

CHAPTER SIXTEEN

Understanding Nonmedical Prescription Drug Use: The Importance of Criminological Theory

Jason A. Ford and Alexis Yohros

Nonmedical prescription drug use (NMPDU) has become a major public health issue in the United States. Because of this, many drug use researchers have focused on documenting prevalence and trends in use, identifying demographic characteristics of those engaged in NMPDU and risk factors for use, and sources of diversion and motives for use. One area with a relative lack of research is examining theoretical explanations of NMPDU. A theory is a statement, or set of principles, about how different things are related. For example, how are interactions between children and their parents related to substance use? Theories are important because they can help us understand why certain people are more likely to use drugs, and they can also be used to create effective prevention and intervention programs.

The study of drug use is interdisciplinary, with academics from medical backgrounds, public health, psychiatry, psychology, social work, sociology, criminal justice, political science, and economics doing research in this area. Given that the use of a prescription drug that has not been prescribed to a person is against the law, some social scientists view NMPDU as a deviant or criminal behavior, just like any other form of drug use. One academic discipline that focuses its efforts on creating theory to understand crime and deviant behavior is criminology. The history of criminological thought has been dominated by three "frames of reference," and these perspectives have driven the development of criminological theory.

First, *classical criminology* argues that human behavior is largely based on intelligence and rationality. This frame of reference argues that humans act in their own self-interest and posits that people engage in a behavior, even criminal ones, when they believe positive outcomes outweigh negative outcomes. The second frame of reference focuses on the criminal law and how certain behaviors come to be illegal and is generally referred to as *theories of the behavior of criminal law*. This frame of reference does not seek to explain individual causes of crime and deviance; rather, the focus is on why society labels certain behaviors as legal (e.g., alcohol use) while others are viewed as illegal (e.g., cocaine or heroin use). Third, *positivist criminology* believes that behavior is largely shaped by factors that individuals cannot control. This frame of reference dominates criminology today, as contemporary criminologists seek to identify factors that place individuals at increased risk for crime and deviance. Some criminologists have a macro orientation and focus of structural characteristics that contribute to crime and deviance, such as neighborhood characteristics. Other criminologists have a micro orientation and focus on important social process, such as family and peer interactions. Given the dominance of positivistic theories today, the theories reviewed in this chapter are positivist.

To date, only a few criminological theories have been used to examine NMPDU. This chapter will outline those theories (social learning, control, strain, and life course) and discuss the research that exists. In addition, this chapter will also present a few other major criminological theories (rational choice, social disorganization, developmental, biosocial, and conflict) to outline how these theories can help us understand NMPDU. Finally, we will discuss the policy implications associated with these theories.

Social Learning Theory

The dominant perspective on social learning in the field of criminology is the theory put forth by Ronald Akers (Akers, 1985). His theory of social learning integrates the sociological concept of differential association (Sutherland, 1947), which focuses on interactions with other people, with concepts from behavioral psychology (Bandura, 1977; Skinner, 1953), which examines how behaviors are reinforced. Akers's social learning theory argues that the causal mechanisms that explain deviant behavior involve interactions with primary group members (i.e., family and friends) who expose individuals to deviant role models and provide normative definitions and reinforcement for behavior.

In outlining social learning theory, Akers relied on four key principles. First, *differential association* focuses on the exposure to others' norms and values that takes place during social interactions. Akers argued that an individual's social networks, especially family and close friends, were of primary importance in the process of learning deviant behavior. Akers believed that the associations with the strongest effects on behavior were those that occurred earlier in life (priority), lasted longer (duration), occupied a lot of time or took place more often (frequency), and involved close or intimate others (intensity).

Second, *imitation* is the modeling of other people's behavior. During social interactions, individuals observe other people being rewarded or punished for behavior. Behavior that is punished is not likely to be imitated, but behaviors that produce a positive outcome for the actor may be imitated. The characteristics of the model, the behavior being observed, and the consequences of the behavior determine whether it will be imitated.

Third, *definitions* are regarded as one's own attitudes or meanings that one gives to a certain behavior, defining it as right or wrong. If one holds favorable definitions of a specific act, they are more likely to engage in it because they view the behavior as acceptable or believe they have something positive to gain by engaging in the behavior.

Finally, *differential reinforcement* examines how behavior is reinforced by examining the received or actual consequences of behavior. Simply stated, individuals engage in a behavior when the rewards outweigh the punishments. Behavior can be reinforced in either positive (when some type of reward is gained) or negative (when a negative stimulus is removed or avoided) ways. Social learning theory is one of the most often tested and empirically supported criminological theories.

Another theory, *techniques of neutralization* (Sykes & Matza, 1957), is closely related to social learning, as it describes in greater detail what types of definitions are conducive to deviant behavior. This theory explains how situational definitions allow individuals to drift back and forth between conventional and deviant behaviors. It argues that individuals utilize certain techniques to justify their criminal actions; this is important, as these techniques neutralize their beliefs that these actions are harmful and protect them from social stigma.

Sykes and Matza outlined five commonly used techniques of neutralization. First, *denial of responsibility* occurs when an individual may claim the act as an accident or due to forces outside one's control (e.g., blaming behavior on growing up in a bad home). Second, *denial of injury* is when an individual claims that the act did not cause any harm (e.g., someone may hit an expensive car and flee, while claiming it is acceptable because the owner has insurance). Third, *denial of victim* is a technique in which an individual believes that the victim got what he or she deserved (e.g., it is okay to assault someone who disrespects you or your family). Fourth, *condemnation of condemners* involves the criminal deflecting blame away from his or her acts by condemning those who disapprove of them (e.g., a petty thief arguing what he has done does not compare to how much financial institutions steal from people). Finally, *appeal to higher loyalties* involves a situation where social controls may be neutralized by surrendering the demands of the larger society for the demands of the groups to which the delinquent belongs (e.g., you engage in a deviant behavior because your friends are doing it and need your help).

Social Learning and NMPDU

A number of researchers have used social learning theory as a framework to understand NMPDU. These studies tend to focus on the importance of drug use among close friends or peers, how individuals define drug use, and the influence of attitudes toward drug use among friends and family members.

Ford and his colleagues have published a number of studies using data from the National Survey on Drug Use and Health (NSDUH), which is a sample of respondents that is representative of the general population of the United States. This research has shown that principles associated with social learning theory are significantly related to nonmedical opioid (Ford & Rigg, 2015) or benzodiazepine use (Rigg & Ford, 2014) and relate to any NMPDU (Ford, 2008; Schroeder & Ford, 2012) among adolescents. A number of studies also use social learning theory to explain NMPDU, especially stimulants, among college and high school students (Ford & Ong, 2014; Higgins, Mahoney, & Ricketts, 2009; Peralta & Steele, 2010; Steele, Peralta, & Elman, 2011; Watkins, 2016). These studies tend to show the importance of drug use among peers, time spent with peers, how friends define behaviors as being deviant, social and nonsocial reinforcement, and perceptions of effectiveness of the drug (to help get better grades) are significantly associated with NMPDU. Finally, a study involving young adults who all misused prescription drugs found support for social learning theory (Mui, Sales, & Murphy, 2014). Specifically, they found that many of those endorsing NMPDU were first exposed to prescription drugs by family members or friends, that many said they used to "fit in" with their friends, and that they believed prescription drugs were a safe alternative to more commonly used "street" drugs.

To date, only one study has looked exclusively at techniques of neutralization in relation to NMPDU among college students (Cutler, 2014). Many different justifications were given for NMPDU: that it was normative in their social group; there was relatively little danger associated with use; it was used for a good reason (to get good grades, not to get high); that their use caused no harm to other people; and many shifted responsibility to health care professionals. Techniques of neutralization may be particularly important when it comes to NMPDU, as these techniques may allow individuals to view themselves as not being "drug users."

Control Theories

Social Bonding

Control theories, in general, argue that people are naturally inclined to be deviant. Because of this, these theories generally seek to explain why people conform to social norms or what mechanisms control deviant behavior. Hirschi's social bonding theory (Hirschi, 1996) argues that people tend to conform when they internalize societal values and norms, or, as Hirschi saw it, they develop a "bond" to society. This social bond has four dimensions. First, *attachment* is the most important element of social bond and involves close relationships to others, such as family, friends, and school. Having close relationships with other people functions to constrain behavior, as involvement in deviant actions may place these important relationships at risk. Second, *commitment* is viewed as an investment in conventional activities and goals and produces a stake in conformity. The more heavily one is invested in conventional activities, the higher the risks and the lower the benefits of engaging in crime. Third, *involvement* or immersion in conventional activities controls crime because it leaves no time or opportunity to commit a criminal act, and such activities expose adolescents to conventional adult role models. Finally, *belief* assumes that each person is socialized to believe in the rules and norms of society. The more one believes that social norms are morally valid and should be obeyed, the less likely one is to violate these rules. Taken together, the stronger an adolescent's bond to society is, the more constrained to conformity they are. It is when social bonds become weak that deviant behavior becomes more likely.

Self-Control

Another control theory argues that behavior is constrained by self-control (Gottfredson & Hirschi, 1990). Their general theory of crime argues that individuals who have low levels of self-control are more likely to engage in a variety of deviant behavior. The source of low self-control is poor parenting, and individuals with low self-control are thought to be impulsive, insensitive to the need of others, physical (as opposed to mental), inclined to take risks, short-sighted, and nonverbal. These characteristics place individuals with low self-control at risk for deviance because it is difficult to resist the immediate gratification that is associated with deviant behavior and they fail to consider the long-term consequences that are associated with their actions.

In sum, given opportunities to engage in deviant behavior, adolescents with lower levels of self-control will be more likely to do so.

Control Theories and NMPDU

A number of studies have examined social bonding and NMPDU. These studies tend to show that adolescents with weak bonds, to either parents or school, are at increased risk for NMPDU. Again, Ford and colleagues used data from the NSDUH to examine social bonding theory among adolescents. They found that elements of social bonding theory were significantly related to the nonmedical use of prescription opioids (Ford & Rigg, 2015); Ambien (Ford & McCutcheon, 2012); and any NMPDU (Ford, 2009; Schroeder & Ford, 2012). Other research has focused on school-based populations. Examining data from the Monitoring the Future study, a national sample of middle and high school students in the United States, Higgins et al. (2009) found a significant link between social bonding and NMPDU. Specifically, they found that adolescents with stronger attachments at school were less likely to report NMPDU. Finally, a study using the College Alcohol Survey, a national sample of college students in the United States, also found support for social bonding (Ford & Arrastia, 2008). College students who reported an attachment to a faculty member were less likely to report NMPDU (Ford & Arrastia, 2008).

To our knowledge, only two studies examined NMPDU using Gottfredson and Hirschi's general theory of crime. Holtfreter et al. (2015) examined the association between low self-control and NMPDU in a sample of individuals aged 60 and older. They found that low self-control, measured as risk-taking and impulsivity, was significantly associated with a greater likelihood of NMPDU. Ford and Blumenstein (2013) examined the relationship between low self-control and various types of drug use among a sample of college students in the southern United States. This research showed that college students with low self-control were more likely to report NMPDU. While there is little research on low self-control and NMPDU, the existing research supports the main principles of the theory.

Strain Theories

The concept of strain is based on the ideas of Emile Durkheim, one of the founding figures of sociology. Durkheim proposed the idea of anomie to describe a state of normlessness, or a situation when the social norms used to control behavior breakdown. Durkheim originally applied the concept of anomie to understand patterns in suicide over time. Simply stated, Durkheim believed that deviant behaviors were more likely when society was in a state of anomie. When thinking about the concept of anomie, an example could be the life of a high school senior and the social controls that parents and teachers may have over the senior's behavior. Generally, parents make sure their children go to school, do their homework, and are not out late on a school night. Once the student graduates and leaves for college, those sources of social control (parents and teachers) are diminished. As a college freshman, one's roommate is not going to make sure one is awake to go to class; one's roommate is also unlikely argue against one going out on a Tuesday night because of classes the next morning. Sociologists would consider the transition to college as a period of anomie, or normlessness, as the social controls provided by parents and other conventional adults are generally weakened. This concept could help us understand the high rates of academic failure and alcohol use among college freshman.

A number of criminologists have expanded on Durkheim's work and have applied the concept of anomie, or strain, to help explain deviant and criminal behavior. For the most part, strain theories state "delinquency results when individuals are unable to achieve their goals through legitimate channels" (Agnew, 2012). Rather than crime being inherent, individuals are pressured into or engage in crime because they are unable to achieve goals, such as monetary success.

Anomie Theory

With a macro focus on elements of the larger social structure, Merton (1938) described *strain* as the gap that existed between cultural goals and the means people had to achieve those goals. Merton argued that society places high emphasis on cultural goals (e.g., monetary success) but low emphasis on the proper norms and rules for achieving those goals (e.g., education and effort). Merton argued that, in American society, it is important to become financially successful, but how one achieves that cultural goal is not that important. Essentially, the ends justify the means. Merton also argued that not everyone has equal access to approved means to achieve cultural goals. Today, an education is an important stepping-stone to financial success, but not all Americans have access to the same quality of education. Thus, strain is created as the cultural goal to be financially successful pushes people to achieve that goal, regardless of the means, but the social structure creates obstacles that make it more difficult for certain groups of people to achieve those goals.

Merton described five "modes of adaptation" people used to adjust to the pressure to achieve certain goals. The most common is *conformity*, when people accept both the culture goals and the legitimate means to accomplishing them. Conformists have little involvement in deviant or criminal behavior. The second type is *innovation*, in which the culture goals are accepted but not the institutionalized means. This is the most common form of deviant adaptations, as individuals turn to criminal acts, such as dealing drugs, as a way to achieve the cultural goal of financial success. The third adaptation is *ritualism*. Here, one knows the goals are unobtainable, but they still follow the legitimate ways of pursuing these goals. Ritualists accept the norms of society and have relatively low levels of deviance and crime. *Retreatism*, the fourth adaptation, occurs when both the goals and means are rejected. Merton described this adaptation as the least common, and people in this category include individuals with psychosis, those who use substances frequently and heavily, and others on the margins of society. Finally, *rebellion* means the cultural goals and means are both rejected and substituted with other goals. Such individuals include rebels and revolutionaries.

General Strain Theory

Building on the work of both Durkheim and Merton, but shifting the focus away from a macro structural orientation, Agnew (1992) proposed a general strain theory that focused on micro social interactions between individuals. Agnew generally describes strain as being treated poorly by other people or as experiencing negative life events and outlines three primary sources of strain. The first type of strain, *failure to achieve positively valued goals*, was very similar to the strain identified by Merton. For instance, a college student who fails an exam (good grades are a valued cultural goal) may use substances to cope. The second type of strain, *removal of positively valued stimuli*, occurs when a person loses something that is important to him or her. For example, having a partner break up with you can be a source of strain; when that occurs, drug use or property damage may result in an attempt to get revenge for being wronged. The third type of strain, *presence of noxious stimuli*, occurs when people experience adverse interactions with others (e.g., living in a poor neighborhood or experiencing child abuse). Deviant or criminal coping is likely in such situations because it allows individuals to avoid or escape these noxious stimuli. Agnew argued that strain increased the likelihood of crime because strain resulted in a range of negative emotions, such as anger, frustration, jealousy, depression, and fear. Experiencing strain and the resulting negative emotions can lead individuals to act dangerously or criminally to correct the situation and alleviate the pressure caused by strain. Thus, Agnew viewed deviance and crime as a coping mechanism to deal with the pressure and negative emotions produced by strain.

Strain Theory and NMPDU

Much of the research involving NMPDU and strain involves general strain theory and identifying different types of strains that may result in NMPDU. Ford and colleagues used data from the NSDUH to examine the relationship between strain and NMPDU. Their measure of strain was based on a series of negative life events (e.g., fights with parents, poor grades, not living with both biological parents, poverty, and poor overall health). This research showed that adolescents who reported strain were more likely to report any NMPDU (Schroeder & Ford, 2012) and nonmedical prescription benzodiazepine use (Rigg & Ford, 2014). Ford et al. (2014) used a similar strategy to examine the relationship between strain NMPDU and gender. This is important, as prior research has shown that adolescent females are at increased risk of NMPDU (Boyd, McCabe, Cranford, & Young, 2006; Ford, 2009; Schepis & Krishnan-Sarin, 2008; Simoni-Wastila & Strickler, 2004; Sung, Richter, Vaughan, Johnson, & Thom, 2005). Research has also shown females and males may respond differently to certain strains (Broidy & Agnew, 1997). In addition to finding support for general strain theory, that strain is related to depression (negative affect) and that both are related to NMPDU, Ford et al. (2014) also found that strain was gendered. That is, males and females have different responses to strain, and "strained" females were at an increased risk for depression compared to "strained" males.

Another study by Ford and Schroeder (2012) applied Agnew's general strain theory to examine whether academic strain was related to nonmedical stimulant use. The study used data from the Harvard School of Public Health's College Alcohol Study and defined academic strain as a disconnect between academic aspirations and actual outcomes. Students who believed academic work was important or very important but had lower GPAs (below 3.0) experienced strain. The results indicated that students who experience academic strain also report higher levels of depression, and those students who report higher levels of depression are more likely to report the nonmedical use of prescription stimulants.

A few other researchers have examined the relationship between strain and NMPDU. Wiegel et al. (2016) looked at the association between work-related stress and cognitive enhancement drug use among a sample of college professors. Although not directly applying general strain theory, the study used many related concepts by looking at the association of work strain and cognitive enhancement use (via stimulant misuse). The results showed a strong association between work-related strains and all measures of cognitive enhancement use. Holtfreter et al. (2015) examined the relationship between strain (poor health), negative affect (depression), and deviant coping (NMPDU). They found that poor health increased the likelihood of NMPDU, in part due to depression.

Life Course Theories

The life course has become a dominant perspective in the field of criminology. While traditional theories of crime and deviance, like those that have been reviewed so far, tend to focus on the initiation of criminal acts among adolescents, life course theories examine a multitude of factors that shape offending behavior from adolescence to adulthood. Life course theories tend to examine developmental trajectories over time, looking at the factors that cause deviance or criminal behavior during the transition from adolescence to adulthood, for example.

This approach argues that events that occur in adolescence are causally related to events that happen later in life. Stability in offending behavior over time is created by a process of cumulative disadvantage, as involvement in deviance or crime at an early age tends to limit future opportunities and options for a conventional life, especially when an individual is arrested. Life course theorists also look for transitions that can redirect developmental trajectories. While most adult criminals began breaking the law when they were adolescents, most adolescents who break the law stop doing so when they become adults. Life course theorists seek to identify important transitions that create turning points and lead to desistance, or the process of the discontinuation of criminal activity.

The leading proponents of the life course approach in criminology are Sampson and Laub (1993), and their theory of age-graded informal social control has been guided by two principles. First, antisocial behavior in adolescence is linked to criminal offending during adulthood. Second, salient life events (e.g., marriage) and social ties embedded in adult transitions explain variations in criminal offending that are unaccounted for by childhood predictors. The significance of the life course approach lies in the study of desistence.

Sampson and Laub argue that change in behavior is possible during the transition to adulthood, if individuals develop strong social bonds. In this, they extend the work of Hirschi's social bonding theory. As adolescents enter adulthood, sources of social bonding shift from family and school to marriage and employment. Their research, which focused on juvenile delinquents, found that those who married and found jobs were more likely to desist from crime as they entered adulthood. Their theory emphasizes the quality and strength of social bonds, so they focused on the level of attachment to spouse and stability of employment. They argued that these social bonds had the ability to produce social capital. Social capital enhances feelings of self-worth and creates a stake in conformity, which is necessary in the desistance process. Much research has supported Sampson and Laub's theory that marriage and work can be important turning points in the life course.

Life Course Theories and NMPDU

Unfortunately, few studies look at life-course theory and NMPDU. A few notable studies, however, look at the link between life events and NMPDU among adults or desistence from NMPDU. A study by Gunter et al. (2012) examined patterns of desistance from nonmedical prescription opioid use to see whether it was similar to illicit drug use. The data they used came from the South Beach Project, a sample of 600 ethnically distinct individuals engaged in polydrug use in Miami-Dade County, Florida. The results found that association with peers with high levels of antisocial traits or drug use hindered the desistence process for nonmedical prescription opioid users. This supports a life-course perspective that emphasizes the significance of social bonds in desistence from drug use trajectories.

Dollar and colleagues have published two studies that examine the relationship between adult social bonds and NMPDU. The first used data from the NSDUH (Dollar & Ray, 2013). The study revealed that marital bonds were significantly and inversely related to all types of NMPDU (with sedatives being an exception), meaning married adults were less likely to report NMPDU. In addition, respondents who were employed were less likely to report the nonmedical opioid use. A second study used data from the National Longitudinal Study of Adolescent Health, a sample of adolescents that was representative of the U.S. population and was interviewed multiple times over numerous years (Dollar & Hendrix, 2015). This research showed that married respondents, respondents who reported higher relationship satisfaction, and respondents with higher levels of work satisfaction were less likely to report NMPDU. This supports Sampson and Laub's contention that the quality of social bonds was more important than simply being married or having a job.

Additional Criminological Theories

There are a number of important theories of crime and deviance that have yet to be used to understand NMPDU. While the previous section outlined what we know about criminological theory and NMPDU, this section will focus on what we do not know. In this section, we will briefly outline a few important criminological theories and discuss how they are relevant to NMPDU.

Rational Choice Theory

Rooted in principles of classical criminology, rational choice theory argues that all humans are rational, have free will, and make decisions based on the consideration of pleasure and pain. The theory is based on the expected utility principle in economics; people make decisions based on the extent to which they expect the choice to maximize benefits and minimize costs. Therefore, as rational actors, an offender will weigh the expected costs and benefits of a criminal act before deciding whether or not to engage in it. For example, a thief may choose not to steal from a specific neighborhood home because the chance of getting caught is higher than the reward that burglarizing the house will bring. These rational decisions involve the initial decision to become engaged in crime to satisfy a need (i.e. money, food); the decision to commit a particular form of crime; and the selection of a suitable target based on costs and benefits. One reason why rational choice is useful to the study of crime and deviance is that the theory focuses on understanding what motivates individuals to engage in criminal acts.

While not explicitly framed as a test of rational choice theory, one study does use concepts close to rational choice to understand NMPDU among college students (Sattler, Sauer, Mehlkop, & Graeff, 2013). This study focused on how social norms, expectations of behavior that are shaped by members of one's social network, influence decision making (weighing the perceived costs and benefits) with regard to the use of cognitive enhancement drugs (i.e., stimulants). This study showed that those who were willing to try such drugs go through a decision-making process. In this process, they consider both the benefits and costs associated with use, including side effects. This is consistent with the principles of rational choice theory.

There are also a number of studies that examine sources of diversion, motives, and perceptions of NMPDU among college and high school students (Ford & Watkins, 2012). This research can help illustrate how NMPDU is a rational decision. Overwhelmingly, the research shows that the most common source of medication is family members and friends. Prescription drugs are not obtained from drug dealers; rather, they are often acquired freely from family members and friends. Adolescents are also as likely to report motives for use that are related to self-treatment (e.g., help concentrate, sleep, relieve pain), as they are to mention recreational motives (e.g., to get high, to experiment) for use. Lastly, the research also shows that adolescents believe that NMPDU is very common among their peers. This research leads to the conclusion that adolescents believe that NMPDU is less harmful than use of traditional street drugs, and this thought likely influences the process described by rational choice theorists.

Social Disorganization Theory

Social disorganization is macro-level theory of crime focused on community trends and patterns rather than individual differences in crime. In their study of rates of delinquency in urban areas, Shaw and McKay (1942) found that certain neighborhoods had higher rates of delinquency than others. Thus, social disorganization theory helps illustrate how neighborhood characteristics influence deviance and crime.

The theory of social disorganization expands on the ecological concept of concentric zone theory, which outlines how urban areas grow through a process of expansion and create separate concentric zones of development that spread from the city center out to suburban neighborhoods. The theory focuses on living conditions in the "zone of transition" that is just outside the central business district of the city but is not entirely residential. It is this area that has the highest rates of delinquency. This transitional zone is characterized by high levels of poverty, physical decay, rapid population growth, and an unstable heterogeneous population. This structural disadvantage has a devastating negative impact on social institutions, such as families and schools. Shaw and McKay did not argue that residents of socially disorganized neighborhoods were inclined to crime; rather, they explained the high crime rates in these areas were a normal response to living in abnormal social conditions.

Simply stated, social disorganization has a negative effect on social control, or the ability to have people follow social norms. Later research on social disorganization examines how collective efficacy, or the ability of neighbors to use informal social control that results in mutual trust and the ability to regulate the behavior of others, and social capital, or strong social ties between community members that create a stake in conformity, link social disorganization to criminal behavior. These concepts recognize that strong ties between members of a socially disorganized neighborhood can work to prevent criminal activity.

As of now, there have been no studies that test the concepts of social disorganization in relation to NMPDU. However, social disorganization researchers have looked at the use of alcohol and other drugs, and that research could be expanded to help illuminate NMPDU processes. Generally speaking, neighborhoods with higher levels of social disorganization also have higher levels of alcohol and other drug use. This research also shows that drugs, both alcohol and traditional "street" drugs, tend to be more available in socially disorganized neighborhoods. These findings are of particular importance, as alcohol and drug use are closely associated with violence and other forms of criminal behavior. A question of particular importance related to NMPDU would be an examination of access to prescription drug based on neighborhood characteristics, particularly if "pill mills," which are pain management clinics that prescribe high rates of commonly misused prescription drugs and are a key medication source, are more likely to be located in socially disorganized neighborhoods.

Developmental Theory

Closely related to the life-course perspective, developmental theories tend to be interdisciplinary and focus on different groups of criminals and unique causal factors. One of the most popular developmental theories in criminology is Moffitt's developmental taxonomy (1993). Her theory describes two types of criminal offenders with distinct patterns of offending and unique causes of offending. Life-course persistent (LCP) offenders constitute a small percentage of the population, but they are highly involved in criminal activity. LCP offenders initiate antisocial behavior early in the life course and continue on a stable path of offending into adulthood. Moffitt argues that a combination of neuropsychological deficits (poor verbal and executive functioning) and a poor social environment (weak social bonds to family and school) are the primary causes of offending for LCP. Simply stated, neuropsychological problems interact with a poor social environment and make it difficult to effectively socialize these individuals, placing them on a deviant path.

In contrast, adolescence-limited (AL) offenders start offending during their teenage years but do not continue offending into adulthood. AL offending can be attributed to a gap between physical and social maturity. That is, adolescents look like and are capable of adult behaviors, but socially they are prohibited from engaging in these types of behaviors. Deviant behavior is a way to break free from this maturity gap, and deviance becomes an act of rebellion, a way for adolescents to cut off ties to parents and assert their independence. AL offenders will often mimic the behavior of their LCP peers, who because of their criminal involvement are viewed more as adults than adolescents. Among AL offenders, the motivation for delinquency begins to diminish once the maturity gap closes and the negative outcomes associated with deviance outweigh the benefits of the behavior.

To date, no research has used developmental perspectives to examine NMPDU. This frame of reference could be used to identify different types of NMPDU. To illustrate, a person who infrequently uses Adderall without a prescription to aid studying is different from a person who uses OxyContin on a daily basis because of dependence symptoms. It is important to understand that not all types of NMPDU are equal. Some people engage in NMPDU occasionally, but others do so daily; some use for instrumental reasons (or to achieve socially approved goals), but others do so to get high; and some people engage in NMPDU and experience few negative outcomes, but others experience use disorder symptoms. The ability of developmental theories to help us understand differences between groups engaged in NMPDU and differences in causes of use can greatly improve our understanding of NMPDU.

Biosocial Theory

There are a number of biological approaches to criminal behavior, but the one most commonly adopted by criminologists today focuses on the interactions between genetic and environmental influences. Such theories are commonly referred to as biosocial theories (Beaver, 2009). This approach takes genetic risk factors for crime and deviance (e.g., dopamine, serotonin, MAOA) and examines how they are shaped by environmental factors (e.g., neighborhoods, family, peers). Some of the research in this area supports a differential susceptibility hypothesis, where an individual's genetic makeup makes him or her more susceptible to environmental influences. So, individuals who possess a certain genetic makeup are more exposed to criminogenic factors from a negative social environment. In sum, biosocial theories argue that a combination of biological (genetic) and social (environmental) factors work together to increase risk for crime and deviance.

In the field of criminology, most research using the biosocial perspective seeks to understand criminal offending, while less research focuses on understanding drug use. Some existing research has examined gene (dopamine, serotonin, MAOA) and environment (social learning theory, social control theory, strain theories, and social disorganization theory) interactions focused on substance use. These studies generally support the biosocial approach. To our knowledge, there are no biosocial studies that specifically focus on NMPDU. Prior criminological research has often ignored biological factors, and research on biosocial factors in NMPDU is important to determine if the social-environmental conditions criminologists have historically relied on to explain crime and deviance remain significant when biological risk factors are considered.

Conflict Theory

Conflict theorists argue that society is best understood by examining conflict between opposing groups over access to important resources and social power. This perspective focuses on how criminal laws are created by those who have power to reflect their own self-interest. This produces a criminal justice system, which was created and controlled by people with power and unfairly labels and punishes the less powerful. An example of this would be how the criminal justice system responds differently to street and white-collar crime. Even though white-collar crime causes more financial harm to society, criminal penalties are more severe for street crime than for white-collar crime.

In addition, conflict theory argues that social groups with little power tend to reject the norms and values of the group in power, resulting in criminal behavior. Those with little power do not believe that living a conventional lifestyle is a possibility given their economical marginalization. They reject the values and norms of mainstream society and live by their own standards of behavior.

Marxist, or critical, theories are closely related to conflict theory. The main difference is that Marxist theories tend to focus on conflict created by capitalism, while conflict theorists argue that there are multiple sources of conflict. Marxist theorists believe in a power-elite model, where social, economic, and political power is controlled by a small ruling class of capitalists. In their view, a capitalist economic system causes a number of problems for society because of its focus on competition, exploitation, and material belongings. It creates a state of egoism where the needs of others are ignored, pitting people against one another. In general, these types of theories focus on how certain behaviors are defined as legal or illegal and argue that the criminal justice system is a tool used by the powerful to control the underclass.

To date, conflict theories have not been applied to NMUPD. Future research could look at the construction of different laws and how punishment differs between illicit drugs and NMUPD. For years, conflict theorists have outlined how certain drugs are connected to certain groups of people and that these drugs are declared illegal as a way to control these groups: for example, opium use among those of Asian descent, marijuana use among those of Mexican descent, alcohol use among Catholics during Prohibition, methamphetamine use by poorer whites, and crack cocaine use among blacks. Given that NMPDU is generally viewed as a problem of the white middle class, conflict theorists would expect a less punitive social response to those who use nonmedically. Conflict theorists would also be interested in the role of capitalism, giving special attention to the role of the medical-industrial complex, the corporations that supply health care services, and products for a profit. The focus here would be on pharmaceutical companies and, to a lesser extent, doctors. Pharmaceutical sales are a billion-dollar industry in the United States. Conflict theorists would look at how pharmaceutical companies have created the idea that prescription drugs are the solution to all health problems and how these corporations profit, regardless of whether the drugs are used medically or nonmedically.

Discussion

Nonmedical prescription drug use has become a major public health issue over the past decade. Most of the academic research on NMPDU focuses on prevalence and trends in NMPDU, sources of diversion and motives for nonmedical use, and identifying demographic characteristics of people engaged in NMPDU and other risk factors for NMPDU. What the discipline of criminology can offer to the study of NMPDU is an examination of theories of crime and deviance. As outlined above, some research examining theories of crime has been conducted, but much more is needed. Applying theory to NMPDU is important because it can help us understand whether NMPDU is similar to other types of drug use. This research can also be used to develop effective prevention and interventions for NMPDU.

Social learning (influence of peers and attitudes of others), control (bonds to family and school as well as self-control), strain (exposure to different types of strain), and life-course (bonds to marriage and employment) theories have all been used successfully to understand NMPDU. What is unknown is how concepts related to rational choice (offender decision making), social disorganization (neighborhood characteristics), developmental (typologies of NMPDU), biosocial (gene-environment interactions), and conflict (power and money) theories are related to NMPDU.

In reality, the criminological study of NMPDU is in its infancy. While criminological theory has allowed us to better understand NMPDU, a number of gaps in the literature remain. Most of the research in this area has focused on individual factors (e.g., peer influence, relationship with parents, school performance, low self-control) that are related to NMPDU. This is surprising, as criminologists also look to neighborhood characteristics when explaining involvement in deviant or criminal behavior. More research rooted in social disorganization theory is needed to understand how the neighborhoods people live in influence the types of drugs they use.

In general, to better understand deviance and crime, criminologists must go beyond the theories discussed in this chapter. These theories simply outline events or conditions that place individuals at increased risk for deviance and crime. Instead, criminologists must examine how individuals perceive and interpret criminogenic events and conditions (Akers, 1985). More simply stated, criminological theories identify important pushes (e.g., strain); pulls (e.g., social learning); and restraints (e.g., social control) that are related to deviance and crime. Future research must identify the factors that make individuals more (e.g., sensation seeking) or less susceptible (e.g., social support) to these criminogenic conditions.

In terms of policy implications, one important finding must be discussed. The various efforts to understand NMPDU using criminological theory have indicated that people do not believe NMPDU is actually drug use. As compared to traditional street drugs, people view prescription drugs as a safe alternative. They believe that NMPDU is widely acceptable in society, that there is little risk of arrest for use, and that use-related consequences and other negative outcomes are unlikely. This does not match the epidemiological data on NMPDU indicating that NMPDU is associated with emergency department utilization, overdose, and a transition to street drugs (as many people who use heroin start out using prescription opioids). Prevention programs must include information on the harms associated with NMPDU to correct this misperception.

References

Agnew, R. (1992). Foundation for a general strain theory of crime and delinquency. *Criminology, 30*(1), 47–88. doi:10.1111/j.1745-9125.1992.tb01093.x.

Agnew, R. (2012). Reflection on "a revised strain theory of delinquency." *Social Forces, 91*(1), 33–38. doi:10.1093/sf/sos117.

Akers, R. L. (1985). *Deviant Behavior: A Social Learning Approach*. Belmont, CA: Wadsworth.

Bandura, A. (1977). *Social Learning Theory*. Englewood Cliffs, NJ: Prentice-Hall, Inc.

Beaver, K. M. (2009). *Biosocial Criminology: A Primer*. Dubuque, IA: Kendall/Hunt.

Boyd, C. J., McCabe, S. E., Cranford, J. A., & Young, A. (2006). Adolescents' motivations to abuse prescription medications. *Pediatrics, 118*(6), 2472–2480. doi:10.1542/peds.2006-1644.

Broidy, L., & Agnew, R. (1997). Gender and crime: A general strain theory perspective. *Journal of Research in Crime and Delinquency, 34*(3), 275–306. doi:10.1177/0022427897034003001.

Cutler, K. A. (2014). Prescription stimulants are "a okay": Applying neutralization theory to college students' nonmedical prescription stimulant use. *Journal of American College Health, 62*(7), 478–486. doi:10.1080/07448481.2014.929578.

Dollar, C. B., & Hendrix, J. A. (2015). The importance of romantic and work relations on nonmedical prescription drug use among adults. *Sociological Spectrum, 35*(5), 465–481. doi:10.1080/02732173.2015.1064800.

Dollar, C. B., & Ray, B. (2013). Adult nonmedical prescription drug use: An examination of bond theory. *Deviant Behavior, 34*(11), 932–949. doi:10.1080/01639625.2013.800406.

Ford, J. A. (2008). Social learning theory and nonmedical prescription drug use among adolescents. *Sociological Spectrum, 28*(3), 299–316. doi:10.1080/02732170801898471.

Ford, J. A. (2009). Nonmedical prescription drug use among adolescents. *Youth & Society, 40*(3), 336–352. doi:10.1177/0044118x08316345.

Ford, J. A., & Arrastia, M. C. (2008). Pill-poppers and dopers: a comparison of non-medical prescription drug use and illicit/street drug use among college students. *Addictive Behaviors, 33*(7), 934–941. doi:10.1016/j.addbeh.2008.02.016.

Ford, J. A., & Blumenstein, L. (2013). Self-control and substance use among college students. *Journal of Drug Issues, 43*(1), 56–68. doi:10.1177/0022042612462216.

Ford, J. A., & McCutcheon, J. (2012). The misuse of Ambien among adolescents: Prevalence and correlates in a national sample. *Addictive Behaviors, 37*(12), 1389–1394. doi:https://doi.org/10.1016/j.addbeh.2012.06.015.

Ford, J. A., & Ong, J. (2014). Non-medical use of prescription stimulants for academic purposes among college students: A test of social learning theory. *Drug and Alcohol Dependence, 144*(Supplement C), 279–282. doi:https://doi.org/10.1016/j.drugalcdep.2014.09.011.

Ford, J. A., Reckdenwald, A., & Marquardt, B. (2014). Prescription drug misuse and gender. *Substance Use & Misuse, 49*(7), 842–851. doi:10.3109/10826084.2014.880723.

Ford, J. A., & Rigg, K. K. (2015). Racial/ethnic differences in factors that place adolescents at risk for prescription opioid misuse. *Prevention Science, 16*(5), 633–641. doi:10.1007/s11121-014-0514-y.

Ford, J. A., & Watkins, W. C. (2012). Adolescent non-medical prescription use. *Prevention Researcher, 19*, 3–7.

Gottfredson, M. R., & Hirschi, T. (1990). *A General Theory of Crime.* Stanford, CA: Stanford University Press.

Gunter, W. D., Kurtz, S. P., Bakken, N. W., & O'Connell, D. J. (2012). Desisting from prescription drug abuse: An application of growth models to Rx opioid users. *Journal of Drug Issues, 42*(1), 82–97. doi:10.1177/0022042612436651.

Higgins, G. E., Mahoney, M., & Ricketts, M. L. (2009). Nonsocial reinforcement of the nonmedical use of prescription drugs: A partial test of social learning and self-control theories. *Journal of Drug Issues, 39*(4), 949–963. doi:10.1177/002204260903900409.

Hirschi, T. (1996). *Causes of Delinquency.* Berkeley: University of California Press.

Holtfreter, K., Reisig, M. D., & O'Neal, E. N. (2015). Prescription drug misuse in late adulthood. *Journal of Drug Issues, 45*(4), 351–367. doi:10.1177/0022042615589405.

Merton, R. K. (1938). Social structure and anomie. *American Sociological Review, 3*(5), 672–682. doi:10.2307/2084686.

Moffitt, T. E. (1993). Adolescence-limited and life-course-persistent antisocial behavior: A developmental taxonomy. *Psychological Review, 100*(4), 674–701.

Mui, H. Z., Sales, P., & Murphy, S. (2014). Everybody's doing it. *Journal of Drug Issues, 44*(3), 236–253. doi:10.1177/0022042613497935.

Peralta, R. L., & Steele, J. L. (2010). Nonmedical prescription drug use among US college students at a Midwest university: A partial test of social learning theory. *Substance Use & Misuse, 45*(6), 865–887. doi:10.3109/10826080903443610.

Rigg, K. K., & Ford, J. A. (2014). The misuse of benzodiazepines among adolescents: Psychosocial risk factors in a national sample. *Drug and Alcohol Dependence, 137*, 137–142. doi:10.1016/j.drugalcdep.2014.01.026.

Sampson, R. J., & Laub, J. H. (1993). *Crime in the Making: Pathways and Turning Points Through Life.* Cambridge, MA: Harvard University Press.

Sattler, S., Sauer, C., Mehlkop, G., & Graeff, P. (2013). The rationale for consuming cognitive enhancement drugs in university students and teachers. *PLoS One, 8*(7), e68821. doi:10.1371/journal.pone.0068821.

Schepis, T. S., & Krishnan-Sarin, S. (2008). Characterizing adolescent prescription misusers: A population-based study. *Journal of the American Academy of Child and Adolescent Psychiatry, 47*(7), 745–754. doi:10.1097/CHI.0b013e318172ef0ld.

Schroeder, R. D., & Ford, J. A. (2012). Prescription drug misuse. *Journal of Drug Issues, 42*(1), 4–27. doi:10.1177/0022042612436654.

Shaw, C. R., & McKay, H. D. (1942). *Juvenile Delinquency and Urban Areas.* Chicago: University of Chicago Press.

Simoni-Wastila, L., & Strickler, G. (2004). Risk factors associated with problem use of prescription drugs. *American Journal of Public Health, 94*(2), 266–268.

Skinner, B. F. (1953). *Science and Human Behavior.* New York: Macmillan.

Steele, J. L., Peralta, R. L., & Elman, C. (2011). The co-ingestion of nonmedical prescription drugs and alcohol: A partial test of social learning theory. *Journal of Drug Issues, 41*(4), 561–585. doi:10.1177/002204261104100406.

Sung, H.-E., Richter, L., Vaughan, R., Johnson, P. B., & Thom, B. (2005). Nonmedical use of prescription opioids among teenagers in the United States: Trends and correlates. *Journal of Adolescent Health, 37*(1), 44–51. doi: https://doi.org/10.1016/j.jadohealth.2005.02.013.

Sutherland, E. H. (1947). *Principles of Criminology* (4th ed.). Philadelphia, PA: Lippincott.

Sykes, G. M., & Matza, D. (1957). Techniques of neutralization: A theory of delinquency. *American Sociological Review, 22,* 664–673.

Watkins, W. C. (2016). A social learning approach to prescription drug misuse among college students. *Deviant Behavior, 37*(6), 601–614. doi:10.1080/01639625.2015.1060799.

Wiegel, C., Sattler, S., Göritz, A. S., & Diewald, M. (2016). Work-related stress and cognitive enhancement among university teachers. *Anxiety, Stress, & Coping, 29*(1), 100–117. doi:10.1080/10615806.2015.1025764.

CHAPTER SEVENTEEN

Conclusions

Ty S. Schepis

In 2016, the Centers for Disease Control and Prevention (CDC) estimated that over 53,000 U.S. residents died as a result of an opioid-related overdose (National Institute on Drug Abuse, 2017). Nearly 8,800 died from a benzodiazepine-related overdose, though the vast majority of those deaths also involved opioid use (National Institute on Drug Abuse, 2017). To illustrate the scale of this tragedy, imagine a mid-sized passenger airplane that seats 150 people, like a Boeing 737 or Airbus 320. Now imagine that one such plane crashes nearly every day, with no survivors. This is the scale of the opioid epidemic.

This example was given by Wilson Compton, the deputy director of the U.S. National Institute on Drug Abuse, in a talk I attended in the summer of 2016. He noted that such a series of tragic airplane accidents would create a massive national effort to solve the problem, and he called for a comparable response to the opioid epidemic. On this, I hope we can all agree. In addition to concrete steps to limit excessive opioid dispensing (while prioritizing appropriate pain treatment) and improve prevention efforts to limit opioid misuse, more research is needed to understand opioid misuse specifically and prescription misuse more broadly.

While I hope this volume provided you, the reader, with a broad overview of prescription misuse, it was not possible to make it more exhaustive because of the preliminary nature of much research into prescription misuse. A number of chapters in the book referred to medication-assisted therapy (MAT) for opioid dependence, which is a well-established and effective treatment. For more on the topic, please see Connery (2015) for a general overview and McCarthy and colleagues (2017) for a review on MAT during pregnancy. Beyond MAT and an increasingly robust literature on public health policies that can help limit opioid misuse (many aspects of which were covered here in chapters 9 through 13), little work has examined psychosocial prevention programs or treatments for opioid misuse specifically and prescription misuse generally. Readers who are interested in prevention should read Hero and coauthors (2016) on the importance of patient education, the statement of the U.S. Preventive Services Task Force (2014), and Crowley and colleagues (2014) on the effectiveness of universal school-based prevention in terms of limiting later prescription misuse.

In addition to research on prevention and treatment, future work will need to adapt to the changing face of the opioid epidemic. While prescription opioids fueled the initial development and entrenchment of the opioid epidemic, the sharp increases in overdose deaths from 2010 have been driven by heroin, initially, and increasingly by illicit fentanyl and derivatives (O'Donnell, Gladden, & Seth, 2017). Fentanyl is also a major public health issue in Canada (Fischer, Vojtila, & Rehm, 2017). There is a strong research literature on heroin use from past heroin crises, though it is not clear that the knowledge derived from those past experiences can be applied to the current epidemic, given that many current heroin users transitioned from opioid misuse (Compton, Jones, & Baldwin, 2016); for fentanyl misuse, there is very little literature to use as a guide. Without neglecting prescription opioids, increasing research will need to focus on heroin and fentanyl use.

Finally, opioid misuse research will need to expand its focus to encompass neglected, but vulnerable, subgroups and more complex processes leading to initial misuse and the development of more severe misuse. As thoroughly covered in chapters 6 and 7, prescription misuse in adolescents and young adults is increasingly well characterized, and research in these age groups should move to better characterize those at risk for initiation and those at highest risk for problematic misuse. In contrast, older adults (examined in chapter 8) are an underexamined subgroup. While they misuse opioids at low rates, they are also more vulnerable than younger individuals to the effects of opioids because of their high rates of polypharmacy and a variety of age-related physical changes that affect the pharmacokinetics and pharmacodynamics of medications. Also, the large population of adults between 25 and 50 years of age are underexamined, and studies in this population of opioid misuse cessation are needed. The natural process (i.e., unassisted by treatment) of ceasing drug use is often an understudied topic, and this also applies to opioid misuse. Discovery of psychosocial characteristics in those who successfully ceased opioid misuse could provide researchers target traits to promote (e.g., social engagement) that aid in natural cessation.

While the focus of this book was largely on opioid misuse, given its outsized contribution to the overall prescription misuse epidemic, the relatively low focus on stimulants, benzodiazepines, and over-the-counter medications was also a result of the much smaller research base on misuse of these medications. For stimulants, a greater relative amount of research on college student misuse exists. This is appropriate given its elevated misuse in this population, but more is needed in young adults in the years following college graduation; preliminary research I conducted with colleagues (Sean Esteban McCabe and Christian Teter) suggests that higher rates of misuse persist in young adult college graduates, and these young adult college graduates are an underexamined group. For benzodiazepines, research on the concurrent use of benzodiazepines and opioids is particularly warranted, given that almost 7,500 (85%) of the nearly 8,800 benzodiazepine-related overdoses noted above involved opioid medication. Generally, more research on benzodiazepine misuse is needed as well as over-the-counter misuse.

In the talk by Wilson Compton that I referenced above, he also mentioned that he believed that we were not at "the beginning of the end" of the opioid epidemic but the "end of the beginning." In other words, the opioid epidemic has moved out of an initial phase where prevalence rates and overdose deaths increased precipitously and into a (likely) more stable phase of elevated overdose deaths and treatment utilization for those with heavy opioid misuse. I hope this book has provided you, the reader, the resources to better understand this initial phase of the opioid misuse epidemic, along with the less studied phenomena of stimulant, benzodiazepine, and over-the-counter medication misuse. With this knowledge, I urge you to engage friends and relatives about prescription misuse; more importantly, I hope you will have conversations with health care providers and elected representatives. Stating your support for measures to limit the damage caused by prescription misuse can push elected representatives to act. These actions can improve policies that must balance legitimate patient needs for these medications with constraints to limit misuse and increase funding for research to better understand the development, prevention, and treatment of prescription misuse. These concrete steps are needed to move the prescription misuse epidemic through its developing middle stage into a stage of terminal decline, and they will save millions of dollars and tens of thousands of lives annually.

References

Compton, W. M., Jones, C. M., & Baldwin, G. T. (2016). Relationship between nonmedical prescription-opioid use and heroin use. *New England Journal of Medicine, 374*(2), 154–163. doi:10.1056/NEJMra1508490.

Connery, H. S. (2015). Medication-assisted treatment of opioid use disorder: Review of the evidence and future directions. *Harvard Review of Psychiatry, 23*(2), 63–75. doi:10.1097/HRP.0000000000000075.

Crowley, D. M., Jones, D. E., Coffman, D. L., & Greenberg, M. T. (2014). Can we build an efficient response to the prescription drug abuse epidemic? Assessing the cost effectiveness of universal prevention in the PROSPER trial. *Preventive Medicine, 62*, 71–77. doi:10.1016/j.ypmed.2014.01.029.

Fischer, B., Vojtila, L., & Rehm, J. (2017). The "fentanyl epidemic" in Canada—Some cautionary observations focusing on opioid-related mortality. *Preventive Medicine.* doi:10.1016/j.ypmed.2017.11.001.

Hero, J. O., McMurtry, C., Benson, J., & Blendon, R. (2016). Discussing opioid risks with patients to reduce misuse and abuse: Evidence from 2 surveys. *Annals of Family Medicine, 14*(6), 575–577. doi:10.1370/afm.1994.

McCarthy, J. J., Leamon, M. H., Finnegan, L. P., & Fassbender, C. (2017). Opioid dependence and pregnancy: Minimizing stress on the fetal brain. *American Journal of Obstetrics and Gynecology, 216*(3), 226–231. doi:10.1016/j.ajog.2016.10.003.

Moyer, V. A., & U. S. Preventive Services Task Force. (2014). Primary care behavioral interventions to reduce illicit drug and nonmedical pharmaceutical use in children and adolescents: U.S. Preventive Services Task Force recommendation statement. *Annals of Internal Medicine, 160*(9), 634–639. doi:10.7326/M14-0334.

National Institute on Drug Abuse. (2017). Overdose death rates. https://www.drugabuse.gov/related-topics/trends-statistics/overdose-death-rates.

O'Donnell, J. K., Gladden, R. M., & Seth, P. (2017). Trends in deaths involving heroin and synthetic opioids excluding methadone, and law enforcement drug product reports, by census region—United States, 2006–2015. *MMWR: Morbidity and Mortality Weekly Report, 66*(34), 897–903. doi:10.15585/mmwr.mm6634a2.

About the Editor and Contributors

Editor

Ty S. Schepis, PhD, is an associate professor of psychology at Texas State University. He obtained his PhD in clinical psychology from the University of Texas Southwestern Medical Center, and he completed a National Institutes of Health-funded Postdoctoral Fellowship in Substance Abuse at Yale School of Medicine. His primary expertise is in nicotine use and prescription misuse in adolescents and young adults, and his work has been published in notable academic journals, including *Addiction, Drug and Alcohol Dependence,* the *Journal of the American Academy of Child and Adolescent Psychiatry,* and the *Journal of Adolescent Health.* He has been principal investigator on four funded National Institutes of Health research grants, all from the National Institute on Drug Abuse, with over $1 million in total research funding.

Contributors

Niloofar Bavarian, PhD, MPH, is an assistant professor in the Health Science Department at California State University, Long Beach. She obtained her PhD and master's in public health from Oregon State University and completed a National Institutes of Health-funded Postdoctoral Fellowship with the Prevention Science Research Training Program at the University of California, Berkeley, and the Prevention Research Center. Dr. Bavarian's research uses theory to examine determinants (intrapersonal, interpersonal, and environmental) of health-promoting and health-compromising behaviors among youth and young adults.

Francesca L. Beaudoin, MD, PhD, is an associate professor of emergency medicine and health services, policy and practice and the director of clinical research for the Department of Emergency Medicine at the Alpert Medical

School of Brown University. She is a board-certified practicing emergency physician at Rhode Island Hospital and the Miriam Hospital, both in Providence, Rhode Island. Dr. Beaudoin is a graduate of the University of Massachusetts Medical School and completed her emergency medicine residency training and doctoral degree in epidemiology at Brown University. Dr. Beaudoin's research focuses on improving opioid-related harms through the investigation of alternatives to opioid analgesics and strategies to improve outcomes in individuals with existing opioid use disorders.

William C. Becker, MD, is a core investigator in the Pain Research, Informatics, Multi-morbidities & Education (PRIME) Center of Innovation at the VA Connecticut Healthcare System and an assistant professor at the Yale University School of Medicine. Dr. Becker is a general internist who is additionally trained in addiction medicine and pain management, and he codirects the Integrated Pain Clinic and Opioid Reassessment Clinic at VA Connecticut and cochairs the Yale School of Medicine's Pain Curriculum Committee. Dr. Becker's VA-, NIH-, FDA-, and PCORI-funded clinical research uses observational and experimental methods to examine and improve the quality of chronic pain treatment in primary care, particularly at the interface between high-impact chronic pain and opioid use disorder. Increasingly, his work focuses on de-implementing high-dose, long-term opioid therapy and improving patient's access to and use of nonpharmacologic pain treatments.

Trevor Bennett, PhD, is emeritus professor of criminology at the University of South Wales Centre for Criminology. Prior to this, he was head of the Centre for Criminology at the University of South Wales and before this acting director of the Institute of Criminology at the University of Cambridge. During this time, he was also a fellow of Wolfson College. Trevor has a long history of conducting research in the field of substance misuse and has secured funds for 37 tendered research projects totaling over £3 million. During his time as head of the Centre for Criminology, he also assisted other Centre colleagues in securing funds for their own research. He has published over 150 articles, book reviews, and book chapters as well as 10 books on drug-related and criminological topics. His recent books include *The Handbook of Crime* (2010) and *Drug–Crime Connections* (2007).

Gregory B. Castelli, PharmD, BCPS, BC-ADM, is a clinical pharmacist and director of the PGY1 Pharmacy Residency at UPMC St. Margaret. He received the PharmD degree from Wilkes University and then completed a PGY1 pharmacy practice residency, PGY2 ambulatory care residency, and faculty development fellowship at UPMC St. Margaret. Following residency, he was a clinical assistant professor at West Virginia University Schools of Pharmacy and Medicine, where he established a clinical practice site with the WVU Department of Family Medicine. Dr. Castelli joined the UPMC St. Margaret Family Medicine and Pharmacy Residencies' faculty in 2016. Dr. Castelli's clinical practice is with the family medicine inpatient service at UPMC St. Margaret and the UPMC St. Margaret Bloomfield-Garfield Family Health Center. His interests include evidence-based medicine, management of diabetes, pain management, and asthma/COPD. Dr. Castelli is active in ACCP and STFM national organizations.

Alvaro Castillo-Carniglia, PhD, MS, is a social epidemiologist with interests in the intersection of substance abuse, violence, and social context, including policy and program evaluation. He has led multiple studies to characterize and measure the national trends in substance use and related problems in the Chilean population. Dr. Castillo-Carniglia is currently a postdoctoral fellow at Violence Prevention Research Program at UC Davis School of Medicine.

Magdalena Cerdá, DrPh, MPH, is the vice chancellor's chair in violence prevention, and associate professor in the Department of Emergency Medicine at the University of California, Davis. Dr. Cerdá integrates approaches from social and psychiatric epidemiology to examine how social contexts shape violent behavior, substance use, and common forms of mental illness. Her research primarily focuses on two areas: (1) the causes, consequences, and prevention of violence; and (2) the social and policy determinants of substance use from childhood to adulthood. Dr. Cerdá has more than 100 publications in peer-reviewed journals in addition to five chapters in major textbooks. Current studies include a simulation of the impact that different types of firearms disqualification criteria could have on rates of firearm-related violence, a national study on the impact that prescription drug monitoring program characteristics have on opioid overdose, and a multicountry study on the health and social consequences of marijuana legalization.

Yu-Ping Chang, PhD, RN, FGSA, is a Patricia H. and Richard E. Garman Professor, associate professor, and the associate dean for research and scholarship at University at Buffalo School of Nursing. She is a fellow of Gerontological Society of America. She has been involved in substance abuse and mental health research since her graduate studies. She has published and coauthored articles and book chapters related to substance abuse and mental health, with a special interest in the older adult population. Her current research focuses on prescription opioid misuse and mental health issues in older chronic pain patients and the effects of brief interventions (e.g., motivational interviewing and mindfulness-based stress reduction) on reducing prescription opioid misuse and improving mental health comorbidities in chronic pain patients receiving care in primary care settings. She has worked with several interdisciplinary teams in various research projects.

Lian-Yu Chen, MD, PhD, is an assistant professor in the Institute of Epidemiology and Preventive Medicine at National Taiwan University, Taiwan. She received her psychiatric residency training in Taipei City Psychiatric Center and later obtained her PhD at the Johns Hopkins Bloomberg School of Public Health. Her expertise is in prescription drug abuse, particularly prescription stimulant abuse. She also has conducted studies on comorbidities of psychiatric and substance use disorders and adolescent substance use. Her work has appeared in several academic journals, including the *Journal of Clinical Psychiatry, Drug and Alcohol Dependence,* and *Addictive Behaviors.* She has served as a principal investigator of several public and national grants in Taiwan, and has received several prestigious awards, including the Lucy Shum Award from Johns Hopkins Bloomberg School of Public Health, the Sartorius Award from World Congress of Asian Psychiatry, and the Best Thesis Award from Taiwanese Society of Addiction Sciences.

Richard Cooper, PhD, is a senior lecturer in public health at the School of Health and Related Research (ScHARR) at the University of Sheffield in the United Kingdom and is also a registered pharmacist. His research and publications span a number of areas and include medical sociology, ethics in health care, health technologies, and different aspects of the supply and misuse of prescribed and over-the-counter medicines. He is a mixed-methods researcher with a particular interest in qualitative approaches. He has presented his work to national and international audiences and through numerous journal articles and chapters. When not doing any of the aforementioned, he plays football, squash, and guitar (all badly).

Sheena Cruz, MPH, is a clinical research coordinator at Veteran Affairs (VA) Long Beach Healthcare System. She obtained her BS in neuroscience from the University of California, Los Angeles, and completed her MPH at California State University, Long Beach. Her current research interests include exploring substance abuse and related diseases in the context of public health theory and medicine.

Chris Delcher, PhD, is an assistant professor in the Department of Health Outcomes and Policy at the University of Florida. He obtained his PhD in epidemiology from the University of Florida, where he focused on understanding the impact of prescription drug monitoring programs on reducing fatal opioid poisonings in Florida. He is a multiyear recipient of federal funding from the Bureau of Justice Assistance (National Institute of Justice) and has published more than 30 papers in high-impact journals such as *Drug and*

Alcohol Dependence, the *American Journal of Epidemiology*, and the *American Journal of Public Health*.

David S. Fink, MPH, MPhil, is interested in the influence of social arrangements and interactions on population health. His primary focus is on (1) the etiology of mental disorders, particularly substance use disorders, and (2) the extension of quantitative methods to estimate the health effects of policies and programs with a goal of (3) improving population health through evidence-based policy. He has published 30 articles, half of which were first-authored, and three book chapters. He is currently a PhD candidate in epidemiology at Mailman School of Public Health at Columbia University.

Jason A. Ford, PhD, is an associate professor in the Department of Sociology at the University of Central Florida. He received his PhD in sociology from Bowling Green State University with a major concentration in crime and deviance. His research interests focus on substance use among adolescents and young adults and factors related to stability and change in offending behavior over the life course. His research on prescription drug misuse focuses on criminological theory, the relationship between misuse and offending behavior, and gender and racial/ethnic variations in misuse.

Winfred T. Frazier, MD, MPH, FAAFP, CPH, is an assistant professor and assistant program director at UTMB Department of Family Medicine. He received his medical degree from Baylor College of Medicine and then completed a family medicine residency at Advocate Illinois Masonic. He completed a faculty development fellowship at UPMC St. Margaret and an MPH at the University of Pittsburgh with a health policy and management focus. He was also a postdoctoral scholar at Pitt, focusing on opioid abuse in the Pennsylvania Medicaid population. Dr. Frazier joined the UTMB Family Medicine Residency Program as faculty in 2017. Dr. Frazier's clinical practice is within the family medicine inpatient and outpatient service at UTMB Jennie Sealy Hospital and the Primary Care Pavilion–Island East. His interests include integration of family medicine and public health, residency education, pharmaceutical policy research, and pain management.

Lilian Ghandour, PhD, MPH, is an associate professor at the Department of Epidemiology and Population Health, Faculty of Health Sciences, American University of Beirut (AUB). She received her PhD from the Johns Hopkins Bloomberg School of Public Health in 2008. Dr. Ghandour has been involved in the design and analyses of various national and international surveys on youth. Her research focuses on youth mental health, particularly the epidemiology of harmful alcohol consumption, and nonmedical use of psychoactive prescription drugs. She is also interested in examining the interplay between youth sexual and mental health. Dr. Ghandour is also involved in translational research, conducting epidemiological research to help inform local national policies and practices. Dr. Ghandour has received several extramural research grants and awards for her work on youth mental health, and she has published extensively in high-tier peer-reviewed journals.

Martin Grabois, MD, is a professor of physical medicine and rehabilitation at the Baylor College of Medicine in Houston, Texas. He completed his doctor of medicine degree at Temple University School of Medicine, where he also completed his residency in physical medicine and rehabilitation. He is a past president of the American Academy of Pain Medicine, the American Congress of Rehabilitation Medicine, the American Pain Society, the American Academy of Physical Medicine and Rehabilitation, and Avondale House. He also served on the editorial boards of three journals and has research interests in pain management, health care access, and treatment costs.

Kiran K. Grover, MPH, is a research associate with the National Institute on Drug Abuse (NIDA) Clinical Trials Network (CTN)–Mid Southern Node at Duke University Medical Center. She coordinates research activities for a study, testing the effectiveness of a buprenorphine physician-pharmacist collaborative care model in the management of patients with opioid use disorder. She is interested in substance abuse and psychiatric epidemiology, with a specific interest in nonmedical prescription opioid abuse among the elderly population. Her goal is to expand her prior research experience and focus on (1) improving the implementation and dissemination of interventions designed to treat substance use disorders among the elderly and (2) preventing prescription opioid use disorders among these populations by addressing the gap in literature on curtailing diversion and abuse of opioid analgesics without jeopardizing pain treatment. Kiran has a MPH from Columbia University, Mailman School of Public Health, and a BASc from Ryerson University.

Travis L. Hase, MD, is an emergency medicine resident physician for the Department of Emergency Medicine at the Warren Alpert Medical School of Brown University. He is a graduate of the George Washington University School of Medicine and Health Sciences. Dr. Hase is a former research fellow and science policy analyst for the White House Office of National Drug Control Policy, where he researched opioid overdose prevention strategies, naloxone use, and policy initiatives focused on opioid-related harm reduction. His research interests broadly include emergency department–based public health interventions.

Stephen G. Henry, MD, MSc, is assistant professor of internal medicine at the University of California Davis School of Medicine in Sacramento,

California. His federally funded research focuses on patient-clinician communication about chronic pain and opioids in primary care as well as opioid epidemiology and use of prescription drug monitoring programs.

Lucas Hill, PharmD, earned his doctor of pharmacy degree from the University of Missouri–Kansas City School of Pharmacy before completing a pharmacy residency and faculty development fellowship in the University of Pittsburgh Medical Center Department of Family Medicine. Dr. Hill is now a clinical assistant professor of health outcomes and pharmacy practice at the University of Texas at Austin College of Pharmacy. He precepts learners and provides comprehensive medication management services for patients with complex chronic diseases at the CommUnityCare Southeast Health & Wellness Center. Dr. Hill is director of Operation Naloxone, an interprofessional collaborative that provides overdose prevention training and resources to health professionals, educational institutions, and the public. He is the principal investigator for the Texas Targeted Opioid Response: Overdose Prevention Project and directs more than $1 million in funding to combat the opioid crisis.

Katy Holloway, PhD, is a professor of criminology at the University of South Wales and director of the Crime, Justice and Society Research Institute. Prior to this, she was a research fellow at the University of Cambridge, where she worked as a data analyst on the New English and Welsh Arrestee Drug Abuse Monitoring Programme. Since then, she has continued to work in the field of substance misuse and has conducted 18 externally funded research projects as well as several unfunded projects. Katy has published widely on substance misuse, including 2 books, more than 20 peer-reviewed journal articles, 15 research reports, 4 book chapters, and in excess of 25 confidential, unpublished reports for police forces and reports for the U.K. government. Katy is currently leading a study on drug and alcohol use among university students in Wales and a study of diversion of opioid substitution medication.

Brian C. Kelly, PhD, is an associate professor in the Department of Sociology at Purdue University. His research examines contextual influences on young people's health, mainly focusing on substance use, sexual health, and mental health. The foci of his recent research projects include prescription drug misuse and risk-taking among young adults, methamphetamine use and HIV risk in China, and the influence of policy contexts on youth substance use. He has received several grants from the National Institute on Drug Abuse to pursue these projects. He is currently editor of the American Sociological Association's *Journal of Health and Social Behavior.*

Kenneth Kemp Jr., MD, is a senior faculty member at the Baylor College of Medicine in Houston, Texas. He has spent his 20-year medical career in both private and academic practice as a physical medicine and rehabilitation physician. He has special interest in nonoperative management of spinal disorders.

June H. Kim, PhD, is currently a postdoctoral fellow at the Behavioral Science Training in Drug Abuse Research at New York University. His prior work includes the role of stressful life events on alcohol craving, differences in nonmedical prescription drug use by educational attainment, and the association between gambling and risky sexual behaviors among inner-city adolescents. He has also been a Communications in Health Epidemiology Fellow (CHEF) at the2x2project.org. His current work involves investigating the role of medical marijuana as an alternative treatment for nonmalignant chronic pain.

Silvia S. Martins, PhD, is an associate professor of epidemiology at the Department of Epidemiology, Columbia University. She is director of the course Principles of Epidemiology and codirector of the Substance Abuse Epidemiology Training program in the institution. She has coauthored more than 135 peer-reviewed epidemiological and substance abuse journal articles and has served as a principal investigator of multiple NIH-funded grants. Her current research focuses on consequences of medical marijuana laws in the United States, recreational marijuana laws in Uruguay, prescription drug monitoring programs, social media and marijuana, gambling and impulsive behaviors among minority adolescents in the United States, and the association of exposure to violence with psychiatric symptoms in preschool children in Brazil. Her research to date has influenced both policy and treatment for substance abuse and addictive disorders. In 2017, Dr. Martins received the Columbia University Mailman's School of Public Health Dean's Award for Excellence in Mentoring.

Tom May, PhD, is a research fellow at the University of South Wales, Centre for Criminology. Prior to this, he worked as a research associate at the University of Bristol and the University of the West of England (UWE), where he contributed to a number of research projects funded by the National Probation Service, National Institute of Health Research (NIHR), and Home Office. He is currently working on a number of substance misuse–related projects with Professors Bennett and Holloway, including the misuse of prescribed-only and over-the-counter medications in Wales, the diversion of opioid substitution medication, and the effectiveness of medically supervised injecting centers. Tom has recently been co-opted onto a subgroup of the Welsh government's Advisory Panel on Substance Misuse to explore the potential benefits of introducing MSICs in Wales.

Mariel Mendez, MPH, is a current premedical postbaccalaureate student at Harvard University. Previously, she received her master's in public health with a certificate in global health at Columbia University Mailman School of Public Health, where she worked on various projects related to immigrant health, child and adolescent health, substance use, and trauma. With a disciplinary framework, Mariel is interested in understanding the immigrant experience (e.g., new migration and return migration) and mental health.

Mark Pawson, MA, is a doctoral student in the sociology department at the CUNY Graduate Center and a project director at the Center for HIV/AIDS Educational Studies and Training (CHEST), where he runs several NIH-funded studies focusing on substance use and sexual health. His research interests mainly include studying drug culture, drug markets, drug policy, and youth subcultures, which have led him to publish empirical work analyzing cannabis consumption, prescription drug misuse, and HIV prevention efforts within gay communities. His dissertation seeks to examine the ongoing processes of medicalization in late modernity as they relate to prescription drug misuse as a meaningful social practice among emerging adults.

Alexander S. Perlmutter, is a doctoral student in Columbia University's Department of Epidemiology after having completed his MPH there in 2016. He has worked with national data sets to explore time trend associations between marijuana use and social experiences, including arrest and knowledge of state medical marijuana laws. He has also used these data to assess associations between prescription drug use and social structures, including employment and age. He also works with the Centre de Recherche d'Épidémiologie et Statistique Sorbonne Paris Cité, where he studied methodological problems in conducting health research. His projects there focused on primary outcome modifications in oncology clinical trials and evaluating the evidence base of mobile health applications. He is interested in methodological issues vis-à-vis addiction studies and the implications of public policy surrounding prescription drug and marijuana use.

Ariadne E. Rivera-Aguirre, MPP, received her BA in economics from Instituto Tecnológico Autónomo de México (ITAM), and she has a master of public policy from Duke University. She currently works as a project coordinator and analyst at the Violence Prevention Research Program (VPRP) at the University of California, Davis. She has been involved in the quantitative analysis of social and policy determinants of substance use. Prior to joining the VPRP, she worked in consulting and policy analysis in developing countries on topics related to reducing the economic and social inequality regarding access and use of information and communication technologies (ICT).

Ariadne's areas of interest include economic development, poverty and inequality, and violence prevention.

Julian Santaella-Tenorio, DVM, MSc, is currently a Fulbright DrPH candidate in the Epidemiology Department at Mailman School of Public Health, Columbia University. His research interests include substance misuse, abuse and dependence, mental health disorders, and the epidemiology of injury and violence prevention. Mr. Santaella-Tenorio is also interested in policy evaluation, including research examining the effects of medical and recreational marijuana laws and prescription drug monitoring programs. He has published multiple manuscripts on these topics and is currently working on a project examining the effects of the prescription opioid epidemic on a variety of health outcomes.

Aaron Sarvet is a PhD student in the public health sciences (epidemiology) at Harvard T.H. Chan School of Public Health. Previously, he worked as a research scientist and biostatistician at the New York State Psychiatric Institute, studying state cannabis policy and also sexual violence on college campuses. His research interests include how state policy can affect the distribution of substance use, violence, and resulting health disparities that fall along the intersections of race, ethnicity, gender, and sexual orientation.

Julia P. Schleimer is a master of public health candidate in epidemiology at Columbia University's Mailman School of Public Health. Previously, she earned a bachelor of science degree in human development and psychology from the University of California, Davis, where she worked on autism research at the Medical Investigation of Neurodevelopmental Disorders (MIND) Institute. Julia now studies the social epidemiology of mental and behavioral health with a particular focus on health disparities. She is currently collaborating with researchers at Columbia University and at the Violence Prevention Research Program at the University of California, Davis, on projects relating to drug policy, marijuana use, and the nonmedical use of prescription opioids.

Luis Segura, MD, MPH, is a doctoral candidate in the Department of Epidemiology at the Columbia University Mailman School of Public Health. He completed his MD at the University Autonomous of Nuevo Leon (UANL) and his MPH at the National Institute of Public Health in Cuernavaca, Mexico. As part of Dr. Silvia S. Martin's research team, he has worked at examining the trends over time in opioid use disorders and heroin use among youth using data from the National Survey on Drug Use and Health (NSDUH). He has examined the trends in intention to smoke cigarettes associated with alternative tobacco product use among adolescents using data from the National

Youth Tobacco Survey (NYTS). Dr. Segura has also been involved in the initial descriptive data analysis of the Boricua Youth Study Gambling cohort. Recently, he has become interested in applying epidemiological causal inference methods in the field of substance abuse and mental health.

Joanna L. Starrels, MD, MS, is an associate professor of medicine at Albert Einstein College of Medicine and Montefiore Medical Center in Bronx, New York. Board certified in both internal medicine and addiction medicine, Dr. Starrels is a physician-investigator and educator who focuses on the safety and effectiveness of opioid analgesics for management of chronic pain. Her research has primarily been funded by grants from the National Institute on Drug Abuse (NIDA). Dr. Starrels has served as expert consultant to the New York City Department of Health and Mental Hygiene and the Centers for Disease Control and Prevention on initiatives to improve opioid prescribing for individuals with chronic pain.

Christian J. Teter, PharmD, BCPP, is an associate professor of psychopharmacology at the University of New England. He obtained his PharmD from the University of Michigan (Ann Arbor) and is board certified in psychiatric pharmacy. Dr. Teter completed a psychiatric pharmacotherapy residency at the University of North Carolina (Chapel Hill) followed by a National Institutes of Health–funded postdoctoral research fellowship in addiction at the University of Michigan (Ann Arbor). His ultimate long-term career goals are to help improve the care of patients at risk or suffering from psychiatric and substance use disorders via research (e.g., pharmacoepidemiology) and community outreach (e.g., mental health education) efforts. He hopes that his scholarly work, in addition to his role as an educator, will result in significant contributions to effective management of patients at risk or suffering from psychiatric and substance use disorders.

Linh Tran, PharmD, is currently a US Medical Affairs Postdoctoral Fellow at Genentech and clinical adjunct faculty for Ernest Mario School of Pharmacy at Rutgers University. He obtained his doctorate of pharmacy from the University of New England College of Pharmacy, and his primary expertise is in bio-oncology. He has been a medical oncology pharmacy consultant for a managed care specialty company, New Century Health. His research interests include motivations for medical and nonmedical misuse of prescription stimulants and value-based health care, exploring the current landscape to identify gaps for opportunities to collaborate with payers and innovations with oncology pharmacotherapy. While training at the University of New England, he worked on an intervention titled "Feasibility Study of a Kindergarten through Grade 12 (K–12) Educational Outreach Intervention: Cannabinoids and the Brain."

Michael Weaver, MD, DFASAM, is a professor in the Department of Psychiatry and Medical Director of the Center for Neurobehavioral Research on Addictions (CNRA) at the McGovern Medical School at the University of Texas Health Science Center at Houston. He received his MD degree from Northeast Ohio Medical University and completed his residency in internal medicine and a fellowship in addiction medicine at the Virginia Commonwealth University Health System. He is currently involved in patient care, medical education, and research. Dr. Weaver sees patients in the Innovations Addiction Treatment Clinic at the Texas Medical Center in Houston. He has extensive experience teaching about addiction to medical students, residents, and community professionals at all levels. He is involved in multiple research projects and collaborates with other researchers on studies involving cocaine, methamphetamine, marijuana, and electronic cigarettes. Dr. Weaver has multiple publications in the field of addiction medicine.

Alexis Yohros, MA, is a current doctoral student in criminology and justice policy at Northeastern University. Previously, she received her master's at the University of Central Florida in Sociology, where she worked on various projects related to intimate partner violence, substance use, and criminological theory. Taking an interdisciplinary approach, Alexis studies the trends, causes, and consequences of violence.

Marcus Zavala, PharmD, is a hospice/long-term care consulting pharmacist and a compounding pharmacist at PerroneRX. He provides a dynamic link between clinical practice and clinical consulting services development to support new models for delivering patient care. His primary expertise is compounding and end-of-life care. He obtained his doctorate of pharmacy from the University of New England College of Pharmacy. His research interests include ketamine for the reduction of suicidality and depression, perceptions of addiction and harm of marijuana, and ocular disease symptom reduction with the use of autologous blood serum eye drops. He is a distinguished recipient of the United States Public Health Services Excellence in Public Health Pharmacy Practice Award. He was presented this honor for leading a team of investigators in developing and promoting public health by spreading evidence-based knowledge and information regarding addiction and the neurological effects of cannabinoids on the developing brain.

Index